Interpreting Epidemiologic Evidence

Interpreting Epidemiologic Evidence

Strategies for Study Design and Analysis

DAVID A. SAVITZ

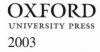
OXFORD
UNIVERSITY PRESS
2003

OXFORD
UNIVERSITY PRESS

Oxford   New York
Auckland   Bangkok   Buenos Aires   Cape Town   Chennai
Dar es Salaam   Delhi   Hong Kong   Istanbul   Karachi   Kolkata
Kuala Lumpur   Madrid   Melbourne   Mexico City   Mumbai
Nairobi   São Paulo   Shanghai   Taipei   Tokyo   Toronto

Published by Oxford University Press, Inc.
198 Madison Avenue, New York, New York, 10016
http://www.oup-usa.org

Oxford is a registered trademark of Oxford University Press

Library of Congress Cataloging-in-Publication Data
Savitz, David A.
Interpreting epidemiologic evidence :
strategies for study design and analysis /
David A. Savitz.
p. ; cm.   Includes bibliographical references and index.
ISBN 0-19-510840-X
1. Epidemiology—Technique. I. Title.
[DNLM: 1. Epidemiologic Research Design.
2. Bias (Epidemiology)
WA 950 S267i 2003]
RA652.4 .S286 2003
614.4—dc21   2002192672

9 8 7 6 5 4 3 2 1
Printed in the United States of America
on acid-free paper

PREFACE

There was no shortage of epidemiology books when I started writing this book in the summer of 1996, and the intervening years have brought many new and very useful ones. Just as it is uninspiring to do a study that ends up as one more dot on a graph or one more line in a table, it was certainly not my goal to merely add one more book to an overcrowded shelf. But there was a particular need that did not seem to be very well addressed in books or journal articles—to bring together concepts and methods with real research findings in order to make informed judgments about the results.

One of the most difficult tasks facing new students and even experienced practitioners of epidemiology is to assess how much confidence one can have in a given set of findings. As I discussed such issues with graduate students and colleagues, and contemplated my own data, it was difficult to find a reasoned, balanced approach. It's easy but uninformative to simply acknowledge epidemiology's many pitfalls, and not much more difficult to mount a generic defense of the credibility of one's findings. What was difficult was to find empirical tools for assessing the study's susceptibility to specific sources of error in ways that could actually change preconceptions and go beyond intuition. This kind of examination is most fruitful when it can give good or bad news about one's study that was unexpected.

I knew that such approaches were out there because I found candidate tools in the work of others. Sometimes our discussions would lead us to a technique applied elsewhere that was applicable to the current situation. Two elements were lacking, however, and I have tried to address them in this book. One is the link between methodological principles and the tools themselves, which involves taking stock of why the strategy for addressing the potential bias may or may not actually be informative, and how it could be misleading. The other is a full listing of the candidates to consider in addressing a potential problem, in the hope of improving our ability to draw upon one tool or another in the appropriate situation. My aspiration was to have a place to turn to when trying to interpret a study that deals with a challenging exposure measure, for example, where you could find a repertoire of tactics to assess how well it was measured as well as a reminder of what the consequences of error would most likely be. Ideally, at the point of planning the study, one would anticipate the challenge and collect the data needed to address the extent of the error upon completion of the study. For every topic in the book, there are chapters in other texts, many of which are excellent, and there are many journal articles on novel aspects of epidemiologic methods, but I could not find a source book of practical guidance on linking methodological principles with research practice. That is what this book aspires to provide.

My original goal in developing the book was to provide a reference that could be used when planning a study or needing to evaluate one. I believe that the book could also be useful in an intermediate or advanced epidemiologic methods course, supplementing a more rigorous methods text. Each chapter is intended to be freestanding, and could be referred to without having read the ones that precede it, but organizing the book along the lines of how research is conceptualized, conducted, and analyzed offers some benefits if the sequence of chapters is followed. Instructors might want to use this book along with evaluation of specific published papers for individual evaluation or group discussion. Using the above example, after considering the underlying algebra of exposure misclassification and its consequences in a methods text, the corresponding chapter in this book and a review of one or more real examples from the literature could help tie the theory to the practice, always a challenge for new (and old) epidemiologists. Making the connection between methodological principles and specific, substantive research applications is the most intellectually stimulating and challenging aspect of the field, in my view.

I thank Abigail Ukwuani for her excellent work in composing the manuscript and Jeff House for his patience and encouragement. I also express my appreciation to a number of distinguished epidemiologists who were kind enough to review various chapters and provide general guidance and encouragement as well: Marilie Gammon, Dana Loomis, Bob Millikan, Andy Olshan, Charlie Poole, Ken Rothman, and Noel Weiss. Joanne Promislow was extremely helpful in going through the manuscript in detail to capture the spirit of the book, and in completing the challenging task of identifying suitable illustrations from the published literature. Nonetheless, these colleagues and others who may read the book will undoubtedly find statements with which they disagree, so their help and acknowledgment should not be seen as a blanket endorsement of the book's contents. Following the spirit espoused in this book, critical evaluation is always needed and I welcome readers' comments on any errors in logic or omissions of potentially valuable strategies that they may find.

CONTENTS

1. Introduction, 1

2. The Nature of Epidemiologic Evidence, 7
   Goals of Epidemiologic Research, 7
   Measurement of Causal Relations Between Exposure and Disease, 10
   Inferences from Epidemiologic Research, 12
   Descriptive Goals and Causal Inference, 15
   Inferences from Epidemiologic Evidence: Efficacy of Breast Cancer Screening, 16
   Inferences from Epidemiologic Evidence: Alcohol and Spontaneous Abortion, 18
   Causal Inference, 20
   Contribution of Epidemiology to Policy Decisions, 24

3. Strategy for Drawing Inferences from Epidemiologic Evidence, 29
   Need for Systematic Evaluation of Sources of Error, 30
   Need for Objective Assessment of Epidemiologic Evidence, 32
   Estimation of Measures of Effect, 34
   Conceptual Framework for the Evaluation of Error, 37
   Identify the Most Important Sources of Error, 39
   Strategies for Specifying Scenarios of Bias, 41

Example: Epidemiologic Research on the Relation Between Dichlorodiphenyltrichloroethane (DDT) Exposure and Breast Cancer, 44

4. Selection Bias in Cohort Studies, 51
   Study Designs, 51
   Purpose of Comparison Groups, 53
   Selection Bias and Confounding, 55
   Evalution of Selection Bias in Cohort Studies, 58
   Integrated Assessment of Potential for Selection Bias in Cohort Studies, 78

5. Selection Bias in Case–Control Studies, 81
   Control Selection, 81
   Evaluation of Selection Bias in Case–Control Studies, 89
   Integrated Assessment of Potential for Selection Bias in Case–Control Studies, 111

6. Bias Due to Loss of Study Participants, 115
   Conceptual Framework for Examining Bias Due to Loss of Study Participants, 115
   Evaluation of Bias Due to Loss of Study Participants, 120
   Integrated Assessment of Potential for Bias Due to Loss of Study Participants, 133

7. Confounding, 137
   Definition and Theoretical Background, 137
   Quantification of Potential Confounding, 141
   Evaluation of Confounding, 145
   Integrated Assessment of Potential Confounding, 157

8. Measurement and Classification of Exposure, 163
   Ideal Versus Operational Measures of Exposure, 164
   Evaluation of Exposure Misclassification, 172
   Assessment of Whether Exposure Misclassification is Differential or Nondifferential, 192
   Integrated Assessment of Potential for Bias Due to Exposure Misclassification, 201

9. Measurement and Classification of Disease, 205
   Framework for Evaluating Disease Misclassification, 205
   Sources of Disease Misclassification, 206

Differential and Nondifferential Disease Misclassification, 212
Assessing Whether Misclassification Is Differential by Exposure, 216
Evaluation of Disease Misclassification, 219
*Integrated Assessment of Potential for Bias Due to Disease
    Misclassification*, 238

10. Random Error, 243
    Sequential Approach to Considering Random and Systematic Error, 245
    *Special Considerations in Evaluating Random Error in
        Observational Studies*, 246
    Statistical Significance Testing, 248
    Multiple Comparisons and Related Issues, 251
    Interpretation of Confidence Intervals, 255
    Integrated Assessment of Random Error, 258

11. Integration of Evidence Across Studies, 261
    Consideration of Random Error and Bias, 262
    Data Pooling and Coordinated Comparative Analysis, 264
    Synthetic and Exploratory Meta-Analysis, 268
    Interpreting Consistency and Inconsistency, 273
    Integrated Assessment from Combining Evidence Across Studies, 281

12. Characterization of Conclusions, 285
    Applications of Epidemiology, 287
    Identification of Key Concerns, 291
    Integrated Consideration of Potential Bias, 293
    Integration of Epidemiologic Evidence with Other Information, 294
    Controversy over Interpretation, 297
    *The Case Against Algorithms for Interpreting
        Epidemiologic Evidence*, 299

Index, 305

Interpreting Epidemiologic Evidence

1

INTRODUCTION

This book was written for both producers and consumers of epidemiologic research, though a basic understanding of epidemiologic principles will be necessary at the outset. Little of the technical material will be new to experienced epidemiologists, but I hope that my perspective on the application of those principles to interpreting research results will be distinctive and useful. For the large and growing group of consumers of epidemiology, which includes attorneys and judges, risk assessors, policy experts, clinicians, and laboratory scientists, the book is intended to go beyond the principles learned in an introductory course or textbook of epidemiology by applying them to concrete issues and findings. Although it is unlikely that ambiguous evidence can be made conclusive or that controversies will be resolved directly by applying these principles, a careful consideration of the underlying reasons for the ambiguity or opposing judgments in a controversy can represent progress. By pinpointing where the evidence falls short of certainty, we can give questions a sharper focus, leading to a clearer description of the state of knowledge at any point in time and thus helping identify the research that could contribute to a resolution of the uncertainty that remains.

Those who are called upon to assess the meaning and persuasiveness of epidemiologic evidence have a variety of approaches to consider. There are formal guidelines for judging causality for an observed association, which is defined as

a statistical dependence of two or more events (Last, 2001). A statistical association by itself does not indicate whether one causes the other, which is the issue
of ultimate interest. The most widely cited framework for assessing the causal
implications of associations is that of Hill (1965), which has been challenged by
others (Rothman & Greenland, 1998) yet continues to be used widely by those
who evaluate research findings in epidemiology. Hill's criteria serve as a means
of reaching conclusions about reported positive associations that can help guide
regulatory or policy decisions. The criteria, however, focus only on the interpretation of *positive* associations, neglecting the need to evaluate the validity of
whatever association was measured or to consider the credibility of an observed
absence of association.

Statistical methods have been used both to evaluate whether observed associations are statistically significant—for example, unlikely to have been observed
if no association is present—and to quantify the strength of an association (Selvin,
1991; Clayton & Hills, 1993). A large methodological literature on confounding
(in which the effect from an exposure of interest is entangled with other contributors), selection bias (in which the individuals who are included in the study
results in erroneous measures of association), and misclassification (error in measurement) contributes importantly to making judgments about the validity of epidemiologic observations (Rothman & Greenland, 1998).

In parallel with the evolution of these more technical methodological considerations, interest in understanding and using epidemiology has grown considerably, reflected in media attention, courtroom applications, and interactions with
scientists in other disciplines. The views of epidemiology within these groups
are not always favorable. Many outside epidemiology have one of two extreme
reactions to the evidence we generate: They may be so impressed with our findings on human beings exposed to the agents that may cause disease that observed
associations are taken as direct reflections of causal effects with little need for
scrutiny or caution. Or they may be more impressed with the lengthy list of potential sources of error, the ubiquitous potential confounders, and the seemingly
unending controversy and flow of criticism among epidemiologists, and may
come to believe that all our observations are hopelessly flawed and cannot be
trusted as indicators of causal relations. Students often start with a naive, optimistic view of the power of the epidemiologic approach, become dismayed with
the many sources of potential error, and then (hopefully) emerge with a sophistication that intelligently balances the promise and the pitfalls. More experienced
epidemiologists appreciate that the truth lies somewhere between the extremes.
Even for those who are familiar with the tools needed to evaluate evidence, however, the integration of that evidence into a global assessment is often a highly
subjective process, and can be a contentious one.

This book is not a step-by-step manual for interpreting epidemiologic data that
guarantees drawing the correct conclusion. It is simply not possible to reduce the

evaluation of evidence to an algorithm for drawing valid inferences. And because the truth is unknown, we could not tell whether any such algorithm worked. A more modest goal is to elucidate the underlying issues involved in the interpretation of evidence so that unbiased, knowledgeable epidemiologists can reach agreement or identify precisely where and why they disagree. In this book, I have tried to develop in some detail the array of considerations that should be taken into account in characterizing the epidemiologic evidence on a given topic, suggest how to identify the key considerations, and most importantly, offer a variety of strategies to determine whether a potential methodologic problem is likely to be influential and if so what magnitude and direction of influence it may have. The methodologic literature, particularly the recent synthesis by Rothman and Greenland (1998), provides the starting point for that evaluation. This book applies some methodological principles in specific and practical ways to the assessment of research findings in an effort to help reach sound judgments. In some cases traditional approaches to evaluating evidence are examined and found to be deficient. Because they are commonly used, however, they warrant careful examination here.

For instance, confounding is rather well-defined in theoretical terms (Greenland & Robins, 1986; Weinberg, 1993). According to Rothman and Greenland (1998), it is "a confusion of effects. Specifically, the apparent effect of the exposure of interest is distorted because the effect of an extraneous factor is mistaken for or mixed with the actual exposure effect" (p. 120). Statistical methods for controlling confounding have been clearly described (Kleinbaum et al., 1982; Rothman & Greenland, 1998), so that if the source of confounding, i.e., the extraneous factor of interest, can be measured accurately, then statistical tools can be used to minimize or eliminate its impact. The potential for confounding is inherent in observational studies where the exposure of interest is often only one of many correlated exposures. In contrast to studies where exposure is assigned randomly and thus isolated from other exposures, the potential for confounding cannot be readily quantified (Greenland, 1990). Nonetheless, in evaluating a measure of association from an observational study, we must judge how likely it is that the association has been distorted by confounding. What are the implications of a lack of knowledge of major risk factors for the disease (and thus candidate confounders) versus having measured and controlled for known strong risk factors? How likely is it that poor measurement of potential confounders has left substantial distortion in the association of interest? How effective is adjustment for indirect markers of potential confounders, such as educational attainment as a proxy for health behaviors? What is the likely direction of confounding, if present? What magnitude of association with disease or exposure would be required to have introduced a given amount of bias? How can we use other studies of the same association to help judge whether confounding is likely to be present?

The product of a careful evaluation of the study itself, drawing on the relevant methodological and substantive literature, is an informed judgment about the plausibility, direction, and strength of confounding, as well as specifying further research that would narrow uncertainty about the impact of confounding. Even when agreement among evaluators cannot be attained, the areas of disagreement should move from global questions about study validity to successively narrower questions that are amenable to empirical evaluation. To move from general disagreement about the credibility of a study's findings to asking such focused, answerable questions as whether a specific potential confounder has a sufficiently large association with disease to have markedly distorted the study results represents real progress. The methodologic principles are needed to refine the questions that give rise to uncertainty and controversy, which must then be integrated with substantive knowledge about the phenomenon of interest to make informed judgments. Much of this book focuses on providing that linkage between methodological principles and substantive knowledge in order to evaluate findings more accurately.

The challenges in interpretation relate to sets of studies of a given topic as well as individual results. For example, consistency across studies is often interpreted as a simple dichotomy: consistency in findings is supportive of a causal association and inconsistency is counter to it. But epidemiologic studies are rarely, if ever, pure replications of one another, and thus differ for reasons other than random error. When studies that have different methodologic features yield similar results, it can be tentatively assumed that the potential biases associated with those aspects of the study that differ have not introduced bias, and a causal inference is thus strengthened. Consistency across studies with features that should, under a causal hypothesis, yield different results suggests that some bias may be operating. There may also be meaningful differences in results from similarly designed studies conducted in different populations, suggesting that some important cofactors, necessary for the exposure to exert its impact, are present in some populations but not others. Clearly, when methodologically stronger studies produce different results than weaker ones, lack of consistency in results does not argue against causality.

The book has been organized to the extent possible in the order that issues arise. Chapter 2 sets the stage for evaluating epidemiologic evidence by clarifying the expected product of epidemiologic research, defining the goals. Next, I propose an overall strategy and philosophy for considering the quality of epidemiologic research findings (Chapter 3). The following chapters systematically cover the design, conduct, and analysis issues that bear on study interpretation.

Beginning with Chapter 4 and continuing through Chapter 9, sources of systematic error in epidemiologic studies are examined. The rationale for dividing the topics as the table of contents does warrants a brief explanation. Selection bias refers to "error due to systematic differences in characteristics between those who take part in a study and those who do not" (Last, 2001). It is the constitution of the study groups that is the potential source of such error. The construction of study groups is different in practice (though not in theory) in cohort and case–control studies. In cohort studies, groups with differing exposure status are identified and monitored for the occurrence of disease in order to compare disease incidence among them. In case–control studies, the sampling is based on health outcome; those who have experienced the disease of interest are compared to a sample from the population that gave rise to those cases of disease. Because the groups are constituted in different ways for different purposes in the two designs, the potential for selection bias is considered in separate chapters (Chapters 4 and 5). Furthermore, given that one particular source of selection bias, that due to non-participation, is so ubiquitous and often so large, Chapter 6 addresses this problem in detail.

Confounding, in which there is a mixing of effects from multiple exposures, is similar in many respects to selection bias, but its origins are natural as opposed to arising from the way the study groups were constituted. Evaluating the presence, magnitude, and direction of confounding is the subject of Chapter 7.

The consideration of measurement error, though algebraically similar regardless of what is being measured, is conceptually different and has different implications depending on whether the exposure, broadly defined as the potential causal factor of interest, the disease, again broadly defined as the health outcome of interest, is measured with error. The processes by which error arises (e.g., memory errors producing exposure misclassification, diagnostic errors producing disease misclassification) and their implications for bias in measures of association make it necessary to separate the discussions of exposure (Chapter 8) and disease (Chapter 9) misclassification.

The complex topic of random error, how it arises, affects study results, and should be characterized is addressed in Chapter 10. The sequence is intentional. Random error is discussed after the other factors to help counter the long-held view that it is the first or automatically the more important issue to consider in evaluating epidemiologic evidence.

There are several increasingly popular approaches to the integration of information from multiple studies, such as meta-analysis [defined as "a statistical synthesis of the data from separate by similar studies" (Last, 2001)] and pooling (combining data from multiple studies for reanalysis). These methods are discussed in Chapter 11. Chapter 12 deals with the integration and summary of information gained from the approaches covered in the previous chapters.

REFERENCES

Clayton D, Hills M. Statistical models in epidemiology. Oxford, England: Oxford University Press, 1993.

Greenland S. Randomization, statistics, and causal inference. Epidemiology 1990;1: 421–429.

Greenland S, Robins JM. Identifiability, exchangeability, and epidemiological confounding. Int J Epidemiol 1986;15:413–419.

Hill AB. The environment and disease: association or causation? Proc R Soc Med 1965;58:295–300.

Kleinbaum DG, Kupper LL, Morgenstern H. Epidemiologic research. Principles and quantitative methods. Belmont, CA: Lifetime Learning Publications, 1982:312–319.

Last JM. A dictionary of epidemiology, Fourth Edition. New York: Oxford University Press, 2001.

Rothman KJ, Greenland S. Modern epidemiology, Second Edition. Philadelphia: Lippincott—Raven, 1998.

Selvin S. Statistical analysis of epidemiologic data. New York: Oxford University Press, 1991.

Weinberg CR. Toward a clearer definition of confounding. Am J Epidemiol 1993;137:1–8.

2

THE NATURE OF EPIDEMIOLOGIC EVIDENCE

GOALS OF EPIDEMIOLOGIC RESEARCH

To evaluate the quality or strength of epidemiologic evidence, we first need to clarify what information we can expect epidemiology to provide (Table 2.1). The effectiveness of epidemiologic research must be defined in relation to attainable, specific benchmarks in order to make judgments about how close the evidence comes to reaching the desired state of perfection. When we examine a study or set of studies, we typically make a statement as to whether those studies have individually or collectively fulfilled their expectations. Broad assessments such as "persuasive" or "inconclusive" are commonly applied to evidence, typically without much consideration of the standard against which it has been judged. It would be unwise to set an unrealistically high goal for epidemiologic research to yield absolute truth that directly benefits society, and equally unproductive to set a low (but readily attained) standard of merely providing clues or suggestions that will be resolved by other scientific approaches. Epidemiology functions somewhere between those extremes.

The highest expectation for epidemiologic research is to generate knowledge that contributes directly to improvements in the health of human populations. Such research would yield new knowledge, and that new knowledge would have beneficial applications to advancing public health. However appropriate this is

TABLE 2–1. Levels of Inference from Epidemiologic Evidence and Attendant Concerns

INFERENCE	REQUIREMENTS
Relations between operational measurements among study measurements	None
Association between measured exposure and disease among study participants	Accurate measurement of exposure; accurate measurement of disease
Causal effect of exposure on disease in study population	Freedom from confounding
Causal effect of exposure on disease in external populations	Generalizability (external validity)
Prevention of disease through elimination or reduction of exposure	Amenability of exposure to modification
Substantial public health impact from elimination or reduction of exposure	Large attributable fraction

as the ultimate goal for epidemiologic inquiry, it would be a mistake to use the criterion of "improvement in public health" as the only test of whether the research effort (from epidemiology or any other scientific discipline) has been successful. Highly informative epidemiologic studies might exonerate agents suspected of doing harm rather than implicate agents that cause disease. Excellent research may show lack of benefit from an ostensibly promising therapeutic measure. Such research unquestionably informs public health practice and should ultimately improve health by directing our energies elsewhere, but the path from information to benefit is not always direct.

Even where epidemiologic studies produce evidence of harm or benefit from such agents as environmental pollutants, dietary constituents, or medications, the link to action is an indirect one. The validity of the evidence is a necessary but not sufficient goal for influencing decisions and policy; societal concerns based on economics and politics, outside the scope of epidemiology, can and sometimes should override even definitive epidemiologic evidence. The goal of public health, not epidemiology, is disease prevention (Savitz et al., 1999). Marketing of the discipline may benefit from claims that epidemiology prevents disease, but many past public health successes have had little to do with epidemiology and many past (and present) failures are not the result of inadequate epidemiologic research. Epidemiology constitutes only one very important component of the knowledge base for public health practice; pertinent data are also contributed by the basic biomedical sciences, sociology, economics, and anthropology, among other disciplines. The metaphor of the community as patient is much more suitable to public health practice than to the scientific discipline of epidemiology. Like clinical medicine, public health practice draws on many scientific disciplines and nonscientific considerations.

At the other extreme, the goals of epidemiologic research ought not to be constrained as so modest and technical in nature that even our successes have no practical value. We could define the goal of epidemiology as the mechanical process of gathering and analyzing data and generating statistical results, such as odds ratios or regression coefficients, divorced from potential inferences and applications. Theoretical and logistical challenges disappear one by one as the benchmark is lowered successively. If a study's intent is defined as assessment of the association between the boxes checked on a questionnaire and the reading on the dial of a machine for those individuals who are willing to provide the information, then success can be guaranteed. We can undoubtedly locate pencils, get some people to check boxes, find a machine that will give a reading, and calculate measures of association. Focusing on the mechanical process of the research is conservative and modest, traits valued by scientists, and averts the criticism that comes when we attempt to make broader inferences from the data. While in no way denigrating the importance of study execution (Sharp pencils may actually help to reduce errors in coding and data entry!), these mechanical components are only a means to the more interesting and challenging end of extending knowledge that has the potential for biomedical and societal benefit.

Beyond the purely mechanical goal of conducting epidemiologic research and generating data, expectations for epidemiology are sometimes couched in terms of "measuring associations" or "producing leads," with the suggestion that scientific knowledge ultimately requires corroborative research in the basic or clinical sciences. The implication is that our research methods are so hopelessly flawed that even at their very best, epidemiology yields only promising leads or hints at truth. In one sense, this view simultaneously undervalues epidemiology and overvalues the other disciplines. Epidemiologic evidence, like that from all scientific disciplines, is subject to error and misinterpretation. Because of compensatory strengths and weaknesses, integrating epidemiologic evidence with that produced by other disciplines is vital to drawing broader inferences regarding causes and prevention of disease. Epidemiologists, however, can and do go well beyond making agnostic statements about associations (ignoring causality) or generating hypotheses for other scientists to pursue. Epidemiology produces evidence, like other scientific disciplines, that contributes to causal inferences about the etiology and prevention of disease in human populations.

For the purposes of this book, I define the goal for epidemiologic research as the quantification of the causal relation between exposure and disease. Although the research itself generates only statistical estimates of association, the standard by which the validity of those measures of association is to be judged is their ability to approximate the causal relation of interest. The utility of those estimated associations in advancing science and ultimately public health generally depends on the extent to which they provide meaningful information on the underlying causal relations. As discussed below, the term *exposure* is really a shorthand notation for agents, interventions, conditions, policies, and anything that might affect health, and *disease* is analogously the broad of array of health conditions that we would seek to be able to understand and ultimately modify, including physiologic states, mental health, and the entire spectrum of human diseases.

The ideal study yields a quantitative measure of association that reflects the causal influence of exposure on disease. Methodologic problems and errors cause a deviation between the study results and this ideal measure, and improvements in research are reflected in bringing the study results closer to a measure of the causal effect. There is no distinction between a study that correctly indicates an absence of a causal association, i.e., an accurate measure of the causal relation indicates none is present, and one that correctly indicates the presence of a causal association; both constitute valid epidemiologic research.

MEASUREMENT OF CAUSAL RELATIONS BETWEEN EXPOSURE AND DISEASE

Estimation of causal effects as the focus of epidemiology was initially emphasized by Rothman (1986), who tried to dislodge epidemiologists from testing statistical hypotheses as a goal and persuade them to focus on quantifying measures of association. With measurement as the goal, assessment of epidemiologic evidence focuses on the aspects of study design, conduct, and analysis that may introduce distortion or enhance the accuracy of measurement. Error, a deviation between the measured result and the true causal relation between exposure and disease, arises from both random and systematic processes. There is no fundamental distinction between accurately measuring a null association and any other association, in direct contrast to the framework of statistical hypothesis testing which focuses on the deviation (or lack thereof) between the study results and those predicted under the null hypothesis. The null hypothesis or lack of association is just another possible state of nature that a valid study seeks to identify. Measurement of a causal relation between exposure and disease focuses on the quantitative index that characterizes the strength of association, which can be a ratio or difference measure, or a regression coefficient in which disease is the dependent variable.

Causality is a complex issue in both philosophical and practical terms (Susser, 1991; Greenland, 1988; Lanes, 1988). Even though causality is an abstraction, not subject to objective determination, it provides a crucial benchmark for discussing the validity of study findings. Epidemiologists or their critics sometimes claim that they do not address causal relations, only statistical associations, perhaps in a well-intentioned effort to acknowledge the limitations in their data. Even more narrowly, we actually measure how questionnaire responses or laboratory assay results relate to other bits of information found in medical records or obtained by using various instruments. The operational activities of epidemiology, like those of other sciences, are far removed from lofty notions like causality. However, the goal of the research is not to check boxes or calculate statistics, but to make inferences about causal relations. If we were satisfied with measuring empirical associations and not interested in causality, there would be no concept of confounding and no interest in identifying exposures that might be manipulated in order to reduce the burden of disease. The recognition of epidemiology's limitations in measuring causal relations should come in the interpretation of the evidence when trying to draw conclusions, not in the statement of research goals or study design and conduct phases. In practice, it is rare to calculate measures of association without interest in the possibility of some causal relation being present. When we calculate a risk ratio of 2.0, the question of whether exposure has doubled the risk of disease is a concern with causality whether or not it is labeled as such.

Epidemiology is well suited to address a wide range of exposures and diseases, not just the prototypic chemical or drug causing a well-defined illness. Exposure includes any potential disease determinant, encompassing age, gender, time period, social conditions, geographic location, and health care in addition to more conventional individual exposures such as diet, stress, or exposure to chemical pollutants. The specific attributes of those diverse exposures pose different challenges, of course, for epidemiologic research. As discussed by Susser (1991), we are interested in many types of determinants of disease, not just exogenous, modifiable causes. The vast literature on gender differences reflects an interest in the causal role of being male or female, with no direct implications for gender modification as a public health intervention.

Similarly, disease is used as shorthand for all health variants of interest, including clinical disease, disability, physiologic alterations, and social disorder. To fit within the framework of epidemiologic inquiry applied in this book, the health measure should be of some ultimate clinical or public health relevance. We would probably exclude from the scope of epidemiology efforts to predict cigarette brand preference, for example, even though it is important to public health, or voting patterns or migration, for example, even though the tools used by marketing researchers, political scientists, and sociologists are very similar to those of epidemiologists. Once the realm of health is defined, exposure constitutes everything that potentially influences it.

The exposures and diseases we wish to study are often abstract constructs that cannot be directly measured. Thus, the data that are collected for study are not direct assessments of the exposure and disease but only operational measures based on available tools such as questionnaires, biological measurements, and findings from physical examination. Some such measures come closer than others to capturing the condition or event of ultimate interest. Nevertheless, it is important to keep in mind that the operational measures are not the entities of interest themselves (e.g., deposition of graphite on a form is not dietary intake, a peak on a mass spectrometer printout is not DDT exposure), but serve as indirect indicators of broader, often more abstract, constructs.

A key issue in evaluating epidemiologic evidence is how effectively the operational definitions approximate the constructs of ultimate interest. The methods of measurement of exposure and disease are critical components of epidemiologic study design. The concept of misclassification applies to all the sources of error between the operational measure and the constructs of interest. The most obvious and easily handled sources of misclassification are clerical error or faulty instrumentation, whereas failure to properly define the relevant constructs, failure to elicit the necessary data to reflect those constructs, and assessment of exposure or disease in the wrong time period illustrate the more subtle and often more important sources of misclassification. We would like to measure causal relations between what is often an abstract construct of exposure and disease, but the study yields a measure of association between an operational measure of exposure and disease. The nature and magnitude of disparity between what we would like and what we have achieved calls for careful scrutiny. Chapters 8 and 9 focus on examination of that gulf between the construct and the operational measures of exposure and disease, respectively.

INFERENCES FROM EPIDEMIOLOGIC RESEARCH

If accurate estimation of causal relations is the goal of epidemiologic studies, then success has been attained when the measure of effect accurately quantifies the causal impact of the exposure on disease in the population under investigation. Even if this goal is completely fulfilled, more is needed. Public health practice and policy requires extrapolation of the findings to other defined populations or to people in general. Such generalization does not result from a single study, nor is it a matter of statistical sampling and inference (Rothman, 1986). Only a series of internally valid studies can result in a body of evidence to help judge (not prove) whether some more universal causal relation is operating that would apply to populations not yet studied.

Extrapolation of findings to previously unstudied populations, by definition, goes beyond the available data, and is thus vulnerable to error in addition to whatever error is contained in the studies that provide the basis for the extrapolation. Universal causal relations (Smoking causes lung cancer.) reflect the ultimate extrapolation, synthesizing a series of individual studies into the untestable assertion about what exposure would do to disease risk in all possible past, present, and future populations. Nonetheless, when we use epidemiologic evidence to guide decisions about individual behavior and public policy, we are implicitly extrapolating a set of research observations to just such new and previously untested situations and populations. Causality is assessed based on judgments about the validity of individual studies, the accumulation of those studies, and extrapolation of the results beyond the study populations that generated the findings.

Application of epidemiologic evidence to other populations, to individual decision-making, or to public health policy requires caution. There are concentric layers of application for epidemiologic evidence. A narrow one might be the use of the data to estimate, within the study population, the quantitative effect of exposure on the occurrence of disease. Somewhat broader would be the use of that evidence to estimate the effect of exposure on disease for a broader population outside the study but otherwise socially and demographically similar to the study population, perhaps to help formulate policy. Assuming that the policy experts are well informed, they will be able to accurately evaluate the strength and clarity of the epidemiologic evidence.

As the information reaches clinicians or the public at large, the questions may go well beyond what can be gleaned directly from epidemiologic data, for example, asking whether a change in clinical practice or individual behavior is *warranted*. It is thus important for epidemiology to examine the full spectrum of potential consequences of a change in policy or practice on the public's health, identifying unanticipated consequences of altered exposure as well as desired outcomes. These are often the most important considerations in setting policy, and epidemiology has a unique role to fulfill in generating critical information.

Beyond the scope of epidemiology comes the feasibility and costs of actually modifying exposure through behavior change, clinical guidelines, or regulation. As the goal is expanded, moving from a characterization of the risks and benefits of alternative courses of action to the question of what *should* be done and how to achieve the desired end, the sufficiency of even impeccable epidemiologic information diminishes and considerations outside of epidemiology often become increasingly prominent. There may be tension between the cautiousness of researchers who wish to ask narrow, modest questions of the data (for which it may be well-suited) and the public who wish to ask the broadest possible questions of ultimate societal interest (for which the data are often deficient).

Even among researchers, different questions can be asked of the same data, and the quality of a given body of data for one type of application may well differ from the same data used for other purposes. Tabulations of cervical cancer mortality in relation to women's occupation (Savitz et al., 1995) have several possible applications, for example. We might ask what guidance such data can provide for cervical cancer screening, making no assumptions whatsoever regarding why some occupational groups have higher risk than others, accepting at face value the observation that they have such elevated risk. If women who work in the manufacturing industry show increased rates of cervical cancer, worksite screening programs in the manufacturing sector might be encouraged. A different application of this observation would be to address the etiologic basis for why some occupational groups show higher risks than others. If we are concerned with the effect of workplace chemical exposures in the etiology of cervical cancer, the exact same data documenting differential risk by employment sector are far less effective since we are lacking needed information on actual workplace exposure. The very same study may answer some questions very effectively, e.g., "Which work sectors are at higher risk?" and others poorly or not at all, e.g., "Do workplace chemicals cause cervical cancer?" Thus, the study's value must be defined relative to a specific application.

The distinctions between the goals of the data generator and data interpreter are especially apparent for descriptive epidemiology, such as demographic patterns, time trends in disease, and to some extent, patterns across groups defined by such broad attributes as gender, social class, and occupation. Such data are often generated for administrative purposes or perhaps to stimulate new ideas about why risks vary across time and populations. Nevertheless, clever interpreters often bring such data to bear in evaluation of causal hypotheses, such as the effect of the introduction or removal of potential causes of disease on time trends in disease occurrence, or the effectiveness of a newly introduced therapy in reducing mortality from a given disease. Even technically accurate data do not guarantee that the inferences that rely on those data are free of error. It depends on the match between the information and the use to which is it put.

The diverse interests of those who evaluate epidemiologic data, including those who generate it, serve as a useful reminder that the data are the object of inquiry rather than the character or intelligence of those who generate it. Individuals of the highest intelligence and moral character can generate flawed information, and those of limited talent can stumble into important and trustworthy findings. The elusive search for objectivity in generating and interpreting epidemiologic evidence is well served by a single-minded focus on the product and application of the information rather than the people who generate or use that product. Efforts to judge evidence based on the track record or mental processes of the investigator can only be a distraction. Although it may sound obvious that it is only the quality of the data that counts, this issue arises in considerations of disclosure of financial support for research that that may bias the investigator (Davidoff et al., 2001), the interpretation of data based on the intent or preconceptions of the investigator (Savitz & Olshan, 1995), and most insidiously, when research is judged based on the track record of those who generated it. As we make use of epidemiologic data to draw inferences, it is necessary to step back not only from the investigators as human beings but even from the original study goals to ask how effectively the information answers a specific question and contributes to a specific inference.

DESCRIPTIVE GOALS AND CAUSAL INFERENCE

Although inferences derived from epidemiologic data are generally concerned with causality, sometimes accurate measurement of the occurrence or pattern of disease is an end in itself. The research is successful to the extent that the measurement is accurate. A classic descriptive goal is to measure disease prevalence or the pattern of disease in demographic subgroups of the population for the purpose of planning and allocating health services. There is no explicit or implicit question about how the pattern of disease came about, only that it is present. The preponderance of women with dementia relative to the number of men with the disease has direct bearing on the provision of extended health care services to the elderly. The fact that this is largely or entirely the result of women's longer survival relative to men's rather than a higher incidence of dementia among women is irrelevant to those who provide care to those with dementia, who must contend with the larger proportion of women than men in need of care. The very concept of *confounding by age* is applicable only to the goal of drawing etiologic inferences regarding the association between gender and dementia, not a concern in meeting health service needs.

Accepting the goal of accurate measurement, avoiding any consideration of causality, there are still several requirements for the research to be valid and therefore useful. Distortion can arise due to problems in subject selection or participation (selection bias). For example, if women with dementia were cared for in institutional settings to a greater extent than men, perhaps due to lack of availability of a spouse as caregiver, an assessment restricted to those receiving institutional care would generate an inaccurate reflection of the true magnitude of gender differences. Similarly, errors in measuring exposure or disease (misclassification) are detrimental to any conceivable use of the data. If the diagnosis of dementia is in error, whether planning health services or studying etiology, the value of the study is diminished. The ill-defined process of *random error* also introduces uncertainty in the study results, independent of any concern with etiologic inference. If instead of conducting a full census of dementia in the service area, a random sample is chosen for enumeration, deviation between the sample and the total population is problematic for optimal service allocation. Each of these processes can result in a measure that is an inaccurate descriptor of the population under study. If we wished to compare dementia prevalence among men and women, non-response, erroneous classification of dementia (or gender), and random error due to sampling would contribute to an inaccurate comparison.

The initial goal of epidemiologic research is accurate measurement of the occurrence of disease or measurement of an association. Selection bias, misclassification, and random error thus reduce accuracy for even these purposes. Going beyond describing associations, epidemiologic studies can address causal relations, placing greater demands on the research and making it more vulnerable to error. Such inferences require consideration of whether the desired constructs have been captured accurately, more challenging for etiologic than descriptive purposes, and whether confounding is present, a concern unique to causal inference.

INFERENCES FROM EPIDEMIOLOGIC EVIDENCE: EFFICACY OF BREAST CANCER SCREENING

A specific example illustrates the range of potential questions that can be applied to epidemiologic data (Table 2.1) and how a given study may answer some questions effectively and others rather poorly. Assume that the exposure under study is participation in a regular mammography screening program and the disease of interest is fatal breast cancer. Such a study has potential relevance to many questions.

1. What is the mortality rate among women who participated in the mammography screening program?

    Answering this question requires, at a minimum, accurate data on participation and mortality. Loss to follow up can interfere with the accurate description of the experience of women enrolled in the program, and accurate measurement of breast cancer mortality is required for the mortality rate to be correct. Note that accurate estimation of mortality does not require consideration of confounding, information on breast cancer risk factors, or concern with self-selection for participation in the program. The goal is largely a descriptive one, accurately estimating a rate.

2. Is breast cancer mortality different in women who participated in the mammography screening program than women who did not participate?

    Beyond the requirement of accurate measurement of participation and mortality is the need to compare participants to nonparticipants. Note that the question as stated does not raise questions of causality, but only makes a comparison of rates. Even if we try to restrain our desire to make inferences about the causal effect of participation, questions arise regarding a suitable comparison group, and the desire to make broader inferences becomes increasingly difficult to escape. Women who did not participate could, under this general statement of the goal, be any women who did not do so, unrestricted by age, geography, breast cancer risk factors, etc. It is rare to make comparisons without some degree of interest in measuring a causal role for the attribute that distinguishes the groups. Claims of agnosticism should be scrutinized carefully—are the investigators just trying to forestall criticism by pretending to be uninterested in a causal inference? Wouldn't they really like to know what the breast cancer mortality rate among participants in the screening program would have been if they had not participated, and isn't that the inference they will make based on the nonparticipants?

3. Has participation in the mammography screening program caused a reduction in breast cancer mortality among those who participated in the program?

This question directly tackles causality and thus encounters a new series of methodologic concerns and questions. In the counterfactual conceptualization of causality (Greenland & Robins, 1986), the goals for this comparison group are much more explicit than in Question 2. Now, we would like to identify a group of women who reflect the breast cancer mortality rate that women who participated in the mammography screening program *would* have had if they had not in fact participated. (The comparison is counterfactual in that the participants, by definition, *did* participate; we wish to estimate the risk for those exact women had they not done so.) We can operationalize the selection of comparison women in a variety of imperfect ways but the conceptual goal is clear. Now, issues of self-selection, baseline risk factors for breast cancer mortality in the two groups, and confounding must be considered, all of which threaten the validity of causal inference.

4. Do mammography screening programs result in reduced mortality from breast cancer?

This question moves beyond causal inference for the study population of women who participated in the screening program, and now seeks a more universal answer for other, larger populations. Even if the answer to Question 3 is affirmative, subject to social and biological modifiers, the very same program may not result in reduced mortality from breast cancer in other populations. For example, the program would likely be ineffective among very young women in whom breast cancer is very rare, and it may be ineffective among women with a history of prior breast cancer where the recurrence risk may demand a more frequent screening interval. In order to address this question, a series of studies would need to be considered, examining the reasons for consistent or inconsistent findings and making inferences about the universality or specificity of the association.

5. Is breast cancer screening an effective public health strategy for reducing breast cancer mortality?

Given that we have been able to generate accurate information to answer the preceding questions, this next level of inference goes well beyond the epidemiologic data deeply into the realm of public health policy. This global question, of paramount interest in applying epidemiology to guiding public policy, requires examination of such issues as the protocol for this screening program in relation to other screening programs we might have adopted, problems in recruiting women for screening programs, financial costs of such programs relative to alternatives, what types of women are expected to benefit from the program, etc.

Answering the first question with confidence is readily within our grasp, and taken literally, the second question as well. The ability to make accurate measurements of exposure and disease is sufficient for addressing those narrow questions, and necessary but not sufficient for addressing the subsequent ones. The second question concerns a comparison but tries at least to defer any causal implications of the comparison—Are the mortality rates different for participants than nonparticipants? The third question is of the nature that much of this book focuses on, namely making causal inferences within a given study, spilling over into the fourth question, which is a broader inference about a series of epidemiologic studies. Question 5 goes well beyond epidemiology alone, though epidemiologic findings are clearly relevant to the broader policy judgment. The specific research question under consideration must be kept in focus, evaluating the quality of evidence for a specific purpose rather than generically. Study designs and data can only be evaluated based on the application of the evidence they generate, and the inferences that are to be made.

INFERENCES FROM EPIDEMIOLOGIC EVIDENCE: ALCOHOL AND SPONTANEOUS ABORTION

Another illustration of the different levels of inference about epidemiologic evidence and the challenges at each level concerns the relation between maternal alcohol intake in early pregnancy and the risk of spontaneous abortion, pregnancy loss prior to 20 weeks' gestation. The initial descriptive goal is to accurately measure alcohol consumption in a population of pregnant women, and then to monitor the incidence of spontaneous abortion. These measurement issues present a substantial challenge for both the exposure and the health endpoint. Generating accurate rates of pregnancy loss across groups with differing alcohol consumption (regardless of the desired application or interest) is fraught with potential error. Alcohol use is notoriously susceptible to erroneous measurement in the form of underreporting, irregular patterns of intake, potentially heterogeneous effects across beverage type, and variability in metabolism. Furthermore, there are no good biological markers of exposure that integrate information over time periods of more than a day. Early pregnancy is also difficult to identify accurately without a rather intensive biological monitoring protocol of daily hormone levels. Inaccuracy in identifying the onset of pregnancy introduces the potential for a differential reported rate of loss simply as a function of the completeness with which pregnancy is recognized in the earliest, most vulnerable period.

To make accurate assessments that extend beyond the individual women enrolled in the study, we need to ask whether those women on whom data are available provide an accurate representation of that segment of the study population that is of interest (freedom from selection bias). For example, do the heavy alcohol users recruited into the study provide an accurate reflection of the risk of spontaneous abortion among the larger target population of heavy alcohol users? Are only the most health-conscious drinkers willing to enroll in such a study, who engage in a series of other, risk-lowering behaviors, yielding spuriously low rates of spontaneous abortion among heavy drinkers relative to the target population of heavy drinkers? Selection among those in the exposure stratum that distorts the rate of spontaneous abortion limits any inferences about the effects of that exposure. Similarly, losses to follow-up may occur in a non-random manner, for example, if those who choose to have elective abortions would have differed in their risk of spontaneous abortion had they allowed their pregnancies to continue, and decisions regarding elective abortion may well differ in relation to alcohol use. These losses may distort the measured rate of spontaneous abortion within a stratum of alcohol use and introduce bias into the evaluation of a potential causal effect of alcohol.

Beyond the potential for misrepresentation of alcohol use, which would distort the results for any conceivable purpose, choices regarding the index and timing of alcohol use must be examined. Even an accurate estimate of the rate of spontaneous abortion in relation to average daily alcohol consumption would not address consumption at specific time intervals around conception, the effects of binge drinking, and the impact of specific beverage types, for example. The inference might be perfectly accurate with respect to one index yet quite inaccurate in fully characterizing the effect of alcohol consumption on risk of spontaneous abortion. If we were only interested in whether alcohol drinkers serve as a suitable population for intensified medical surveillance for pregnancy loss during prenatal care, for example, average daily alcohol intake might be quite adequate even if it is not the index most relevant to etiology. Misclassification and information bias are assessed relative to the etiologic hypothesis regarding an effect of alcohol on spontaneous abortion.

Technically, the study can only examine the statistical association between verbal or written response to questions on alcohol use and hormonal, clinical, or self-reported information pertinent to identifying spontaneous abortion. A truly agnostic interpretation of such measures is almost unattainable, given that the very act of making the comparisons suggests some desire to draw inferences about the groups being compared. To make such inferences correctly about whether alcohol *causes* spontaneous abortion, epidemiologic studies must be scrutinized to assess the relationship between the operational definitions of exposure and disease and the more abstract entities of interest. Criticism cannot be avoided by claiming that a study of questionnaire responses and pathology records has been conducted. Rather, the effectiveness of the operational measures as proxies for the constructs of interests is a critical component of interpreting epidemiologic evidence.

Our ultimate interest in many instances is in whether alterations in alcohol consumption would result in alterations in risk of spontaneous abortion. That is, would women who are high alcohol consumers during pregnancy assume the risk of low alcohol consumers if they had reduced their alcohol consumption? To address this question of causality, we would like to compare the risk among high alcohol consumers to what their risk would have been had they been otherwise identical but nondrinkers or low consumers of alcohol (Greenland & Robins, 1986). Our best estimate of that comparison is derived from the actual non-alcohol consumers with some additional statistical adjustments to take into account factors thought to be related to spontaneous abortion that distinguish the groups. Beyond all the measurement and selection issues within groups of differing alcohol use, we now have to ask about the comparability of the groups to one another. Confounding is a concern that only arises when we wish to go beyond a description of the data and make hypothetical inferences about what would happen if the exposed had not been exposed. The burden on the data rises incrementally as the goal progresses from pure description to causal inference.

CAUSAL INFERENCE

Others have discussed the philosophical issues underlying causal inference in some detail, including the challenges of making such inferences from observational studies (Lanes, 1988; Susser, 1977, 1991; Rothman & Poole, 1996). The key point is that causal inference is just that—an inference by the interpreter of the data, not a product of the study or something that is found within the evidence generated by the study. Given its nature, formulaic approaches to defining when it has been attained, as though the evidence were dichotomous instead of distributed continuously, and affirmative proof of causality should be avoided. Even the widely used criteria for causality (US Surgeon General, 1964; Hill, 1965) have limited value except as a broad set of guidelines of indirect value in assessing the potential for biased measures of association.

Causal inference in epidemiology is based on exclusion of non-causal explanations for observed associations. There are many possible reasons for the reported measures of association obtained in epidemiologic studies to be inaccurately reflecting the causal impact of exposure on disease. Random error and the familiar epidemiologic concepts of confounding, selection bias, and information bias are mechanisms for producing data that do not correctly quantify the causal component of the association of interest. Although researchers are sometimes reluctant to use the word *causality* because of modesty or the realization that their study falls short of definitively resolving the presence or absence of causality (and they are always right), articulating the goal of measuring the magnitude of causal effects helps to guide discussion of the evidence that has been obtained. With the exception of studies that seek a pure description, most epidemiologic research has an explicit or implicit goal of contributing toward a broader, causal inference. Making the goal explicit and ambitious helps to focus the evaluation of the evidence that was obtained.

The cliché that epidemiologic studies generate only measures of association, not causation is meaningless. The same is true of experimental studies, of course, even though the opportunity to randomly allocate exposure provides important advantages in making inferences beyond the immediate results. Nevertheless, even experiments just generate measures of association as well. We could just as accurately say that epidemiologic studies just generate numbers or binary codes in computers. It would be technically true, but not at all helpful in assessing what can be done with those numbers. Perhaps what is intended by emphasizing the inability of epidemiologic studies to address causality is that in epidemiology, like other sciences, we generate inferences from the data, trying to impose a meaning that is not inherent in the data. The data yield measures of association and those who examine the data make inferences about causality.

Drawing inferences is a speculative process, and acknowledging that fact advances rather than detracts from the value of epidemiologic research. Intelligent speculation is precisely the way to make complete, maximally useful assessments of epidemiologic research—Has the study accurately measured the constructs of interest? Does the measure of association accurately reflect the experience of the study population? Did the exposure contribute to an increased risk of disease in this population? Would the elimination of exposure reduce the risk of disease? Would exposure have the same effect in other populations? Without using the word causal, answers to each of these questions bear directly on causal inference. All questions concerning distortion of the measure of association help to accurately assess the causal effect of exposure, and any questions about whether the observed relation would hold in other populations and how much impact there would be from reducing the exposure make use of the presumed causal association that has been measured.

We ought not set the bar too high for studies to serve as the basis for considering causality—it is not required that the studies be flawless to justify such scrutiny. Once causal inference is recognized to fall along a continuum of interpretation, even descriptive or methodologically weak studies are fodder for the assessment of causality. There is no basis for setting a threshold of effect size or study quality as a prerequisite to enter the realm of causal inference. Studies that contribute modestly to a causal evaluation should be recognized and valued as doing exactly that.

Those who conduct the research need not even provide a comprehensive or definitive interpretation of their own data, an elusive goal as well. A perfectly complete, unbiased, accurate representation of the study results is also unattainable. The principal goal of the investigators should be to reveal as much as possible about their study methods and results in order to help themselves and others make appropriate use of their research findings. Given that the challenges to causal inference can often be anticipated, data that bear on the threats to such inference are needed to interpret the results. Many of the strategies suggested in this book require anticipation of such a challenge at the time of study design and execution. If a key confounder is known to be present, e.g., tobacco use in assessing alcohol effects on bladder cancer, detailed cross-tabulations may be desirable to help assess whether confounding has been successfully eliminated. If the assessment of a construct poses special challenges, e.g., measurement of workplace stress, then the instrument needs to be described in great detail along with relevant data that bear on its validity. Ideally, this complete description of methods and results is conducted with the goal of sharing as much of the information as possible that will assist in the interpretation by the investigators and others. The formal discussion of those results in the published version of the study provides an evaluation of what the study means to the authors of the report. Although the investigators have the first opportunity to make such an evaluation, it would not be surprising if others among the thousands of reviewers of the published evidence have more helpful insights or can bring greater objectivity to bear in making the assessment. Rather than stacking the deck in providing results to ensure that the only possible inferences are concordant with those of the original researchers, those who can provide enough raw material for readers to make different inferences should be commended for their full disclosure rather than criticized for having produced findings that are subject to varying interpretations. This pertains to revealing flaws in the study as well as fully elucidating the pattern of findings. In the conventional structure of publication, the *Methods* and *Results* are the basis for evaluation and inference; the *Discussion* is just a point of view that the investigators happen to hold.

We sometimes have the opportunity to directly evaluate the role of potential biases, for example, assessing whether a given measure of association has been distorted by a specific confounding factor. Generating an adjusted measure of association tells us whether potential confounding has actually occurred, and also provides an estimate of what the association would be if confounding were absent. Note that the exercise of calculating a confounder-adjusted result is also inherently speculative and subject to error, for example, if the confounder is poorly measured. An example of a concern that is typically less amenable to direct evaluation is the potential for selection bias due to non-response, usually evaluated by comparing participants to nonparticipants. The hypothesis that the association has been distorted by confounding or non-response is evaluated by generating relevant data to guide those who review the evidence, including the authors, in making an assessment of the likelihood and extent of such distortion.

In an ideal world, causal inference would be the end product of systematic evaluation of alternative explanations for the data, with an unambiguous conclusion regarding the extent to which the measured association accurately reflects the magnitude of the causal relationship. In practice, a series of uncertainties preclude doing so with great confidence. The list of alternative explanations is limited only by the imagination of critics, with insightful future reviewers always having the potential to change the status of the evidence. Judgment of whether a particular alternative explanation has truly been eliminated (or confirmed) is itself subjective. Hypotheses of bias may be more directly testable than the hypothesis of causality, but they remain challenging to definitively prove or disprove. The culmination of the examination of individual contributors to bias is a judgment of how plausible or strong the distortion is likely to be and how confidently such an assertion can be made rather than a simple dichotomy of present or absent. Thus, the answer to the ultimate question of whether the reported association correctly measures the etiologic relationship will always be "maybe," with the goal of making an accurate assessment of where the evidence fits within the wide spectrum that extends from the unattainable benchmarks of "yes" or "no."

The array of potential biases that limit certainty regarding whether an etiologic association (or its absence) has been measured accurately is valuable in specifying the frontier for advancement of research. If the major concerns remaining after the most recent study or series of studies can be clearly articulated, the agenda for refinement in the next round of studies has been properly defined. If the somewhat mundane but real problem were one of small study size and imprecision, then a larger study with the strengths of the previous ones would be suggested. If uncertainty regarding the role of a key confounder contributes importantly to a lack of resolution, then identifying a population free of such confounding (by randomization or identifying favorable circumstances in which the exposure and confounder are uncoupled) or accurate measurement and control of the confounder may be needed. Precisely the same process that is needed to judge the strength of evidence yields insights into key features needed for subsequent studies to make progress.

The most challenging and intellectually stimulating aspect of interpreting epidemiologic evidence is in the process of assessing causality. A wide array of methodological concerns must be considered, integrating the data from the study or studies of interest with relevant substantive knowledge and theoretical principles. We are rarely able to fully dispose of threats to validity or find fatal flaws that negate the evidence, leaving a list of potential biases falling somewhere along the continuum of possibility. With this array of such considerations in mind, a balanced, explicit judgment must be made. On the one hand, the need to make such complex assessments is threatening and all but guarantees disagreement among experts. On the other hand, viewed in this manner, each increment in knowledge of the methodological and substantive issues yields benefits in making wiser judgments. Whether moving from a point of near certainty toward certainty or from complete ignorance to slightly more informed speculation, progress made by research can be appreciated.

CONTRIBUTION OF EPIDEMIOLOGY TO POLICY DECISIONS

Viewing causal inference in epidemiology as falling on a continuum of certainty, never reaching a clearly defined point of resolution, may sound like a formula for inaction. If tobacco use has not actually been *proven*, beyond all possible doubt, to cause disease based on epidemiologic studies, then how can actions to curtail or eliminate use of tobacco be justified? In fact, the spectrum of scientific certainty has been used cynically at times to argue that control of tobacco or other hazards should await definitive proof, quite possibly with the knowledge that such proof will never come. It would be much easier to explain and market epidemiologic evidence to outsiders if we set a quantitative threshold for proven as is done in court (more probable than not). In opposition to such an approach is the inability to measure certainty in such formal, quantitative terms, the incentive it would create to understate or exaggerate the certainty of epidemiologic evidence, and the real possibility that errors of overinterpretation and underinterpretation of epidemiologic research would become more rather than less common.

Policy decisions or individual behavioral decisions can be viewed as an integrated assessment of the risks and benefits among alternative courses of action. There are always a variety of options available, including inaction, whether or not such lists are formally articulated. In the case of tobacco, three simple options are *(1)* lack of regulation, *(2)* complete banning, and *(3)* policies to discourage its use. Among the components of such a decision are economic concerns with tobacco farmers, cigarette manufacturers, and the retail trade industry, the value placed on individual freedom, the magnitude of health harm from tobacco use, and the burden on the health care system from tobacco-related disease. Note that the policy decision is not based solely on epidemiologic evidence, though epidemiology contributes importantly to the decision. Even if we had some accepted threshold for proven, reaching that threshold would not make the appropriate policy clear.

Restricting discussion to the epidemiologic component of the information needed for wise decision-making, a variety of issues must be considered. The probability that tobacco contributes to specific diseases and the quantitative assessment of such effects is critical to policy makers. Because the ultimate decision integrates epidemiology with many other lines of evidence, however, a given amount of epidemiologic evidence may be sufficient for some purposes and insufficient for others. That is, the definition of "sufficient epidemiologic evidence" is specific to the situation, depending on the weight of other factors promoting or discouraging the different policy options. For a given level of epidemiologic evidence, extraneous considerations define whether the balance tips in favor of one action or another. In a simple illustration, assume the epidemiologic evidence of potential adverse effects is identical for two food additives, one of which prevents life-threatening microbial contamination and the other merely enhances the visual appeal of the product. The epidemiologic evidence could be appropriately viewed as insufficient to warrant elimination of the first product but sufficient to warrant elimination of the second, but what really differs is the competing considerations outside of the epidemiologic evidence concerning the food additive's potential for harm.

A clearer, more honest appraisal of the role of epidemiologic evidence as the basis for action has several benefits, in spite of the potential for abuse resulting from a more open acknowledgment of the uncertainties. Full evaluation of risks and benefits should, in principle, lead to wiser actions than attempts to oversimplify the decision, e.g., "health harm must be avoided at any costs" or "the epidemiologic evidence demands action." Acknowledging the subtle balance among the various considerations that influence policy can help to define where further epidemiologic evidence would be most helpful. Research priorities in epidemiology should be influenced by an appreciation of those situations in which more definitive answers would tip the balance on important policy issues, focusing investment of resources on those situations in which the balance is fragile and can be shifted with refined epidemiologic information.

In some instances, even a wide range of inferences from epidemiologic evidence all fall in a range that would have the same policy implications. In examining the influence on public policy regarding tobacco use, the ongoing controversies about differential effects on lung cancer by cell type, different effects among men and women, and quantification of the interaction with diet or occupational exposures are of scientific importance and may yield important insights regarding mechanisms of disease causation, but their resolution is unlikely to affect the key message for those who must decide tobacco policy. A wide range of reasonable interpretations of the epidemiologic evidence all lead to the same policy choice.

Recognizing that epidemiology is but one of many scientific approaches to informing policy (Savitz et al., 1999) might liberate epidemiologists somewhat from their fear of overinterpretaion or unwarranted speculation. Weak or preliminary epidemiologic findings might well be injected into the policy discussion and correctly limited in their impact. There is great concern about fearmongering and rapidly changing evidence at early stages of the evolution of research (Taubes, 1995). However, if correctly interpreted, those early findings often are and should be superseded at the policy level by other scientific and non-scientific concerns. Weak contributory evidence is not the same as no evidence or counterproductive evidence.

It is important for epidemiologists to recognize that scientific disciplines such as toxicology contribute independent evidence to be used in assessing health risks and benefits, not just assisting in the interpretation of epidemiology. Absolved of the fear that their data might be taken too literally and isolated from other important scientific and non-scientific considerations, epidemiologists might be less inhibited about generating evidence on matters of public controversy such as health risks and benefits of medically induced abortion or the identification of risk factors associated with intentional injury.

A perceived drawback to the use of epidemiologic evidence is the highly visible and persistent controversies that surround it, which can be inconvenient for policy makers and at times, disconcerting to the public at large (Taubes, 1995). There is no evidence that the proportion of published findings from epidemiology that are inaccurate or misleading differs from that in other scientific disciplines. The cold fusion story illustrates that even in physics, science does not follow straight lines of progress, building one accurate, and properly interpreted finding on top of the other.

Most associations reported in the epidemiologic literature probably do not provide an accurate reflection of the exact causal relation they are intended to address. Perusal of any issue of an epidemiology journal contains dozens, sometimes hundreds, of estimates of association regarding how diet, medications, and workplace exposures might affect health, and few readers would take those individual findings and interpret them as quantitative reflections of the underlying causal effects. Capturing causal relations with accuracy is tremendously challenging. Epidemiologic measures of association are distorted to varying extent by random error or bias, or perhaps reflect a real phenomenon that is not exactly what it purports to be. By and large, researchers appropriately treat those findings as leads to be challenged and pursued. Whereas experimental approaches may well have a better rate of success in having their observed associations reflect causality, the challenge there is often one of applicability to the human health conditions of ultimate interest.

Perhaps the unique feature of epidemiology is how amenable it is to overinterpretation and sensationalism in the media. Most publications in physics and molecular biology, right or wrong, reach others in the field and do not engage media or public interest. When the alarms are found to be false alarms, the science moves forward without shame. The same phenomenon in epidemiology, played out in a much more public arena, yields an impression of incompetence, exaggeration of the value of research findings, and endless acrimony among competing factions.

There are two possible solutions to this dilemma: *(1)* The optimal, infeasible solution is to ensure that published epidemiologic evidence is valid. *(2)* The alternative is to continue to put forward fallible observations, debate their merits, and seek a systematic, objective appraisal of the value of the information. The remaining chapters of this book are devoted to that goal of organizing the scrutiny and interpretation of epidemiologic evidence.

The importance of epidemiologic evidence in decision-making at a societal and personal level is generally recognized, sometimes excessively so, but the unique strengths of epidemiology in that regard are worth reiterating. Study of the species of interest, humans, in its natural environment with all the associated biological and behavioral diversity markedly reduces the need for extrapolation relative to many experimental approaches with laboratory animals or cell cultures. It has been suggested that experimental approaches to understanding human health obtain precise answers to the wrong questions whereas epidemiology obtains imprecise answers to the right questions. Just as those who design experiments seek to make the inferences as relevant as possible to the ultimate applications in public health and clinical medicine, epidemiologists must strive to make their information as valid as possible, not losing the inherent strength of studying free-living human populations.

REFERENCES

Davidoff F, DeAngelis CD, Drazen JM, Hoey J, Hʼjgaard L, Horton R, Kotzin S, Nicholls MG, Nylenna M, Overbeke AJPM, Sox HC, Van der Weyden MB, Wilkes MS. Sponsorship, authorship, and accountability. N Engl J Med 2001;345:825–827.

Greenland S. Probability versus Popper: An elaboration of the insufficiency of current Popperian approaches for epidemiologic analysis. In Rothman KJ (ed), Causal inference. Chestnut Hill, MA: Epidemiology Resources Inc., 1988:95–104.

Greenland S, Robins JM. Identifiability, exchangeability, and epidemiologic confounding. Int J Epidemiol 1986;15:413–419.

Hill AB. The environment and disease: association or causation? Proc Roy Soc Med 1965 ;58:295–300.

Lanes SF. The logic of causal inference. In Rothman KJ (ed), Causal inference. Chestnut Hill, MA: Epidemiology Resources Inc., 1988:59–75.

Rothman KJ. Modern Epidemiology. Boston: Little, Brown and Co., 1986.

Rothman KJ, Poole C. Causation and causal inference. In D Schottenfeld, JF Fraumeni Jr (eds), Cancer Epidemiology and Prevention, Second Edition. New York: Oxford University Press, 1996:3–10.

Savitz DA, Andrews KW, Brinton LA. Occupation and cervical cancer. J Occup Envir Med 1995;37:357–361.

Savitz DA, Olshan AF. Multiple comparisons and related issues in the interpretation of epidemiologic data. Am J Epidemiol 1995;142:904–908.

Savitz DA, Poole C, Miller WC. Reassessing the role of epidemiology in public health. Am J Pub Health 1999;89:1158–1161.

Susser M. Judgment and causal inference: criteria in epidemiologic studies. Am J Epidemiol 1977;105:1–15.

Susser M. What is a cause and how do we know one? A grammar for pragmatic epidemiology. Am J Epidemiol 1991;133:635–648.

Taubes G. Epidemiology faces its limits (news report). Science 1995;269:164–169.

US Department of Health, Education, and Welfare. Smoking and health. Report of the Advisory Committee to the Surgeon General. Public Health Service Publication No. 1103. Washington, DC: US Government Printing Office, 1964.

3

STRATEGY FOR DRAWING INFERENCES
FROM EPIDEMIOLOGIC EVIDENCE

Validity of epidemiologic results refers broadly to the degree to which the inferences drawn from a study are warranted (Last, 2001). The central goal in evaluating epidemiologic evidence is to accurately define the sources of uncertainty and the probability of errors of varying magnitude affecting the results. Validity cannot be established by affirmatively demonstrating its presence but rather by systematically considering and eliminating, or more often reducing, the sources of bias that detract from validity. The goal of this scrutiny is to quantify the uncertainty resulting from potential biases, considering the probability that the different sources of potential bias have introduced varying magnitudes of distortion. Part of this assessment can be made on theoretical grounds, but whenever possible, pertinent data should be sought both inside and outside the study to assess the likely magnitude of error. Sometimes the information needed to evaluate a potential source of error is readily available, but in other instances research has to be undertaken to determine to what extent the hypothesized source of error actually may have affected the study results. In fact, an important feature of the data collection and data analysis effort should be to generate the information needed to fairly and fully assess the validity of the results. In principle, with all relevant data in hand from the set of pertinent studies, a comprehensive evaluation of sources of uncertainty would yield a clear and accurate inference regarding the present state of knowledge and identify specific methodologic issues that need to be addressed to advance knowledge in future studies. This ideal comprehensive, quantitative, objective assessment of evidence is, of course, unattainable in practice, but serves as a standard to which interpreters of epidemiologic evidence should aspire.

An easier and perhaps more commonly used approach to assessing evidence is to rely on a summary judgment of experts, either individually or as a committee. Peer review of manuscripts submitted for publication, informal assessment by colleagues, and consensus conferences typically fall into this category. Although the experts can and often do apply objective criteria, in practice the summary pronouncements are often sweeping and lacking in statements of probability: the data are inconclusive or causal inference is justified or the evidence is weak. The advantages of relying on authoritative individuals or groups are the speed with which a summary of the evidence can be generated, the ease of explaining the process (at least at a superficial level) to outsiders, and the credibility that authorities have among both experts and nonexperts. In the absence of information on the basis for such assessments however, there is no assurance that the evidence was considered comprehensively, quantitatively, or objectively. Decomposing the evaluation into its component parts allows others to understand and challenge the steps that led to the final conclusion. By revealing the process by which conclusions were drawn, the assumptions, evidence, and inferences are made clear for all to understand (and criticize). In principle, the conclusion that evidence is convincing could only come from having considered and determined that potential sources of bias have little impact, and the evidence that led to that conclusion is essential to assess whether it is likely to be correct. Similarly, the assessment that the evidence from reported associations is weak or inconclusive must arise from having identified sources of bias and evidence that those biases have distorted the results to a substantial degree. The underlying pieces of information that led to the final evaluation are as important as the conclusion itself.

NEED FOR SYSTEMATIC EVALUATION OF SOURCES OF ERROR

To serve the goal of accurate interpretation of epidemiologic evidence, there are substantial intellectual and practical advantages to a systematic, component-by-component evaluation:

1. Conclusions drawn from the results of epidemiologic studies are more likely to be valid if the evaluation is truly comprehensive, enumerating and carefully considering all potentially important sources of bias. Although this thorough examination may make the ultimate inferences more, not less, equivocal, the conclusions will be more accurately linked to the evidence.

Even (especially?) experts have preconceptions and blind spots, and may well be prone to evaluating evidence based on an initial, subjective overview and then maintaining consistency with their initial gut impressions. For example, a study done by talented investigators at a prominent institution and published in a prestigious journal may convey an initial image of certain validity, but none of those characteristics provide assurance of accuracy nor does their absence provide evidence that the results are in error. Systematic scrutiny helps to ensure that important limitations are not overlooked and ostensibly important limitations are examined to determine whether they really are likely to have had a substantial impact on the study results.

2. Intellectual understanding of the phenomenon of interest and methodologic issues is enhanced by a detailed, evidence-based examination. Even if experts were capable of taking unexplained shortcuts to reach an accurate assessment of the state of knowledge (epidemiologic intuition), without understanding of the process by which the judgment was reached, the rest of us would be deprived of the opportunity to develop those skills. Furthermore, the field of epidemiology makes progress based on the experience of new applications, so that the scholarly foundations of the discipline are advanced only by methodically working through these steps over and over again. Reaching the right conclusion about the meaning and certainty of the evidence is of paramount importance, but it is also vital to understand *why* it is correct and to elucidate the principles that should be applied to other such issues that will inevitably arise in the future.

3. Research needs are revealed by describing specific deficiencies and uncertainties in previous studies that can be remedied. Bottom line conclusions reveal little about what should be done next—What constructive action follows from a global assessment that the evidence is weak or strong? By explaining the reasoning used to draw conclusions, a natural by-product is a menu of candidate refinements for new studies. Quantifying the probability and impact of sources of potential error helps to establish priorities for research. The most plausible sources of bias that are the most capable of producing substantial error are precisely the issues that need to be tackled with the highest priority in future studies, whatever the current state of knowledge. In practice, it is often only a few methodological issues that predominate to limit the conclusiveness of a study or set of studies, but this becomes clear only through systematic review and evaluation.

4. Reasons for disagreement among evaluators will only be revealed by defining the basis for their judgments. Multiple experts often examine the same body of evidence and come to radically different conclusions, puzzling other scholars and the public at large. If those who held opposing views would articulate the component steps in their evaluations that generated their summary views, and characterize their interpretations of the evidence bearing

on each of those issues, the points of disagreement would be much better understood. Whether the disagreement concerns substantive or methodologic issues, narrower issues are more amenable to resolution than sweeping, summary evaluations. The discourse is much more informative for others as well when the argument is in specific terms (e.g., "Is a particular confounder associated strongly enough with disease to have yielded a relative risk of 2.0 under the null hypothesis?"), as opposed to one reviewer claiming the evidence for an association is convincing and the other asserting that it is weak.

NEED FOR OBJECTIVE ASSESSMENT OF EPIDEMIOLOGIC EVIDENCE

The need to strive for impartiality in the evaluation of evidence must be stressed, partly because there are strong forces encouraging subjectivity. Among the most vital, exciting aspects of epidemiology are its value in understanding how the world we live in operates to affect health and the applicability of epidemiologic evidence to policy. Epidemiologic research bears on the foods we eat, the medications we take, our physical activity levels, and the most intimate aspects of our sexual behavior, emotional ties, and whether there are health benefits to having pets. Putting aside the scholarly arguments made in this book, I am sure every reader "knows" something about what is beneficial and harmful, and it is difficult to overcome such insights with scientific evidence. (I don't need epidemiologic research to convince me that there are profound health benefits from owning pet dogs, and I am equally certain that pet cats are lacking in such value.) Epidemiologic evidence bearing on such issues is not interpreted in a vacuum, but rather intrudes on deeply held preconceptions based on our cultures, religions, and lifestyles. Judgments about epidemiologic evidence pertinent to policy inevitably collide with our political philosophy and social values. In fact, suspicion regarding the objectivity of the interpretation of evidence should arise when researchers generate findings that are consistently seen as supporting strongly held ideology.

Beyond the more global context for epidemiologic evidence, other challenges to impartiality arise in the professional workplace. On a personal level, we may not always welcome criticism of the quality of our own work or that of valued colleagues and friends, or be quite as willing as we should be to accept the excellent work done by those we dislike. The ultimate revelation of an ad hominem assessment of evidence lies in the statement that "I didn't believe it until we saw it in our own data." Such self-esteem may have great psychological value but is worrisome with regard to objectivity. Epidemiologists may also be motivated to protect the prestige of the discipline, which can encourage us to overstate or understate the conclusiveness of a given research product. We may be tempted to close ranks and defend our department or research team in the face of criticism, especially from outsiders. Such behavior is admirable in many ways, but counter to scientific neutrality.

Perhaps most significant for epidemiologists, who are often drawn to the field by their strong conviction to promote public health agendas, is the temptation to promote those public health agendas in part through their interpretations of scientific evidence (Savitz et al., 1999). The often influential, practical implications of epidemiology, the greatest strength of the discipline, can also be its greatest pitfall to the extent that it detracts from dispassionate evaluation. The implications of the findings (quite separate from the scientific merits of the research itself) create incentives to reach a particular conclusion or at least to lean one way or another in the face of true ambiguity. The greatest service epidemiologists can provide those who must make policy decisions or just decide how to live their lives is to offer an objective evaluation of the state of knowledge and let the many other pertinent factors that bear on such decisions be distilled by the policy maker or individual in the community, without being predigested by the epidemiologist.

For example, advocates of restrictions on exposure to environmental tobacco smoke may be inclined to interpret the evidence linking such exposures to lung cancer as strong whereas the same evidence, viewed by those who oppose such restrictions, is viewed as weak. A recent review of funding sources and conclusions in overviews of the epidemiologic evidence on this topic finds, not surprisingly, that tobacco industry sponsorship is associated with a more skeptical point of view (Barnes & Bero, 1998). Whereas judgment of the epidemiologic evidence is (or should be) a matter for science, a position on the policy of restricting public smoking is, by definition, in the realm of advocacy—public policy decisions require taking sides. However, the goal of establishing sound public policy that advances public health is not well served by distorting the epidemiologic evidence.

Fallible epidemiologic evidence on the health effects of environmental tobacco smoke may well be combined with other lines of evidence and principles to justify restricted public smoking. Believing that public smoking should be curtailed is a perfectly reasonable policy position but should not be used to retrofit the epidemiologic evidence linking environmental tobacco smoke to adverse health effects and exaggerate its strength. Similarly, strongly held views about individual liberties may legitimately outweigh epidemiologic evidence supporting adverse health effects of environmental tobacco smoke in some settings, and there is no need to distort the epidemiologic evidence to justify such a policy position. As discussed in Chapter 2, epidemiologic evidence is only one among many sources of information to consider, so that limited epidemiologic evidence or even an absence of epidemiologic evidence does not preclude support for a policy of such restriction nor does strong epidemiologic evidence dictate that such a policy must be adopted. Cleanly separating evaluation of epidemiology from applications of that evidence to policy encourages a more dispassionate assessment of the epidemiology and ultimately more rational, informed policy.

A primary goal of this book is to help make the evaluation of epidemiologic evidence more objective, in large part by making the criticisms and credibility of those criticisms more explicit, quantitative, comprehensive, and testable through empirical evaluation. Even when scientists disagree about the proper course of action, which they inevitably will do, just as nonscientists disagree, they may still agree about the key sources of uncertainty in the epidemiologic literature and the direction and magnitude of the potential biases.

At first glance, revealing epidemiology's "dirty laundry" by exposing and dwelling on the sources and magnitude of error may be seen as threatening to its credibility among other scientists and the public at large. Elevating the debate to focus on concrete, testable hypotheses of bias is more likely to have the beneficial by-product of enhancing the image of epidemiology in the broader scientific community. There seems to be the impression that epidemiologists have limitless criticisms of every study and thus they are unable to present a clear consensus to other scientists, policy makers, and the public. Such criticism and debate should not be restrained for public relations purposes, but to be useful the debate should focus on important issues in the interpretation of the evidence, explain why those issues are important, and point toward research to resolve those concerns. If those who held opposing viewpoints were better able to reach agreement on the specific points of contention that underlie their differences, work to encourage the research that would resolve their disagreements, and accept the results of that improved research, other scientists and the public could better understand that epidemiologists engage in the same process of successive approximations of the truth as other scientific disciplines. The disagreements would be clearly seen as constructive debate that helps to refine the study methods and reach greater clarity in the results and encourages the investment of resources in the research to resolve important controversies, not as personal bickering or petty disagreements over arcane, inconsequential issues. The ultimate test of the value of the disagreement is in whether it leads to improvements in the research and advancements in knowledge.

ESTIMATION OF MEASURES OF EFFECT

The starting point for evaluating the validity of results is to calculate and present estimates of the effect measure or measures of primary interest. This estimate might be disease prevalence, a risk ratio or risk difference, or a quantitative estimate of the dose-response function relating exposure to a health outcome. In order to consider the extent to which the study has successfully measured what it sought to measure, the key outcomes must be isolated for the most intense scrutiny. The question of validity is operationalized by asking the degree to which the estimated measure of effect is accurately representing what it purports to measure.

The measure of interest is quantitative, not qualitative. Thus, the object of evaluation is not a statement of a conclusion, e.g., exposure does or does not cause disease, or an association is or is not present. Instead, the product of the study is a measurement of effect and quantification of the uncertainty in that estimate, e.g., we estimate that the risk of disease is 2.2 times greater among exposed than unexposed persons (with a 95% confidence interval of 1.3 to 3.7), or for each unit change in exposure, the risk of disease rises by a 5 cases per 1000 persons per year (95% confidence interval of 1.2 to 8.8). Statement of the result in quantitative terms correctly presents the study as an effort to produce an accurate measurement rather than to create the impression that studies generate dichotomous results, e.g., the presence or absence of an association (Rothman, 1986). The simplification into a dichotomous result, based either on statistical tests or some arbitrary, subjective judgments about what magnitude of association is real or important hinders the goal of quantitative, objective evaluation.

The alternative approach, driven by conventional frequentist statistical concepts, is to focus on the benchmark of the null hypothesis, motivated perhaps by a desire for neutral, restrained interpretation of evidence. In this framework, study results are viewed solely to determine whether the data are sufficiently improbable under the null hypothesis to lead to rejection of the null hypothesis or a failure to reject the null hypothesis. For studies that generate ratio measures of effect, this is equivalent to asking whether we reject or fail to reject the null hypothesis that the relative risk is 1.0. Rejecting the null hypothesis implies that the relative risk takes on some other value but tells us no more than that. The null value is just one hypothetical true value among many with which the data can be contrasted, not the only or necessarily the most important one. The magnitude of uncertainty in an estimated relative risk of 1.0 is not conceptually different than the uncertainty in estimates of 0.5 or 5.0. Also, focusing on the measure as the study product avoids the inaccurate impression that successful studies yield large measures of effect and unsuccessful studies do not. Successful studies yield accurate measures of effect, as close as possible to the truth with less uncertainty than unsuccessful ones.

The measure of interest is determined by the substantive study question, presented in common language rather than statistical jargon. For example, a study may suggest that persons who drink 4 or more cups of coffee per day have 1.5 times the risk of a myocardial infarction compared to persons who drink fewer than 4 cups of coffee per day, with a 95% confidence interval of 0.8 to 2.6. Study products are not expressed in terms of well-fitting models or regression coefficients, nor should the results be distilled into test statistics such as t-statistics or chi-squared statistics or as p-values. In the above example, an indication that the comparison of the risk of myocardial infarction among persons drinking 4 or more cups of coffee versus those drinking fewer than 4 cups of coffee yielded a chi-square statistic of 8.37 or a p-value of 0.074 is not a result that can be directly related to the substantive question driving the study. These statistical measures are generated only to serve as tools to aid in the interpretation of epidemiologic evidence about disease or relations between exposure and disease, not as the primary study product. The product of the study is the quantitative estimate of effect and accompanying uncertainty, which is generated by statistical analysis, but the statistical analysis is not the product in its own right. In some instances, the translation of a statistical to a substantive measure is trivial, such as converting a logistic regression coefficient into an adjusted odds ratio as a measure of effect. In other instances, particularly when viewed from a rigid statistical testing framework or from the perspective of fitting statistical models, the quantitative measure of interest can become obscure. In one example, a key result was that a term did not enter the model in a stepwise regression (Joffe & Li, 1994) so that the reader could only infer the estimate of effect must be small and/or imprecise (Savitz & Olshan, 1995a). "Not entering the model" is a rather indirect statement about the magnitude and precision of the effect estimate. Similarly, a statistically significant p-value is not a measure of direct interest any more than a response proportion or a measure of reliability. They are all tools to assist in assessing the validity of the truly important measure, the one that quantifies the relation of interest. In serving that purpose, some statistical products are more valuable than others.

Many intermediate and peripheral statistical results are typically generated in addition to the primary estimate of effect and those can certainly help in the interpretation of the primary result. All the preliminary efforts to describe the study population, characterize respondents and nonrespondents, and evaluate associations between exposure or disease and potential confounders are important for assessing validity. However, they play a supporting, not the leading role as products of the study. Except for methodologic efforts in which the primary aim is to examine a hypothesized source of bias rather than a causal relation between exposure and disease, studies are not typically undertaken to measure response proportions or quantify confounding. When statistical procedures are used in an attempt to remove bias, such as adjustment for confounders or corrections for measurement error, the study result that constitutes the object of scrutiny may then become the adjusted measure of effect. Therefore, the process by which the measure was generated, including statistical adjustments intended to make it more accurate, needs to be examined to assess the validity of the final result. In asking if the study generated an accurate measure of effect, it is important to know whether confounding or measurement error was successfully addressed. If a potential source of bias in the measure has been identified and corrected, then obviously it is no longer a source of bias. On the other hand, attempts to make such corrections can be ineffective or, at worst, harmful.

Data collection efforts often yield numerous analyses and contribute substantively to many different lines of research (Savitz & Olshan, 1995b). For the purposes of examining and discussing validity of measurement, each analysis and each key measure must be considered separately. While there are techniques for refining individual estimates based on an array of results that address random error (Greenland & Robins, 1991), for evaluating systematic biases, the focus is not the study or the data set but rather the result, since a given study may well yield accurate results for one question but erroneous results for others. Features of the study uncovered through one analysis may bear positively or negatively on the validity of other analyses using the same data set, in that the same sources of bias can affect multiple estimates. However, the question of whether the study product is accurate must be asked for each such product of the study.

Some confusion can arise in discussing accurate measurement of individual variables versus accurate measures of association. If the study is designed to measure disease prevalence, for example, the study product and object of scrutiny is the prevalence measure. We ask about sources of distortion in the observed relative to the unknown true value of disease prevalence. When the focus is on measures of association, the measure of association is the key study product. Errors in measurement of the pertinent exposure, disease, or confounders all may produce distortion of the measure of association, but the focus is not on the measurement of individual variables; it is on the estimate of the association itself.

CONCEPTUAL FRAMEWORK FOR THE EVALUATION OF ERROR

Viewing the study product as a quantitative measure makes the evaluation of the accuracy of the study equivalent to a quantitative evaluation of the accuracy of the measure. Just as studies are not good or bad but fall along a continuum, the accuracy of the study's findings are not correct or incorrect but simultaneously informative and fallible to varying degrees. This quantitative approach to the examination of bias is contrasted with an evaluation that treats biases as all-or-none phenomena. If the product of a study is presented as a dichotomy, e.g., exposure is/is not associated with disease, then sources of potential error are naturally examined with respect to whether or not they negate that association: Is the association (or lack of association) due to random error? Is the association due to response bias? Is the association due to confounding? The search for error is viewed as an effort to implicate or exonerate a series of potentially fatal flaws that could negate the results of the study. Such an approach simplifies the discussion but it does not make full use of the information available to draw the most appropriate inference from the findings.

A more constructive approach to the consideration of bias would consider the role of systematic error in much the same way that random error is viewed—as a ubiquitous source of some amount of error, but for which the focus is on how much error is present with what probability. In fact, to consider biases as having all-or-none effects on the results is just as inappropriate as considering random error to be present or absent. Just as larger studies have less random error than small studies, soundly designed and conducted studies have less systematic error than less well designed and conducted studies.

Another important parallel is the magnitude of potential error. Random error may cause small deviations between the estimated measure of effect and the underlying parameter value, but becomes increasingly improbable as a cause of more substantial deviations. Similarly, it is generally reasonable to assume that biases may cause small amounts of measurement error more readily than large amounts of such error. Unfortunately, the underlying theoretical and quantitative framework for characterizing the impact of sampling error or error that arises in the randomization of subjects does not apply so readily to observational studies (Greenland, 1990), and the extension of that framework to non-random error is even less readily translated into formal quantitative terms even though it remains a useful goal.

A more quantitative assessment of bias has two distinct components, both taking on a spectrum of possible values: How *probable* is it that a specific source of bias has yielded distortion of a given *magnitude*? It would be possible for a candidate bias to be very likely or even certain to be present and introduce a small amount of error, for example, selection bias from non-response, but to be very unlikely to introduce a large amount of error. Rather than asking, "How likely is it that selection bias from non-response introduced error?" we would like to know, "How much does selection bias shift the position and change the width of the confidence interval around the estimated measure of effect?"

For example, initially ignoring the contribution of selection bias or misclassification, it may be inferred that an observed relative risk of 2.0 under the null hypothesis seems highly unlikely to result from random error, whereas once the information on these sources of bias are incorporated, such a disparity becomes much more plausible. The interpretation for other candidate deviations between estimated effects and hypothesized true values would also shift with the incorporation of an understanding of the potential for selection bias, the strength of the study's results for some candidate hypotheses becoming stronger and for other candidate hypotheses becoming weaker. There are families of questions that correspond to probabilities of distortion of specified amounts, and assessing the potential for such distortion requires an integration of the probability and magnitude of the phenomenon.

The ideal form of an answer to the series of questions regarding bias would be a revised point estimate and confidence interval for the estimated measure of effect that is now positioned to account for the distortion resulting from each bias and has a width that takes into account the possibility that the source of bias yields varying magnitudes of error. Starting with the conventionally constructed confidence interval derived solely from considerations of random error, there might be a shift in the general placement of the interval to account for a given form of bias to be more likely to shift results upward than downward, but there would also be a widening of the confidence interval, perhaps asymmetrically, depending on how probable it is that varying magnitudes of distortion are present. Additional sources of bias could, in principle, be brought into consideration, each one providing a more accurate reflection of the estimate of the measure of effect, integrating considerations of bias and precision.

In practice, the ability to quantify sources of bias other than random error poses a great challenge, but the conceptual benchmark remains useful. This attempt at quantification reminds us that even in an ideal world, hypothetical biases would not be proven present or absent, but their possible effect would be quantified, and the estimated measure of effect would shift as a result. In some instances, we may have the good fortune of finding that the range of plausible effects of the bias are all negligible, enabling us to focus our energies elsewhere. When we find that the bias is capable or even likely to introduce substantial distortion, those are the biases that need to be countered in subsequent studies in order to remove their effect or at least to more accurately account for their impact and reduce uncertainty. The strategies of the following chapters are intended to help in estimating the direction and magnitude of distortion resulting from various biases, focusing wherever possible on the use of empirical evaluation to help bridge the gap between the ideal quantitative, probabilistic insights and what is often a largely intuitive, informal characterization of the impact of bias that is commonly applied at present. Collecting and analyzing additional data, conducting sensitivity analyses, and incorporating information from outside the study of interest are among the strategies that are proposed to help in this challenging mission.

IDENTIFY THE MOST IMPORTANT SOURCES OF ERROR

Examination and critical evaluation of a study result should begin with an enumeration of the *primary* sources of vulnerability to error, either by the authors as the first ones to see and evaluate the findings, or by the users of such information. Although this seems obvious, there may be a temptation to focus on the sources that are more easily quantified (e.g., nondifferential misclassification) or to enumerate all conceivable biases, giving equal attention to all. Instead, the first stage of evaluation, to ensure that the scrutiny is optimally allocated, should be to identify the few possibilities for introducing large amounts of error. Projecting forward to conceptualize that unknown but ideal integrated measure of effect that incorporates all sources of distortion, we are trying to anticipate as best we can which sources of error, both random and systematic, will dominate the overall, integrated function. Those potential biases that are either not likely to be present at all, or if present are unlikely to have a major quantitative impact, will have minimal influence on the position and degree of dispersion in the estimate and need not be given much attention.

Perhaps the most common misallocation of attention is the traditional focus on random error, analogous to looking for a lost key near the lamppost solely because the light is brightest there. Just because the conceptual and quantitative framework is most advanced for considering random error (though actually only for experiments), there is no reason to overemphasize its importance relative to concerns for which the technology is less advanced. Interpreting study results based on whether they are statistically significant or whether a confidence interval includes or excludes some particular value of interest gives undue attention to random error. In small studies, imprecision may indeed be one of the principal sources of uncertainty and deserves primary attention, but in many cases there is no justification for a primary focus on random error rather than bias. The temptation to focus on random error may arise from copying the approach applied to experimental studies, in which random allocation and the ability to control experimental conditions isolates random error as the principle concern if the other features of the study are conducted optimally. Similarly, the algebra of misclassification has advanced to the point that correction formulae are widely available (Copeland et al., 1977; Kleinbaum et al., 1982; Flanders et al., 1995), making it relatively easy to consider simple scenarios of misclassification patterns and their effect on the study results. Although these techniques for quantification of the impact of misclassification are of tremendous value and the repertoire of such techniques needs to be markedly expanded and used more often, their availability should not unduly influence the focus of the evaluation of study results on misclassification. Mundane and often intractable problems such as non-response or the conceptual inaccuracy of measurement tools should be given the priority they warrant, not downplayed solely because they are more difficult to address in a rigorous, quantitative manner. The importance of a given issue is not necessarily correlated with the availability of tools to address it.

Although each study will have distinctive attributes that define its strengths and vulnerabilities, a subset of candidate biases can often be expected to be near the top of the list. Structural features of the study that directly rather than indirectly influence the estimated measure of interest are of particular concern. Generally, selection factors (e.g., non-comparability of controls and cases, underlying reasons why some persons are and are not exposed) and measurement errors in the primary exposure or disease variables (often based on a limited correspondence between the available data and the desired data) will be of importance. Confounding and related issues (e.g., incomplete control of confounding) are often not as compelling unless there are rather strong risk factors that are likely to be associated with the exposure of interest. This situation is perhaps less universal than the problems of non-response and measurement error. In small studies, where some of the cells of interest contain fewer than 10 subjects, random error may be the overwhelming concern that limits the strength of study results.

For each study or set of studies under review, the critical issues, which are generally few in number, should be specified for close scrutiny to avoid superficial treatment of an extensive list of issues that mixes trivial with profound concerns. These critical issues are distinguished by having a sufficiently high probability of having a quantitatively important influence on the estimated measure of effect. If such candidates are considered in detail and found not to produce distortion, the strength of the evidence would be markedly enhanced. These issues are important enough to justify conducting new studies in which the potential bias can be eliminated, sometimes simply requiring larger studies of similar quality, or to suggest methodological research that would determine whether these hypothetical problems have, in fact, distorted past studies.

STRATEGIES FOR SPECIFYING SCENARIOS OF BIAS

Specifying hypotheses about biases is analogous to specifying substantive hypotheses in that they should address important phenomena, be specific (in order to be testable), and be quantitative in their predictions (Hertz-Picciotto, 2000). The conditions by which the estimated measure of effect could provide an inaccurate reflection of the causal relation between exposure and disease must be stated clearly so that the plausibility of those conditions that would produce such bias can be evaluated. In the case of random error, ill-defined random processes are invoked (see Chapter 10), though the anticipated effect on the results can be postulated with clarity. The probability of at least some random error influencing the measured results is always 100%, but there is no direct way to determine where the observed data fit in the distribution of possible values.

For hypotheses of systematic error, specific relationships or patterns of error in measurement can be proposed and evaluated. For non-response to have biased the exposure–disease association, for example, a pattern of response in which exposure and disease jointly influence the probability of responding must occur (Greenland, 1977; Greenland & Criqui, 1981). If information bias or misclassification is suggested, then the hypothesis pertains to the source of measurement error, how it operates among subsets of study subjects, and its quantitative impact in contributing to the disparity between the causal parameter of interest and the estimated measure of effect.

Some degree of error due to confounding, selection bias, and misclassification will be present based solely on random processes. For example, in the same way that randomized exposure assignment inevitably leaves some confounding due to non-comparability (which becomes smaller as study size becomes larger), a random contribution to confounding is surely present in observational studies as well. Similarly, even when a perfectly suitable mechanism of control selection is chosen for a case–control study, some selection bias will be present due to random processes alone, a result of sampling. Aside from the systematic reasons that misclassification may occur, there is a random element to assigning the incorrect value (whether based on a laboratory technique, human memory, or written records) that causes some amount of error to be ubiquitous. On *average*, there may be no error, but a given study is likely to contain some amount. These manifestations of random error may be viewed as the source of the random error that we routinely consider in our analyses and interpretation, and as expected, the predicted impact diminishes as study size becomes larger.

On the other hand, there are sources of error that have a structural explanation, that do not diminish in size as study size becomes larger, and that can be examined and tested like other hypothesized explanations for study findings. The first issue to be examined in evaluating whether a potential bias has affected the results should focus on the likely direction of potential error—is it symmetrical on either side of the observed value or more likely to make the estimated measure of effect an overestimate or underestimate of its correct value? For some biases such as those resulting from exposure misclassification, movement in relation to the null value provides the basis for predictions, i.e., starting from the true value, is our estimate likely to be closer or further from the null? Random error is generally presumed to be symmetrical around the true value, on the appropriate scale of measurement. Non-response biases are typically described in terms of the direction from the true value. If non-response is independent of exposure and disease status, or related to exposure and disease but independently, no bias is expected in measures of association even though precision is lost (Greenland & Criqui, 1981). If non-response were thought to be greater among exposed persons with disease or unexposed persons without disease, then the bias would be toward a spurious reduction in measures of effect, whereas if non-response were greater among exposed persons without disease or unexposed persons with disease, the bias would be toward an increased observed measure of effect. These various scenarios serve to define the array of possibilities for explaining how, given candidate true values for the measure of association, the observed results may have been obtained. Some candidate biases serve to raise the deviations from the true values only to one side or another of the observed measure, whereas others increase the probabilities on both sides of the observed value, as occurs for random error.

The second step in the specification of bias scenarios requires consideration of the magnitude of distortion. For selected hypothetical true values for the parameter of interest, we ask about the probability that bias has introduced varying magnitudes of distortion. When considering random error, this estimate of the disparity between true and measured values is asked in terms of the probability of a random sampling process having yielded a sample which is as or more deviant under the null (or some other specific) hypothesis. The same type of assessment needs to be made for other sources of error. In the case of non-response, for example, varying degrees and patterns of non-response associated with exposure and disease status yield predictable amounts of distortion. Specifying the pattern of response in relation to exposure and disease directly determines the magnitude of disparity between some assumed true value and the observed measure (Kleinbaum et al., 1982). Although many different combinations of circumstances would lead to the same magnitude of bias, we can view them in principle as a set of scenarios for which the probability of occurrence should be considered.

Another way to quantify the magnitude of bias is to evaluate the probability that deviations of a specified magnitude from the true value of the measure of effect have resulted from the specific source of bias. That is, starting from some benchmark of interest for the correct measure, we can ask about the probability of there having been enough error from specified sources to generate the results we obtained. In contrast to sampling theory, which serves as the basis for evaluating random error generically, in evaluating the probability of biases of varying magnitudes, we would like to make use of all relevant substantive information bearing on the scenario of bias. This includes evidence from within the study, methodological research that addresses the problem more generically, and studies similar to the one of interest that may provide information concerning the potential bias. Integrating these diverse sources of information into a comprehensive, quantitative assessment requires judgment about the underlying process by which bias is thought to have been produced and the relevance or weight assigned to the various lines of evidence. Such an assessment should strive to integrate the statistical, biologic, and epidemiologic evidence that bear on the issue.

In assessing the potential for a given magnitude of bias from non-response, for example, one might consider the most directly applicable information first. The absolute magnitude of non-response is clearly critical. Any evidence regarding patterns of non-response in the specific study from a more intensively recruited subset or available data on nonparticipants would contribute substantially to the inferences about the probability of bias of a given magnitude. The reasons for non-response, such as patient refusal, physician refusal, or being untraceable would enter into the evaluation, considering whatever is known about the people lost through such processes. Comparison of results of the study under scrutiny to results from similarly designed studies that had a better response could be helpful in making an assessment, but the evidence must be extrapolated. Generic information about nonrespondents in other study settings and influence of non-response more generally would also be of interest but even less directly applicable. Integration of these diverse threads of information into an overall assessment is a challenge and may well lead to discordant judgments.

A natural by-product of this effort is the identification of gaps in knowledge that would help describe and quantify probabilities of biases that would distort the findings in a specific direction of some specified magnitude. That is, in attempting to implement the ambitious strategy of specifying, quantifying, and assessing the probabilities of specific types of bias, limitations in our knowledge will be revealed. Sometimes those limitations will be in the conceptual understanding of the phenomenon that precludes assessment of the potential bias, pointing toward need for further methodological work. Questions may arise regarding such issues as the pattern of non-response typically associated with random-digit dialing, which points toward empirical methodological research to evaluate this technique in order to produce generalizable information. Often, the solution must be found within the specific study, pointing toward further analyses or additional data collection. Finally, and perhaps most importantly, the largest and most likely potential biases in one study or in the set of studies suggests refinement required in the next attempt to address the hypothesized causal relationship.

Even though the ambitious attempt to delineate and quantify biases as proposed above will always fall short of success, the uncertainties revealed by the effort will be constructive and specific. Instead of being left with such unhelpful conclusions as "the evidence is weak" or "further studies are needed," we are more likely to end up with statements such as "the pattern of non-response is not known with certainty, but if exposed, non-diseased persons are underrepresented to a sizable extent, the true measure of association could be markedly smaller than what was measured." Moving from global, descriptive statements to specific, quantitative ones provides direction to the original investigators, future researchers, and to those who must consider the literature as a basis for policy decisions.

EXAMPLE: EPIDEMIOLOGIC RESEARCH ON THE RELATION BETWEEN DICHLORODIPHENYLTRICHLOROETHANE (DDT) EXPOSURE AND BREAST CANCER

To illustrate the strategy, if not the complete implementation, of an evaluation of sources of error in epidemiologic studies, the first major epidemiologic study on persistent organochlorides and breast cancer by Wolff and colleagues (1993) is examined. The hypothesis they considered was that persistent organochloride compounds, including the pesticide DDT, its metabolite dichlorodiphenyldichloroethane (DDE), and the industrial pollutant, polychlorinated biphenyls

(PCBs), might increase the risk of developing breast cancer. A major motivation for such inquiry is the experimental evidence of carcinogenicity of these compounds and the postulated effects of such compounds on estrogenic activity in humans and other species (Davis et al., 1993). Prior to 1993, studies in humans had generally been small and were based largely on comparisons of normal and diseased breast *tissue* rather than on an evaluation of exposure levels in *women* with and without breast cancer. Because the report by Wolff et al. (1993) was a major milestone in the literature and stood essentially in isolation, it provides a realistic illustration of the interpretive issues surrounding a specific epidemiologic study. The fact that a series of subsequent evaluations have been largely negative (Hunter et al., 1997; Moysich et al., 1998; Millikan et al., 2000) does not detract from the methodologic issues posed at the time when the initial study was first published and evaluated.

In order to evaluate the possible association between exposure to persistent organochloride compounds and breast cancer, Wolff et al. (1993) identified over 14,000 women who had been enrolled in a prospective cohort study between 1985 and 1991 that included collection of blood samples for long-term storage. From this cohort, all 58 women who developed breast cancer and a sample of 171 controls who remained free of cancer had their sera analyzed for levels of DDT, DDE, and PCBs. After adjustment for potential confounders (family history of breast cancer, lifetime history of lactation, and age at first full-term pregnancy), relative risks for the five quintiles of DDE were 1.0 (referent), 1.7, 4.4, 2.3, and 3.7. Confidence intervals were rather wide (e.g., for quintile 2, approximately 0.4–6.8 as estimated from the graph, and for quintile 5, 1.0–13.5).

The focus here is on the critical interpretation of these results in terms of epidemiologic methods, but the contribution of this study to expanding interest in the potential environmental influences on breast cancer generally is a notable achievement with implications yet to be fully realized. The first step in examining these data is to define the result that is to be scrutinized for potential error. Although PCBs were examined as well as DDT and DDE, we will focus on DDE and breast cancer, for which the evidence was most suggestive of a positive association. An entirely different set of criticisms might arise in evaluating the validity of the measured absence of association (or very small association) identified for PCBs.

There were three main calculations undertaken for DDE: a comparison of means among cases versus controls (of dubious value as a measure of association), adjusted odds ratios calculated across the five quintiles (as provided above), and an estimated adjusted odds ratio for increasing exposure from the 10th to 90th percentile of 4.1 (95% confidence interval: 1.5–11.2), corresponding to an assumed increase from 2.0 ng/mL to 19.1 ng/mL. Although the latter number smoothes out the irregularities in the dose–response gradient that were seen across the quintiles, and may mask non-linearity in the relationship, it provides a convenient single number for scrutiny. The question we focus on is whether changing a woman's serum DDE level from 2.0 to 19.1 ng/mL would actually cause her risk of breast cancer to rise by a factor of 4.1.

What are the primary sources of uncertainty in judging whether the reported association accurately reflects the causal relationship between DDE and the development of breast cancer? We ask first whether the association between the study variables was likely to have been measured accurately, deferring any consideration of whether the association is causal. The underlying study design is a cohort, in which healthy women were identified and followed prospectively over time for the occurrence of breast cancer. Given the identification of all cases and appropriate sampling of controls from within this well-defined cohort, selection bias is unlikely. The constitution of the study groups being compared is thus not likely to have distorted the measure of association other than by having drawn an aberrant sample of the cohort to serve as controls, which is accounted for in the measures of precision. Although there is always some degree of laboratory error in the assays of DDE given the technical challenges in measuring the low levels of interest, the masking of case–control status suggests that such errors would be similar for cases with breast cancer as for controls without breast cancer. As discussed at length in Chapter 8 and elsewhere (Kleinbaum et al., 1982), nondifferential misclassification of this nature is most likely to be associated with some shift in the relative risk toward the null value. Furthermore, quality control procedures described in the manuscript make laboratory error an unlikely source of major distortion.

Random error is an important concern, as reflected by the wide confidence intervals. Based on the confidence interval reported for the point estimate of a relative risk of 4.1, 1.5 to 11.2, true values of 3 to 6 or 7 could readily have yielded the observed estimate of 4.1 through random error. The data are not likely to have arisen however, under assumptions about more extreme values that would markedly change the substantive interpretation of the study, such as the null value or relative risks of 10 or 15.

Accepting the observed association as a reasonable if imprecise estimate, the possibility of an association being present without reflecting a causal relation between DDE and breast cancer must be considered. Two key concerns are as follows:

1. Is there some metabolic consequence of early breast cancer that increases the serum level of DDE among cases? Given that serum was collected in the six months or more prior to breast cancer diagnosis, latent disease may have affected the balance between fat stores and serum levels of DDE in a manner that artifactually raised (or lowered) the serum DDE level of cases. A detailed evaluation of the metabolism of DDE in serum is beyond the scope of this discussion, but any such effect on cases would

directly distort the measured relative risk given that the controls did not experience the disease of concern. Assessment of the validity of this hypothesis requires examination of the literature on metabolism, storage, and excretion of persistent organochlorides and an understanding of the physiologic changes associated with the early stages of breast cancer. Independent of this study, examining patterns of association for cases with varying stages of disease might help to evaluate whether such bias occurred, with the expectation that the bias would result in stronger influence among cases with more advanced disease and little or no influence among cases with carcinoma *in situ* of the breast (Millikan et al., 1995). Such a bias might also be expected to be strongest for cases diagnosed close to the time of serum collection (when latent disease is more likely to be present) as compared to cases diagnosed later relative to serum collection.

2. Has lactation or childbearing confounded the measured association between serum DDE and breast cancer? The investigators reported that lactation was associated with a decreased risk of breast cancer (Wolff et al., 1993) as reported by others, and that adjustment for lactation markedly *increased* the relative risk. Lactation is known to be a major pathway to eliminating stored organochlorides and thus causes lower measured levels of these compounds in the body. Whatever exposure level was truly present prior to the period of lactation, the level measured after lactation would be lower. If adjustment affected the reported relative risk for the comparison of 10th to 90th percentile of DDE to the same extent as it affected their categorical measure of relative risk of DDE, the odds ratio without adjustment for lactation would have been around 2.4 instead of 4.1. Thus, the validity of the lactation-adjusted estimate warrants careful scrutiny (Longnecker & London, 1993).

If early-life DDE levels are etiologically important, lactation presumably has artificially lowered later-life serum levels and introduced error relative to the exposure of interest (prelactation levels). If lactation reduced the risk of breast cancer (independent of its DDE-lowering influence), then lactation would be expected to introduce positive confounding and falsely elevate the relative risk (Longnecker & London, 1993). Lactation would lower the measure of exposure and lower breast cancer risk, so that failure to adjust for lactation would result in a spuriously elevated relative risk for DDE and breast cancer, and adjustment for lactation would therefore lower the relative risk. The reason for the opposite effect of adjustment for lactation is not clear (Dubin et al., 1993), but it suggests that lactation history was associated with a higher level of DDE rather than a lower level of DDE in this population. The high proportion of nulliparous (and thus never-lactating) women in the Wolff et al. (1993) study may influence the observed impact of lactation in comparisons of those with and without such a history.

On the other hand, focusing on lactation as a means of reducing body burden (unfortunately, through exposure to the infant), if later-life DDE levels are critical, and lactation's beneficial impact on breast cancer risk is mediated by reduced DDE levels, then adjustment for lactation is inappropriate given that it is an exposure determinant but not a confounder. The preferred relative risk for estimating the causal effect of DDE would not include adjustment for lactation history. Lactation would be no different than working on a farm or consuming DDT-contaminated fish in that it affects merely the DDE levels but has no independent effects on breast cancer.

Resolution of these uncertainties regarding the role of lactation in the DDE/breast cancer association requires further evaluation of the temporal relationship between exposure and disease, improved understanding of the epidemiology of lactation and breast cancer, and a methodological appreciation of the subtleties of confounding and effect measure modification. If we were able to have measurements available from both early life (e.g., prereproduction and lactation) as well as later life but prior to the development of disease, we could empirically assess the relationship of those measurements to one another and to the risk of breast cancer. The resolution of the role of lactation and breast cancer is also complex (e.g., Newcomb et al., 1994; Furberg et al., 1999), but is an active area of investigation.

Each of these issues could affect the true (unknown) measure of the relative risk in comparison to the observed value of 4.1. We would like to be able to assign probabilities to these alternative scenarios given that they have implications for the interpretation of the study results. If these potential biases were incorporated, the distribution of values around the point estimate would not necessarily be symmetrical, as is presumed for random error, but may take other shapes. For example, metabolic effects of early disease seem more likely to artificially elevate case serum DDE levels relative to controls rather than lower them, so that the confidence interval might be weighted more on the lower relative risk end. Lactation may require several curves to address its potential role according to the alternative hypotheses. Insofar as it reflects a true confounder of the DDE/breast cancer association, more refined measurement and adjustment for the relevant aspects of lactation might be predicted to further elevate the DDE/breast cancer association in the Wolff et al. (1993) study (Greenland & Robins, 1985; Savitz & Barón, 1989). As a marker only of reduced body burden of DDE, it should not have been adjusted and thus the smaller relative risks reported without adjustment may be more valid, making true values below 4.1 more compatible with the observed results than values above 4.1. On the other hand, since the confounding influence of lactation was counter to the expected direction (Longnecker & London, 1993), we may wish to raise questions about the assessment of lactation or DDE, and spread the probability curve more broadly in both directions.

Evaluation of results through specifying and working through the consequences of a series of potential biases, focusing on two principal ones in some detail, has not answered the question of whether the measured association of DDT/DDE and breast cancer was accurate, but it helped to refine the question. Instead of asking whether the study's results are valid, we instead ask a series of more focused and answerable questions that bear on the overall result. Does preclinical breast cancer distort measured levels of serum DDE, and if so, in which direction? Is lactation inversely related to breast cancer, independent of DDE? Is serum DDE level a more accurate reflection of early-life exposure among non-lactating women? Some of these questions point toward research outside of the scope of epidemiology, but other approaches to addressing these questions would involve identifying populations in which the threat to validity is much reduced. The lactation issue could be examined in a population in which breastfeeding is absent, not resolving the questions about lactation, DDE, and breast cancer, but addressing DDE and breast cancer without vulnerability to distortion by lactation. These refined questions are, in principle, testable and would help to resolve the questions raised by the Wolff et al. (1993) study. The critical evaluation of study results should enhance intellectual grasp of the state of the literature, help us judge the credibility of the measured association, and identify testable hypotheses that would clarify a study's results and advance knowledge of the issue.

REFERENCES

Barnes DE, Bero LA. Why review articles on the health effects of passive smoking reach different conclusions. JAMA 1998;279:1566–1570.

Copeland KT, Checkoway H, McMichael AJ, Holbrook RH. Bias due to misclassification in the estimation of relative risk. Am J Epidemiol 1977;105:488–495.

Davis DL, Bradlow HL, Wolff M, Woodruff T, Hoel DG, Anton-Culver H. Medical hypothesis: xenoestrogens as preventable causes of breast cancer. Environ Health Perspect 1993;101:372–377.

Dubin N, Toniolo PG, Lee EW, Wolff MS. Response "Re: Blood levels of organochlorine residues and risk of breast cancer." J Natl Cancer Inst 1993;85:1696–1697.

Flanders WD, Drews CD, Kosinski AS. Methodology to correct for differential misclassification. Epidemiology 1995;6:152–156.

Furberg H, Newman B, Moorman P, Millikan R. Lactation and breast cancer risk. Int J Epidemiol 1999;28:396–402.

Greenland S. Response and follow-up bias in cohort studies. Am J Epidemiol 1977; 106:184–187.

Greenland S. Randomization, statistics, and causal inference. Epidemiology 1990;1: 421–429.

Greenland S, Criqui MH. Are case-control studies more vulnerable to response bias? Am J Epidemiol 1981;114:175–177.

Greenland S, Robins JM. Confounding and misclassification. Am J Epidemiol 1985; 122:495–506.

Greenland S, Robins JM. Empirical-Bayes adjustments fo rmultiple comparisons are sometimes useful. Epidemiology 1991;2:244–251.

Hertz-Picciotto I. Invited Commentary Shifting the burden of proof regarding biases and low-magnitude associations. Am J Epidemiol 2000;151:946–948.

Hunter DJ, Hankinson SE, Laden F, et al. Plasma organochlorine levels and risk of breast cancer in a prospective study. N Engl J Med 1997;337:1253–1258.

Joffe M, Li Z. Male and female factors in fertility. Am J Epidemiol 1994;140:921–929.

Kleinbaum DG, Kupper LL, Morgenstern H. Epidemiologic research: principles and quantitative methods. Belmont, CA: Lifetime Learning Publications, 1982.

Last JM. A Dictionary of Epidemiology, Fourth Edition. New York: Oxford University Press, 2001;184–185.

Longnecker MP, London SJ. Re: Blood levels of organochlorine residues and risk of breast cancer. J Natl Cancer Inst 1993;85:1696.

Millikan R, DeVoto E, Duell EJ, Tse C-K, Savitz DA, Beach J, Edmiston S, Jackson S, Newman B. Dichlorodiphenyldicholoroethane, polychlorinated biphenyls, and breast cancer among African-American and white women in North Carolina. Cancer Epidemiol, Biomarkers Prev 2000;9:1233–1240.

Millikan R, Dressler L, Geradts J, Graham M. The importance of epidemiologic studies of in-situ carcinoma of the breast. Breast Cancer Res Treat 1995;34:65–77.

Moysich KB, Ambrosone CB, Vena JE, et al. Environmental organochlorine exposure and postmenopausal breast cancer risk. Cancer Epidemiol Biomarkers Prev 1998;7:181–188.

Newcomb PA, Storer BE, Longnecker MP, et al. Cancer of the breast in relation to lactation history. N Engl J Med 1994;330:81–87.

Rothman KJ. Modern Epidemiology. Boston: Little, Brown, and Company, 1986:77.

Savitz DA, Barón AE. Estimating and correcting for confounder misclassification. Am J Epidemiol 1989;129:1062–1071.

Savitz DA, Olshan AF. Re: "Male and female factors in infertility." Am J Epidemiol 1995;141:1107–1108.

Savitz DA, Olshan AF. Multiple comparisons and related issues in the interpretation of epidemiologic data. Am J Epidemiol 1995b;142:904–908.

Savitz DA, Poole C, Miller WC. Reassessing the role of epidemiology in public health. Am J Pub Health 1999;89:1158–1161.

Wolff MS, Toniolo PG, Lee EW, Rivera M, Dubin N. Blood levels of organochlorine residues and risk of breast cancer. J Natl Cancer Inst 1993;85:648–652.

4

SELECTION BIAS IN COHORT STUDIES

STUDY DESIGNS

Except for research that seeks simply to characterize the frequency of disease occurrence in a population, epidemiologic studies make comparisons between two or more groups. The goal is to draw inferences about possible causal relations between some attribute that may affect health, generically called *exposure*, and some health outcome or state, generically called *disease*. The exposure may be a biological property, such as a genotype or hormone level; an individual behavior, such as drug use or diet; or a social or environmental characteristic, such as living in a high-crime neighborhood or belonging to a particular ethnic group. Disease also covers many types of health events, including a biochemical or physiologic state, for example, elevated low density lipoprotein cholesterol, a clinical disease, for example, gout, or an impairment in daily living, for example, the inability to walk without assistance.

The study designs used to examine exposure–disease associations were clearly organized by Morgenstern et al. (1993). All designs are intended to allow inferences about whether exposure influences the occurrence of disease. Two axes serve to define the universe of possible study designs. The first concerns the way in which the health outcome is measured. The health event can be assessed in the form of disease incidence, defined as the occurrence of disease in persons previously free of the condition, or prevalence, defined as the proportion of the population affected by disease at a given point in time. The second axis concerns the approach to selecting study subjects, specifically whether or not sampling is based on the health outcome. Health outcome-dependent sampling occurs when inclusion in the study is based at least in part on whether or not the disease has already occurred in the subjects, for example, selecting all cases of disease but only evaluating a fraction of the population at risk. Sampling without regard to health outcome will be referred to as a cohort study, and sampling based on health outcome as a case–control study. Thus, there are cohort studies of disease incidence, cohort studies of disease prevalence, case–control studies based on incident cases, and case–control studies based on prevalent cases.

In contrast to some past views that case–control studies are fundamentally different in their logic or structure, their only defining characteristic is sampling for inclusion based in part on having experienced the health outcome of interest. Selection for study that does not depend on health status results in a cohort design, where participants may constitute the whole population, may be chosen randomly, or may be selected based on their exposure status or other attributes that are related to disease but not of primary interest, such as age or gender. The defining feature is that there is not selective sampling based on the health outcome of interest. Once chosen, the health experience of the entire population that generates the cases is characterized, whereas in case–control studies, only a segment of the population experience that produced the cases is monitored for exposure or other factors of interest.

Note that this terminology eliminates the notion of a cross-sectional study, since selection of a population without regard to exposure or disease status, typically used to define cross-sectional studies, constitutes a cohort design because there is no selection based on the health outcome. In practice, the efficiency of a cohort study can often be enhanced by manipulating the distribution of exposure that naturally occurs in the population. Often, there is value in oversampling the most (or least) exposed, relatively rare groups, to ensure adequate numbers in the limiting part of the exposure spectrum. If interested in the long-term impact of dietary fat on the development of prostate cancer, we could simply select all men in some source population, e.g., retired members of a labor union, or we could selectively oversample men who have especially low and especially high levels of fat consumption. Either design is referred to as a cohort study.

With or without selective sampling based on exposure status, we can expect to have a full continuum of dietary fat intakes in the population in the above example concerning dietary fat and prostate cancer. Though contrasts in exposure groups are emphasized for conceptual clarity throughout this chapter, most exposures are not true dichotomies. Exposures may be measured in the form of nominal categories (e.g., ethnicity of Asian, African-American, or European ancestry), ordinal categories (e.g., nonsmoker, light smoker, heavy smoker), or on a truly continuous scale (e.g., dietary intake of folate). Nonetheless, it is conceptually easier to consider contrasts among groups than to consider differences along a continuum. There are statistical models that fully accommodate the spectrum of exposure, imposing varying degrees of assumptions on the shape of the dose-response curve, but it is difficult to grasp the underlying principles without considering exposure groups, even when those groups have to be formed from continuous measures of exposure.

PURPOSE OF COMPARISON GROUPS

The purpose of making comparisons of disease occurrence among groups of differing exposure, as is done in cohort studies, is entirely different than the purpose of making comparisons of exposure prevalence between cases and a sample of the study base, as is done in case–control studies. There is the temptation to draw false parallels because both are steps toward estimating measures of association.

In case–control studies, the controls are selected to provide an estimate of exposure prevalence in the study base that gave rise to the cases. The goal for achieving a coherent study, or the manifestation of a problem in subject selection, is a disparity not between the cases and the controls, but rather between the controls who were chosen and the study base that generated the cases (Miettinen, 1985). This is discussed at some length in Chapter 5.

In cohort studies, the purpose of the unexposed group is to provide an estimate of the disease rate that the exposed group would have had, had they not been exposed (Greenland & Robins, 1986). That is, the ideal comparison would be the counterfactual one in which the same individuals would be monitored for disease occurrence under one exposure condition and simultaneously monitored for disease occurrence under another exposure condition. Under that scenario, the comparison of disease rates among subjects with and without exposure would indicate precisely the causal effect of the exposure. Obviously we cannot do this. Even in the most favorable situation, in which subjects can be observed for the outcome under both exposed and unexposed conditions in sequence, there is still an order to the treatments to be balanced and considered, and there are unintentional but inevitable changes in conditions with the passage of time. More importantly, there are few health endpoints that are ethically and feasibly studied in this manner, requiring a brief time course for etiology, complete reversibility of effects, and minimal severity of the health endpoint being evaluated. Inability to study the same subjects simultaneously exposed to contrasting exposures (impossible) or even the same subjects under different conditions imposed at different times (rarely feasible) calls for alternative strategies for making comparisons of health outcomes among groups with differing exposures.

Experiments or randomized controlled trials are built on the assumption that randomized assignment of exposure generates groups that are interchangeable with respect to baseline risk of disease. These provide a far clearer basis for isolating the causal effect of exposure than can typically be achieved in observational studies, even though there are often compromises required in randomized studies with regard to the inclusion of subjects or range of exposure that can be considered. The randomization process is intended to produce groups that would, in the absence of intervention, have identical health experiences.

Thus, after randomization, the incidence of disease among those who are unexposed is thought to be a very good estimate of the incidence that would have occurred among the exposed, had they not been exposed. In large studies in which the randomization is effectively implemented and maintained, the comparison between those who get the treatment (exposed) and those who do not get the treatment (unexposed) should approximate the causal effect of exposure, with deviations resulting solely from random error. In this design, random error results from an effective random allocation process yielding groups that are not, in fact, perfectly balanced with respect to baseline disease risk. If the randomization process were to be repeated over and over, there would be a distribution of values for the baseline disparity in disease risk, clustered around the absence of any difference, but a bell-shaped curve with small differences commonly observed and large differences more rarely produced. In a single randomized allocation, there is no way to know where the chosen sample fits on that distribution. Note, however, that the process itself is assumed to be conceptually and operationally perfect, with the only deviations caused by random error.

As we move to a purely observational design, in which exposure states are observed rather than assigned randomly, we still make the same inference about causal effects of exposure. The challenges in doing so however, are far more profound. We would like to be able to claim that the unexposed provide a good estimate of the disease risk that the exposed persons would have experienced had they not been exposed. The confidence in our ability to constitute groups at equal baseline risk of the health outcome due to randomized allocation is lost, and we must carefully scrutinize the actual mechanism by which the groups are created. The potential for random error that is present even with a perfect allocation process remains, as described above, but we must add to this a concern with the distortion that results from the non-random allocation of exposure. The goal remains to compare disease incidence in two groups defined by their exposure, e.g., exposed and unexposed, and isolate the causal effect of that exposure. To argue that the disease rate among the unexposed reflects what the disease rate among the exposed would have been in the absence of exposure requires the assumption that the groups would have had identical disease experience had it not been for the exposure.

In practice, it is common for the design of a cohort study to begin with an identified exposed group, e.g., oral contraceptive users or marathon runners. Establishment of the exposed group places the burden on the investigator to identify an unexposed group that approximates the disease incidence that the exposed group would have had if they had not been exposed. In the absence of any true influence of the exposure on disease occurrence, the exposed and unexposed groups should have equal disease incidence and confounding or selection bias is said to be present if this condition is not met. Distinguishing between differences in disease incidence due to the causal effect of exposure and differences in disease incidence due to selection bias or confounding is an essential challenge in the interpretation of cohort studies. There is no direct way of isolating these contributors to the observed differences (or lack of differences) in disease occurrence, but this chapter offers a number of tools to help in this assessment.

Because the key issue is comparability between two groups with varying exposure rather than the actual constitution of either group, it is somewhat arbitrary to "blame" one of the groups when the two are not comparable. The discussion of cohort studies focuses on obtaining a non-exposed group that is comparable to the exposed group, but the challenge could be viewed with equal legitimacy as identifying an exposed group that is comparable to the non-exposed one. Whether beginning with an exposed group and seeking a suitable unexposed group or the reverse, what matters is their comparability.

The focus in this chapter is on examining whether the method by which the groups were constituted has produced selection bias. The algorithm for generating the comparison groups is the subject of evaluation, though the actual constitution of the group depends on both the algorithm as it is defined and the process of implementing it to form the study groups. No matter how good the theoretical properties of the selection mechanism, non-response or loss to follow up can introduce distortion or, under rather optimistic scenarios, correct errors resulting from a faulty group definition. Non-response is a form of selection bias, but because it is so pervasive and important in epidemiologic studies, a separate chapter (Chapter 6) addresses that issue alone. Another source of error in constituting the study groups, which is not discussed in this chapter, is when the mechanism for selection of subjects does not perform as intended due to random processes. This possibility is accounted for in generating variance estimates and confidence intervals, with random selection of subjects one of the few sources of readily quantifiable sampling error in epidemiologic studies (Greenland, 1990) (Chapter 10). In asking whether selection bias has arisen, it is useful to distinguish between a faulty mechanism for selection and a good mechanism that generated an aberrant result. This chapter focuses on the mechanism.

SELECTION BIAS AND CONFOUNDING

There are two closely related processes that introduce bias into the comparison of exposed and unexposed subjects in cohort studies. When there is a distortion due to the natural distribution of exposures in the population, the mixing of effects is referred to as confounding. When there is a distortion because of the way in which our study groups were constituted, it is referred to as selection bias. In our hypothetical cohort study of dietary fat intake and prostate cancer, we may find that the highest consumers of dietary fat tend to be less physically active than those who consume lower amounts of dietary fat. To the extent that physical activity influences the risk of disease, confounding would be present not because we have chosen the groups in some faulty manner, but simply because these attributes go together in the study population. In contrast, if we chose our high dietary fat consumers from the labor union retirees, and identified low fat consumers from the local Sierra Club, men who are quite likely to be physically active, there would be selection bias that results in part from the imbalance between the two groups with respect to physical activity, but also quite possibly through a range of other less readily identified characteristics.

Confounding tends to be the focus when the source of non-comparability is measurable at least in principle and can therefore be adjusted statistically. To the extent that the source of non-comparability can be identified, whether it arises naturally (confounding) or as the result of the manner in which the study groups were chosen (selection bias), its effects can be mitigated by statistical adjustment. When the concern is with more fundamental features of the groups to be compared and seems unlikely to be resolved through measurement of covariates and statistical control, we usually refer to the consequence of this non-comparability as selection bias.

The potential for selection bias depends entirely on the specific exposures and diseases under investigation, since it is the relation between exposure and disease that is of interest. Groups that seem on intuitive grounds to be non-comparable could still yield valid inferences regarding a particular exposure and disease, and groups that seem as though they would be almost perfectly suited for comparison could be problematic. Similarly, there are some health outcomes that seem almost invariant with respect to the social and behavioral factors that influence many types of disease and other diseases subject to a myriad of subtle (and obvious) influences.

For example, incidence of acute lymphocytic leukemia in childhood varies at most modestly in relation to social class, parental smoking, or any other exposures or life circumstances examined to date (Chow et al., 1996). If we wished to assess whether the incidence of childhood leukemia in the offspring of men who received therapeutic ionizing radiation as treatment for cancer was increased, the selection of an unexposed group of men might be less daunting since the variability in disease incidence appears to be independent of most potential determinants studied thus far. That is, we might be reasonably confident that rates from general population registries would be adequate or that data from men who received medical treatments other than ionizing radiation would be suitable for comparison. In other words, the sources of non-comparability in the exposed and unexposed populations are unlikely to have much effect, if any, on the acute lymphocytic leukemia rates in the offspring.

In contrast, if we were interested in neural tube defects among the offspring of these men, we would have to contend with substantial variation associated with social class (Little & Elwood, 1992a), ethnicity (Little & Elwood, 1992b), and diet (Elwood et al., 1992). The same exposure in the same men would vary substantially in vulnerability to selection bias depending on the outcome of interest and what factors influence the risk of that outcome. Selection bias is a property of a specific exposure–disease association of interest, not an inherent property of the groups.

Despite the danger of relying solely on intuition, we often start with intuitive notions of group comparability based on geography, demographic characteristics, or time periods. Do the exposed and unexposed groups seem comparable? Social or demographic attributes are related to many health outcomes, so achieving comparability on these indicators may help to reduce the chance that the groups will be non-comparable in disease risk. If location, time period, and demography effectively predict comparability for a wide range of other unmeasured attributes, then the similarity is likely to be beneficial, on average, even if it provides no absolute assurance that the many unmeasured factors that might distinguish exposure groups are also balanced.

Sociodemographic or geographic comparability helps to ensure balance with respect to many known and unknown determinants of disease, but does non-comparability with regard to sociodemographic or other broad characteristics make it likely that selection bias is present? The answer depends entirely on the exposure and disease outcomes of interest and whether adjustment is made for readily identified determinants of disease risk. In fact, the more general question of whether imbalance between groups matters, i.e., whether it introduces bias, is most conveniently interpreted as a question of whether the imbalance introduces confounding. Is the attribute on which the groups are non-comparable associated with exposure, whether naturally (as in confounding) or due to the investigator's methods of constituting the study groups (as in selection bias)? Is the attribute associated with the disease of interest, conditional on adjusting for measured confounders? Just as natural imbalance on some attributes does not introduce confounding and imbalance in others does, some forms of inequality in the constitution of the study groups can be ignored and other forms cannot.

Continuing to focus on whether the selection of study groups introduces confounding, some sources of non-comparability are readily measured and controlled, such as gender or age, whereas others are quite difficult to measure and control in the analysis, such as health-care seeking or nutrient intake. The challenges, discussed in more detail in the chapter on confounding (Chapter 7), are to anticipate, measure, and control for factors that are independently related to exposure and disease. Whether non-comparability between the exposure groups based on measurable attributes is viewed as confounding or selection bias is somewhat arbitrary in cohort studies. In general, epidemiologists pay little attention to asking why the exposure and the confounder are associated, only asking whether they are. A true confounder could be controlled or exacerbated by the manner in which study groups are selected, as in matching (Rothman, 1986). What is critical to evaluating selection bias is to recognize that if the sources of potential bias can be measured and controlled as confounding factors, the bias that they introduce is removed. Some forms of selection that lead to non-comparability in the study groups can be eliminated by statistical adjustments that make the study groups comparable.

EVALUATION OF SELECTION BIAS IN COHORT STUDIES

Multiple sources of information, both within and outside the study, can help in the assessment of whether selection bias is likely to be present. These indicators do not provide definitive answers regarding the probability that selection bias of a given direction and magnitude is present, which is the desired goal. Nonetheless, by drawing upon multiple threads of information, the ability to address these critical questions is markedly enhanced. While the goal is a fully defined distribution of probabilities for bias of varying magnitude, a more realistic expectation for these tools is to begin to sketch out that information and use the disparate pieces of information as fully and appropriately as possible. Not all the tools suggested below are applicable in every study, but a more systematic consideration of the repertoire of these approaches should yield insights that would not otherwise be obtained. In some instances, the very lack of information needed to apply the tool provides relevant information to help characterize the certainty of the study's findings and suggests approaches to develop better resources for addressing the potential bias.

Compare Unexposed Disease Rates to External Populations

Comparison of the absolute rate of disease occurrence in the unexposed portion of the cohort with the rate of disease in an appropriate external reference population may help to determine whether the unexposed group is likely to provide a suitable benchmark of comparison for the exposed study group. The purpose of this strategy is to evaluate whether the unexposed group is likely to be effective in its role of measuring what the disease rate would have been in the exposed group had they not been exposed. The scrutiny of the unexposed group could help to reveal whether some unidentified peculiarity caused an anomalous deviation in disease occurrence, upward or downward, that would translate directly into a distortion in the measure of association between exposure and disease. The reason to focus on the unexposed group is that the exposed group's disease rates may differ from an external population either due to a true effect of the exposure or to the same sort of idiosyncrasies alluded to above with regard to the unexposed group. If the rate of disease in the unexposed group differs substantially from an external reference population, however, it is clearly not due to the exposure but due to some other characteristics of the unexposed population.

An important challenge to implementing this approach is that only a few diseases have standardized ascertainment protocols and readily available information on frequency of disease occurrence in populations external to the study. For example, cancer registries comprehensively document the occurrence of diagnosed disease using rigorous protocols and publish rates of disease on a regular basis (Ries et al., 1996). When conducting a study of the possible carcinogenicity of an industrial chemical, for example, in which the strategy is to compare cancer incidence in exposed workers to workers without that exposure, it would be informative to compare the cancer incidence observed among the unexposed workers to the incidence in populations under surveillance as part of the Surveillance, Epidemiology, and End Results (SEER) Program or other geographically suitable cancer registries. Some assurance that the rate difference or ratio comparing the exposed to unexposed workers is valid would be provided if the cancer rate in the unexposed workers were roughly comparable to that of the general population. If a notable discrepancy were found between the unexposed workers and the community's incidence rate more generally, the suitability of the unexposed workers serving as the referent for the exposed workers might be called into question.

A critical assumption in applying this strategy is that the methods of ascertainment need to be comparable between the unexposed group in the study and the external referent population. For some outcomes, for example, overall mortality rates, comparisons can be made with some confidence in that the diagnosis and comprehensiveness of ascertainment is likely to be comparable between the unexposed subset of the cohort and an external population. However, for many diseases, the frequency of occurrence depends heavily on the ascertainment protocol, and the sophistication of methods in a focused research enterprise will often exceed the quality of routinely collected data. Comparing an unexposed segment of the cohort in which disease is ascertained using one method with an external referent population with a substantially different method of disease ascertainment is of little value, and observing discrepancies has little or no bearing on the suitability of the unexposed as a referent. If the direction and ideally the magnitude of the disparity between the methods of disease ascertainment were well understood, such a comparison might help to provide some assurance that the disparity in the disease occurrence across groups is at least in the expected direction.

As an illustration of the strategy and some of the complexity that can arise in implementation, consider a study of the relationship between pesticide exposure and reproductive outcomes in Colombia (Rostrepo et al., 1990). Using questionnaires to elicit self-reported reproductive health outcomes for female workers and the wives of male workers, the prevalence of various adverse outcomes was tabulated, comparing reproductive experiences before exposure onset to their experiences after exposure onset (Table 4.1). In principle, the prevalence before exposure should reflect a baseline risk, with the prevalence after onset of exposure reflecting the potential effect of pesticides.

A number of the odds ratios are elevated, but concerns were raised by the authors regarding the credibility of the findings based on the anomalously low frequency of certain outcomes, most notably spontaneous abortion. Whereas one would generally expect a risk of approximately 8%–12% based on self-reported data, the results here show only 3.6% of pregnancies ending in spontaneous abortions among female workers prior to exposure and 1.9% among wives of male workers prior to their partners' exposure. This could reflect in part the very low risk expected for a selectively healthly population, by definition younger than those individuals after exposure onset. Much of the aberrantly low prevalence of spontaneous abortion is likely due to erroneous underreporting of events in both groups, however, an issue of disease misclassification. Regardless, the strategy of comparing outcome frequency among the unexposed to that of an external population was informative.

In selected areas of the country, congenital malformations are comprehensively tabulated and data on prevalence at birth are published. Information from vital records, including birth records (birth weight, duration of gestation) and death data used to generate cause-specific mortality, constitutes a national registry for the United States and provides a readily available benchmark for studying health events that can be identified in such records. Yet the ascertainment methods even for these relatively well-defined conditions can differ markedly between a given research protocol and the vital records protocol. For example, identification of congenital malformations depends strongly on whether medically indicated abortions are included or excluded as well as the frequency of such abortions, how systematically newborn infants are examined, how far into life ascertainment is continued (many malformations only become manifest some time after birth), etc. Cumulatively, those differences can cause substantial differences between groups that would be identical if monitored using a consistent protocol. Even for monitoring gestational age or birth weight of infants, differences can arise based on the algorithm for estimating conception date (e.g., the use of ultrasound versus reliance on last menstrual period for dating), and inclusion or exclusion of marginally viable births.

For many chronic health conditions of interest, both diagnosed diseases and less clearly defined symptoms, data from comparable populations may be un-

TABLE 4.1. Comparison of Prevalence Ratios for Reproductive Outcomes Before and After Onset of Potential Pesticide Exposure, Colombia

	Female Workers				Wives of Male Workers			
	Risks (%)				Risks (%)			
PREGNANCY OUTCOME	BEFORE EXPOSURE	AFTER EXPOSURE	OR	95% CI	BEFORE EXPOSURE	AFTER EXPOSURE	OR	95% CI
Induced abortion	1.46	2.84	1.96	1.47–2.67	0.29	1.06	3.63	1.51–8.70
Spontaneous abortion	3.55	7.50	2.20	1.82–2.66	1.85	3.27	1.79	1.16–2.77
Premature baby	6.20	10.95	1.86	1.59–2.17	2.91	7.61	2.75	2.01–3.76
Stillbirth	1.35	1.34	0.99	0.66–1.48	1.01	0.89	0.87	0.42–1.83
Malformed baby	3.78	5.00	1.34	1.07–1.68	2.76	4.16	1.53	1.04–2.25

OR, odds ratio; CI, confidence interval.

Rostrepo et al., 1990.

available or insufficiently comparable for making informative comparisons. For example, in a study of physical activity and incidence of diabetes, comparisons of diagnosed diabetes in an external population with comprehensively ascertained diabetes based on screening in a cohort are likely to be uninformative since differences are likely to arise as a result of the thoroughness of medical care in detecting marginal cases of disease. Even when we know that differences in ascertainment protocols are likely to produce differences in measures of incidence, however, we may be comforted somewhat by finding that the application of a more comprehensive protocol for identifying cases in the cohort study results in the expected higher incidence of diabetes than is found in the external population.

Rarely will such outside populations provide a perfectly suitable comparison without some adjustment for basic social and demographic determinants of disease such as age, gender, and race. The more relevant question then is comparability within and across more homogeneous subsets of the population. If the study of physical activity and diabetes had a different age or gender composition or a different distribution of body mass index than the external referent population, we would need to stratify on gender, age, and body mass index to make the comparison informative. Criteria for establishing cutpoints for the diagnosis of diabetes would need to be comparable, or diagnoses of one of the populations might need to be truncated by restriction to make them comparable. We would also need to ensure that a comparable protocol for measuring glucose levels was applied in the two settings. One approach to ensuring that a valid comparison can be made between the unexposed and the external referent is to anticipate the desire to make this comparison in the planning stage of the study, and to ensure that comparable methods are used or at least can be reconstructed from the data obtained so that the outcome occurrence can be legitimately compared once the study is completed.

When disease rates are at least approximately comparable between the unexposed and outside population, some comfort can be taken in that selection bias is less likely than if the rates vary considerably for inexplicable reasons. If they differ because of applying different diagnostic protocols, then the comparison is uninformative. Even when similar outcome rates are observed, it is, of course, still possible for the unexposed group in the study to provide a poor estimate of the disease frequency that the exposed population would have experienced in the absence of exposure. Both the unexposed group and the external population may be aberrant in a similar manner and both may be poorly reflective of the experience the exposed group would have had absent the exposure.

Where the unexposed population differs for unexplained reasons from the external population, selection bias becomes more plausible, but such differences do not prove that the unexposed group is an inappropriate comparison population. The contrast between the unexposed group and the external population is motivated by an interest in detecting some problem in the constitution of the unexposed group that yields an aberrant disease rate. In addition to that possible basis for a disparity between the unexposed group and an external referent, the unexposed group may differ because they provide a superior referent for the exposed group and the differences simply reflect the unsuitability of the external referent population for comparisons. The main reason for including an unexposed group in the study when external population disease rates are available is to tailor the unexposed group to be most useful for making a counterfactual comparison with the exposed population. Even after taking into account simple sociodemographic factors to make the external population as comparable as possible to the unexposed group, there may well be characteristics of the study populations that make them comparable to one another but different from the external population.

In the example above, if there were some regional effect on the occurrence of diabetes, perhaps related to the ethnic composition of both the exposed and unexposed populations or distinctive dietary habits in the region, then a disparity in diabetes incidence between the unexposed population (persons with low physical activity) and the U.S. population would be expected and the unexposed population would remain a suitable group for generating baseline disease rates for comparison to the exposed (highly physically active) individuals. Despite efforts to ensure comparable methods of ascertainment of disease, the subtleties of the methods for measuring and classifying diabetes might differ between the unexposed segment of the cohort and the external population whereas we would have imposed an identical protocol for measurement on the exposed and unexposed cohort members. If the external referent population were certain to be the more suitable comparison population for the exposed individuals, there would have been no point in generating disease rates for an unexposed population in the first place. The unexposed study population is thought to be the preferred group for generating baseline disease rates, and the comparison to external populations provides a point of reference and can add some information to support a more thorough evaluation of the potential for selection bias, but not a definitive test for its presence or absence.

Assess Whether Expected Patterns of Disease are Present

For most diseases, epidemiologic understanding has advanced to the point that we can make predictions with some confidence about patterns of risk in relation to certain attributes and exposures. Many diseases rise with age, vary in predictable ways with gender or social class, or are known to be associated with tobacco or alcohol use. For example, if studying the influence of a drug that may prevent osteoporosis in middle-aged and elderly women, we would expect to observe decreased risk of osteoporosis among African-American women and among those who are most physically active as has been found in many previous studies. Verification that such expected patterns are present within the study cohort provides indirect evidence against some forms of selection bias as well as some evidence against extreme measurement error.

This strategy is illustrated in a recent study of the possible role of anxiety and depression in the etiology of spontaneous labor and delivery (Dayan et al., 2002), a topic for which results of previous studies have not led to firm conclusions. A cohort of 634 pregnancies was identified during 1997–1998 in France, and women were administered instruments to measure anxiety and depression as well as a range of other known and suspected risk factors for preterm birth. In addition to examining and presenting results for anxiety and depression, exposures of un-known etiologic significance, the authors presented results for a range of factors for which the associations are well established (Table 4.2). Despite the impreci-sion in this relatively small cohort, increased risk associated with heavy smok-ing, low prepregnancy body mass index, prior preterm delivery, and genitouri-nary tract infection was confirmed. This does not guarantee that the results found for anxiety and depression are certain to be correct, but it increases confidence somewhat that the cohort is capable of generating results compatible with those of most previous studies for other, more extensively examined, predictors of risk.

For demographic and social predictors, the internal comparisons help to assess whether there has been some differential selection that has markedly distorted the patterns of disease. If we conducted a study of osteoporosis in which African-American women experienced comparable rates of osteoporosis or higher rates than white women, we would be motivated to ask whether there had been some unintended selection that yielded an aberrant group of African Americans or whites or both. When men and women or young and old persons show the ex-pected pattern of disease risk relative to one another, then it is less likely that the pattern of selection differed dramatically in relation to gender or age. That is, the young men who were enrolled show the disease patterns expected of young men, and the older women who were enrolled show the disease patterns expected of older women.

It is possible, of course, to select an entire cohort that has aberrant disease rates but ones that are uniformly aberrant across all subgroups. We would thus find the expected pattern by making such comparisons within the cohort. We may find that all enrolled persons show a lower or higher than expected rate of disease, but that subgroups differ as expected relative to one another. A uniformly elevated or depressed rate of disease occurrence may well be less worrisome in that the goal of the study is to make internal comparisons, i.e., among exposed versus unexposed persons. The choice of the study setting or population may yield groups with atypically high or low overall rates. For example, in almost any randomized clinical trial the high degree of selectivity for enrollment in the trial does not negate the validity of the comparison of those randomized to dif-ferent treatment arms.

TABLE 4.2. Sociodemographic and Biomedical Characteristics of Pregnant Women, France, 1987–1989

CHARACTERISTICS	NO.	%
Age (years)		
< 20	31	4.9
20–34	516	81.4
≥ 35	87	13.7
Marital status		
Living alone	71	11.2
Married or cohabiting	563	88.8
Ethnicity		
Europe	598	94.3
Others	36	5.7
School education		
Primary school	50	7.9
Secondary school	420	66.2
Higher education	164	25.9
Occupation		
Not employed	243	38.3
Lower level of employment	262	41.3
Middle and higher level of employment	129	20.3
Smoking habits during pregnancy		
Nonsmoking	416	65.6
1–9 cigarettes daily	142	22.4
10 cigarettes or more daily	76	12.0
Parity		
0	236	37.2
1–2	333	52.5
≥ 3	65	10.3
Prepregnancy body mass index*		
< 19	93	14.7
19–< 25	398	62.8
≥ 25	143	22.6
Prior preterm labor		
No	575	90.7
Yes	59	9.3

(*continued*)

TABLE 4.2. Sociodemographic and Biomedical Characteristics of Pregnant Women, France, 1987–1989 (*continued*)

CHARACTERISTICS	NO.	%
Prior preterm birth		
No	600	94.6
Yes	34	5.4
Prior miscarriage		
No	494	77.9
Yes	140	22.1
Prior elective termination		
No	517	81.5
Yes	117	18.5
Other complications in previous pregnancies		
No	565	89.1
Yes	69	10.9
Conception		
Natural	589	92.9
Contraceptive failure	21	3.3
Medically assisted	24	3.8
Gestational age at the first consultation		
≤ 12 weeks	573	90.4
> 12 weeks	61	9.6
Vaginal bleeding		
No	558	88.0
Yes	76	12.0
Urinary tract infection		
No	579	91.3
Yes	55	8.7
Cervical and vaginal infection		
No	533	84.1
Yes	101	15.9
Other medical risk factors		
No	595	93.8
Yes	39	6.2
Consultation		
Not stressful	558	88.0
Stressful	78	12.0

*Weight (kg)/height (m)^2.

Dayan et al., 2002.

Note that the known determinants of disease patterns in relation to sociodemographic attributes or established etiologic exposures are not, of course, the ones under study. The primary interest is rarely in documenting that the expected, established bases for differences in disease are found in a particular population. Rather, some suspected but unproved determinant of disease incidence is typically the object of the study. The critical assumption is that observing expected patterns for *known* predictors increases confidence in the validity of patterns for the *unknown* effects of the exposure of interest. Failure to find the expected patterns of disease would raise substantial concern, whereas observing the expected patterns provides only limited reassurance.

Assess Pattern of Results in Relation to Markers of Susceptibility to Selection Bias

Although the actual amount of selection bias cannot readily be measured since that would require independent knowledge of the true causal effect, under an hypothesized mechanism for the production of selection bias, subsets of the cohort may be identified in which the amount of that bias is likely to be more severe or less severe. Stratifying the cohort into groups with greater and lesser potential for distortion due to selection bias, and calculating the estimated measure of effect within those subgroups, can yield two important observations: *(1)* the stratum that is most likely to be free of the source of bias, or in which the bias is weakest, should yield the most valid results, all other conditions equal, and *(2)* by assessing the gradient of results in relation to the hypothesized levels of selection bias, the overall importance of the source of bias in affecting the study can be better understood. If the results differ little or not at all across groups in which the bias is very likely to be more or less severe, it is probably not having a major influence on the results at all. In contrast, if the results show a strong dose-response gradient in relation to the amount of selection bias thought to be present, the source of bias is likely to be an important influence on study results. Even if no subgroup that is completely free of the source of bias can be isolated, it may be possible to extrapolate based on the gradation that is created. If the magnitude of the measure of association is diminishing steadily as the dose of the hypothesized bias decreases, one might speculate that the association would be even weaker than it is in the stratum least susceptible to bias if the bias were fully eliminated.

For example, one might postulate that the challenges of recruiting elderly participants in research would lead to a greater vulnerability to selection bias in the upper age strata compared to the lower age strata. Stratifying on age as a potential marker of the magnitude of such bias, and assessing the magnitude of association in subgroups defined by age, would provide information on selection bias that differs by age. If elderly participants show a stronger or weaker association than younger study participants, that deviation may be an indicator of the operation of selection bias, with the younger group generating the more valid result.

The challenge in interpretation is that selection bias across strata would produce the exact same pattern as effect measure modification across the same strata. For example, although selection bias that is more extreme for elderly participants would produce different measures of association than among younger participants, the stronger or weaker association among the elderly may reflect true effect modification in the absence of any bias. Elderly people may truly respond to the putative causal agent differently than younger people. Of course, both selection bias and effect measure modification can be operating, either in the same direction or in opposite directions. Thus, the absence of such a pattern does not persuasively rule out the potential for selection bias. Perhaps the elderly really do experience a weaker association between exposure and disease, and selection bias masks that pattern by increasing the strength of association among the elderly and thereby eliminating the appearance of effect measure modification.

In some instances, the mechanism thought to underlie selection bias may be directly amenable to empirical evaluation. A classic selection bias is the healthy worker effect in studies that compare health and mortality among industrial workers with health and mortality patterns in the community population. The demand for fitness at the time of hire and for sustained work in physically demanding jobs gives rise to an employed group that is at lower risk of mortality from a range of causes as compared to the general population (Checkoway et al., 1989), literally through selection for employment. Consistent with the approach suggested for examining selection bias, the more highly selected subgroups are in regard to the physical or other demands of their job that predict favorable health, such as education or talent, the more extreme the discrepancy tends to be (Checkoway et al., 1989). One might expect the magnitude of selection to be greater for a job requiring intense physical labor, such as longshoreman, or one that requires specialized talents, such as carpenter, as compared to jobs that are less demanding physically (e.g., clerk) or professionally (e.g., janitor).

The effect of this selection for hire tends to diminish over time, presumably because the good health that was required at the time of hire has faded. Those chosen to be fit have become less fit relative to their peers, even though there is typically still some level of selectivity for sustained employment (Checkoway et al., 1989). Those who leave work before retirement age show evidence of selectively unfavorable mortality, for example, in comparison to those who sustain their employment. By elucidating the pattern and extent of the healthy worker effect, our understanding of the phenomenon has markedly increased and therefore our ability to recognize and control its effects has been greatly enhanced. It is difficult to identify any other form of selection bias that is so well understood because addressing the healthy worker effect over the past 30 years has been fundamental to progress in studies of occupational disease. This elucidation of the healthy worker effect has required extensive effort to dissect the process (Choi, 1992; Arrighi & Hertz-Picciotto, 1994), develop specialized analytic approaches to minimize its impact (Steenland & Stayner, 1991), and recognize that failure to account for the phenomenon adequately substantially weakens the validity of research in occupational epidemiology.

In studies of prevalence, a particular form of selection bias concerns the loss of potentially eligible individuals prior to the time of assessment. A study of female garment workers compared the prevalence of musculoskeletal disorders to that of hospital workers who did not have jobs associated with the putative ergonomic stressors (Punnett, 1996). She reported a crude prevalence ratio of 1.9, but was concerned with the possibility of a stronger causal effect that was masked by the more affected garment workers selectively leaving employment, with those remaining to be included in the prevalence study showing a lower prevalence of the disorder. To address this possibility, she examined the incidence of new onset of pain in relation to the number of years prior to the survey (Fig. 4.1). This figure demonstrates that the onset of musculoskeletal pain among garment workers was markedly greater in the period proximal to the survey and rare in the earlier years, consistent with the hypothesized attrition of workers whose pain onset was earlier. No such pattern was found among hospital workers. The magnitude of selection, and thus selection bias, is least for the recent period prior to the survey and much greater for the more temporally remote time period.

Like other approaches to identifying bias, stratifying on indicators of severity of selection bias is fallible, but can yield informative clues. Even in the absence of a mechanistic understanding of the underlying process, hypothesizing a plausible pathway for selection bias, examining results within strata of differing vulnerability to the hypothesized selection, and observing whether there are

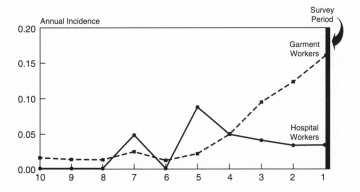

FIGURE 4.1. Conditional incidence density of musculoskeletal pain by calendar year, among 158 female garment assembly workers and 69 female hospital employees, Massachusetts, 1972–1981 (Punnett, 1996).

differences in the pattern of association across those strata provides valuable evidence to assess the probability and magnitude of selection bias.

Assess Rates for Diseases Known Not to Be Affected by the Exposure

For most exposures of possible health relevance, we have sufficient background knowledge to delineate some health outcomes that are likely to be affected (typically the ones that motivate the study and similar diseases) and other health outcomes that are highly unlikely to be affected. The conventional wisdom is fallible, of course. There are notable historical examples of erroneous assumptions about health outcomes that were certain to be unaffected by a given exposure. For example, men with chronic bronchitis were selected as controls in early case–control studies of lung cancer because chronic bronchitis was believed to be unaffected by tobacco smoking. Humans have a way of surprising epidemiologists with unanticipated associations, but in general, we can specify some diseases that are very likely to be affected by the exposure of interest based on current knowledge and diseases that are very unlikely to be affected by that exposure. Within the bounds of random error, and in the absence of selection bias, we would expect rates of disease that are not causally related to the exposure to be similar among exposed and unexposed groups. In other words, should differences be found in the rates of certain diseases in relation to exposure, and the possibility that such differences result from a causal effect of the exposure is remote, random error and selection bias become the most plausible candidate explanations.

For example, in a study of the effects of sunscreen use on risk of developing melanoma (an illustration from an oral presentation by Diana Petitti, Kaiser Permanente of Southern California), we would not expect sunscreen use to influence the risk of myocardial infarction, breast cancer, or motor vehicle injury. To determine whether our group of nonusers of sunscreen is a good counterfactual comparison group to the sunscreen users, reflecting the risk that the sunscreen users would have had in the absence of sunscreen use, we might find it useful to examine an array of causes of death that include some that should not differ due to a causal impact of sunscreen use. Even if our assumptions are incorrect in some of the diseases thought to be unrelated to sunscreen use, examination of the overall pattern of results across a range of presumably unrelated diseases would reveal whether a systematic tendency is present for exposed and unexposed groups to differ. If, for example, we observed consistently depressed disease rates across a series of causes of death thought not to be causally related to sunscreen use, the comparability of the groups for studying melanoma might be called into question. We may well find that users experience a lower risk of myocardial infarction, for example, due to other manifestations of the health consciousness that led them to be sunscreen users and may have lower rates of motor vehicle injury due to seat belt use, likely correlated with sunscreen use as a preventive health measure. We would be reminded to look carefully for other, correlated preventive health measures that may lead to more (or less) favorable patterns of melanoma incidence among sunscreen users, such as more frequent examination by a physician. If the sunscreen users had disease patterns similar to nonusers, except for the one of interest, i.e., melanoma, the potential for selection bias would be reduced.

A recent report on the impact of fine particulate air pollution on mortality from respiratory and cardiovascular disease, plausible consequences of such exposure, also considered a residual set of deaths from other causes (Pope et al., 2002). The extraordinarily large study of volunteers enrolled by the American Cancer Society into the Cancer Prevention II Study, 1.2 million adults, provided the basis for this investigation. As is often the case with studies of this issue, the measures of association between pollutants and mortality are modest in magnitude but highly precise, given the large population (Table 4.3). The categories of particular interest and plausibility, lung cancer and cardiopulmonary disease, showed increments in risk of 6% to 13% per 10 μg/m^3 over the time intervals examined, contributing to an association with all-cause mortality that was present but lower in magnitude. Once deaths from lung cancer and cardiopulmonary disease are removed, the residual category showed essentially no association, as one might expect from a conglomeration of other cancers, infectious diseases, injury mortality, etc. That is, observing an association between fine particular air pollution and deaths from causes other than those most plausible would raise the serious possibility that some selection bias for persons living in high exposure communities was operating and would suggest that the apparent effect of particulates on lung cancer and cardiopulmonary diseases might be due to some non-specific aspect of living in more highly exposed communities.

TABLE 4.3. Adjusted Mortality Relative Risk Associated with a 10 μg/m^3 Change in Fine Particles Measuring Less Than 2.5 μm in Diameter, American Cancer Society Cancer Prevention II Study

	Adjusted RR (95% CI)*		
CAUSE OF MORTALITY	1979–1983	1999–2000	AVERAGE
All-cause	1.04 (1.01–1.08)	1.06 (1.02–1.10)	1.06 (1.02–1.11)
Cardiopulmonary	1.06 (1.02–1.10)	1.08 (1.02–1.14)	1.09 (1.03–1.16)
Lung cancer	1.08 (1.01–1.16)	1.13 (1.04–1.22)	1.14 (1.04–1.23)
All other cause	1.01 (0.97–1.05)	1.01 (0.97–1.06)	1.01 (0.95–1.06)

*Estimated and adjusted based on the baseline random-effects Cox proportional hazards model, controlling for age, sex, race, smoking, education, marital status, body mass, alcohol consumption, occupational exposure, and diet.

RR, relative risk; CI, confidence interval.

Pope et al., 2002.

Like all criteria for assessing selection bias, this approach can also be misleading. As already noted, diseases thought to be unrelated to exposure may turn out to be causally related to the exposure, so that we would erroneously infer selection bias when it is not present. Many if not all known causes of disease affect more than one specific entity. Conversely, comparability for diseases other than the one of interest is only indirectly pertinent to whether the exposure groups are comparable for the disease of interest. A selection bias may be present or absent solely for the health outcome of interest, so that reassuring patterns for other outcomes are misinterpreted as indicative of valid results for the outcome of interest. The patterns of disease other than the one of interest are a flag to examine the issue further, not a definitive marker of the presence or absence of bias.

Assess and Adjust for Baseline Differences in Risk of Disease

As noted previously, differences between the exposed and unexposed groups that affect risk of disease can sometimes be measured and statistically adjusted as confounding factors. In the case of selection bias, those differences arise or are modified based on the way in which the study groups were constituted. Specifically, the link between exposure and the confounding factor is a result of selection bias instead of occurring naturally as in classical confounding. The means of identifying and controlling such markers of selection bias is identical to that for other sources of confounding (Rothman & Greenland, 1998).

The nature of the selection bias that introduces confounding should be examined to yield insights into the mechanism by which the bias was produced. By enhancing understanding of the origins of the selection bias that can be controlled statistically, we will be better able to evaluate the potential for differences in exposure groups that cannot be so readily controlled, including residual selection bias related to the influences that we have attempted to remove in the analysis. The phenomenon is exactly analogous to that of residual confounding—when there are large differences between groups, and the measure of the determinant of those differences is imperfect, then adjustment for that imperfect measure will yield incompletely adjusted results (Greenland & Robins, 1985). Empirically, we might expect that large baseline differences in important risk factors for disease will be more likely to leave residual selection bias after adjustment as compared to smaller baseline differences or weaker risk factors for disease. As with residual confounding (Savitz & Barón, 1989), we can observe the impact of adjusting using the best available indicators, and speculate (even speculate quantitatively) about what the result would be with a more complete adjustment.

Consider the example of trying to isolate the independent effect of physical exertion on coronary heart disease from other determinants of this health outcome. If the highly active members of the cohort are recruited from running clubs and fitness facilities, and the low or normal exertion group is chosen from a health care provider roster, the high exertion group may well have other distinctive attributes that predict a reduced risk of coronary heart disease, beyond any influence of their regimen of physical exertion. In an effort to isolate the effect of physical exertion and control for confounding, we would measure and adjust for suspected influential differences in diet, medication use, preventive health care, etc. The goal is to make this group, which has been self-selected to be physically active, less deviant and better approximate the group that would have resulted from randomized assignment of intense exercise. It seems likely that the proposed adjustments would help to move the results in the desired direction, but unlikely that the adjustments would be completely successful given that such self-selection is an elusive construct. By observing the change in pattern of results with successive adjustments, information is generated to speculate about the impact of the unattainable complete adjustment for the selection bias. If adjustment diminishes the observed benefits of intense physical activity substantially compared to the crude results, then the possibility that complete adjustment would fully eliminate observed benefits is more plausible. We might infer that the observed benefits in the unadjusted comparison are a result of incomplete control for selection bias. In some instances, this problem of baseline comparability is so severe as to demand a randomized study, despite the daunting logistical aspects of such an undertaking for exposures such as physical exercise. Short of eliminating the problem, the goals of understanding its origins, reducing it, and speculating about the impact of its elimination must suffice.

Similarly, understanding the health risks and benefits for women using postmenopausal estrogen therapy has been extremely challenging, in that the women who do and do not elect to use such therapy are not comparable in baseline risk of cardiovascular disease. Matthews et al. (1996) compared future users of estrogen replacement therapy with future nonusers, and users were shown to have a consistently favorable profile on a number of attributes (Table 4.4). Cohorts of users and nonusers clearly would not reflect women at equal baseline risk of coronary heart disease. Investigators who address the risks and benefits of estrogen replacement therapy are aware of this threat to validity, and make attempts to adjust for a wide array of factors. For example, analyses of the Nurses Health Study data (Stampfer et al., 1991) adjusted for a long list of candidate baseline differences and still found a marked reduction in heart disease incidence among users (Table 4.5). Whether comparability was truly achieved despite these efforts is open to debate; recent findings from the Women's Health Initiative suggest the observational studies were in error (Writing Group for the Women's Health Initiative Investigators, 2002).

Restrict Study Groups to Enhance Comparability

The fact that groups naturally differ in exposure provides the opportunity to conduct observational studies, but is also the basis for selection bias. The ideal study is one in which those exposure differences arise from random or effectively ran-

TABLE 4.4. Mean ± Standard Error Levels of Other Biologic Characteristics and Health Behaviors of Premenopausal Examination of Subsequent Users and Nonusers of Estrogen Replacement Therapy, Pittsburgh, Pennsylvania, 1983–1992.

CHARACTERISTIC	SUBSEQUENT USER	NONUSER	T-TEST OR X^2	P VALUE
Blood pressure (mmHg)				
Systolic	107.1 ± 0.8	112.1 ± 1.1	3.73	< 0.001
Diastolic	71.4 ± 0.6	73.8 ± 0.7	2.68	0.008
Glucose (mmol/liter)				
Fasting	4.81 ± 0.05	4.88 ± 0.07	0.95	0.35
Two-hour	5.03 ± 0.10	5.27 ± 0.14	1.43	0.15
Fasting insulin (μU/liter)	7.66 ± 0.44	9.10 ± 0.55	2.13	0.03
Height (m)	1.64 ± 0.005	1.63 ± 0.005	0.24	0.81
Weight (kg)	64.2 ± 0.9	68.5 ± 1.1	3.01	0.003
Alcohol intake (g/day)	9.7 ± 0.8	7.5 ± 0.8	2.01	0.05
Weekly physical activity (Kjoules)	7158 ± 791	5122 ± 369	2.33	0.02
Ever smoker (%)	61.8	55.0	1.53	0.22
Current smokers (%)	28.7	34.1	1.13	0.29

Matthews et al., 1996.

dom assignment, of course. In non-randomized studies, exposure differences arise in diverse ways, and the vulnerability to selection bias differs as a function of how the exposure differences arose. A link between the reasons for being exposed or unexposed and the risk of disease suggests susceptibility to selection bias. For that reason, studies of medical interventions, including drugs, are especially susceptible to such bias. Treatments are not randomly assigned by clinicians, one would hope, but given in response to a specific condition in a particular individual. Interventions are provided for medical conditions, of course, and those medical conditions may themselves influence the occurrence of the disease of interest. As always, randomized exposure assignment is the optimal way to overcome such bias, but there are alternative strategies to consider.

Where there are distinctive, multiple pathways by which exposure occurs, separation of exposed subjects based on the reasons for exposure into those distinct pathways may help to understand and control selection bias. Some of the reasons for exposure may be very unlikely to have an independent effect on disease risk, and thus be free of such bias, whereas others are hopelessly confounded by the indications for exposure and therefore ill-suited to measure the causal effect of exposure. Instead of simply aggregating all exposed persons as a single entity, we would create subgroups defined by the reasons for exposure. Just as it was proposed to stratify by vulnerability to selection bias to assess whether the patterns of results differed across strata, we would stratify by reasons for exposure to determine whether the groups with the greater risk of selection bias yield

Used Postmenopausal Hormones, After Adjustment for Age and Multiple Risk Factors, Nurses Health Study

GROUP*	NO. OF PERSON-YEARS	Major Coronary Disease		Fatal Cardiovascular Disease		Total Stroke		Ischemic Stroke		Subarachnoid Hemorrhage	
		NO. OF CASES	RR (95% CI)	NO. OF CASES	RR (95% CI)	NO. OF CASES	RR (95% CI)	NO. OF CASES	RR (95% CI)	NO. OF CASES	RR (95% CI)
No hormone use	179,194	250	1.0	129	1.0	123	1.0	56	1.0	19	1.0
Current hormone use	73,532										
Adjusted for age	—	45	0.51 (0.37–0.70)	21	0.48 (0.31–0.74)	39	0.96 (0.67–1.37)	23	1.26 (0.78–2.02)	5	0.80 (0.30–2.10)
Adjusted for age and risk factors	—		0.56 (0.40–0.80)		0.61 (0.37–1.00)		0.97 (0.65–1.45)		1.46 (0.85–2.51)		0.53 (0.18–1.57)
Former hormone use	85,128										
Adjusted for age	—	110	0.91 (0.73–1.14)	55	0.84 (0.61–1.15)	62	1.00 (0.74–1.36)	34	1.14 (0.75–1.74)	12	1.42 (0.70–2.90)
Adjusted for age and risk factors	—		0.83 (0.65–1.05)		0.79 (0.56–1.10)		0.99 (0.72–1.36)		1.19 (0.77–1.86)		1.03 (0.47–2.25)

*Women with no hormone use served as the reference category in this analysis. The risk factors included in the multivariate models were age (in five-year categories), cigarette smoking (none, former, current [1 to 14, 15 to 24, and ≥ 25 cigarettes per day]), hypertension (yes, no), diabetes (yes, no), high serum cholesterol level (yes, no), parental myocardial infarction before the age of 60 (yes, no), Quetelet index (in five categories), past use of oral contraceptives (yes, no), and time period (in five two-year periods).

RR, relative risk; CI, confidence interval.

Stampfer et al., 1991.

measures of association that differ from groups that are less susceptible. If we find such a pattern, more stock should be placed in the findings for the exposed group that is less vulnerable, and if we do not, then there is some evidence that the hypothesized selection bias has not materialized and we can be somewhat more confident that there is no need to subdivide the exposed group in that manner.

For example, the potential effect of sexual activity in late pregnancy on risk of preterm birth has been considered in a number of studies (Read & Klebanoff, 1993; Sayle et al., 2001). The comparison of sexually active to sexually inactive women is fraught with potential for selection bias. Some women undoubtedly refrain from sexual activity due to discomfort or irritation associated with genital tract infection, which may well be a marker of increased risk of preterm birth (French & McGregor, 1997). Others may refrain from sexual activity because of concerns associated with a history of previous poor pregnancy outcomes, a strong predictor of subsequent adverse pregnancy outcome. For some women, the lack of a partner may be the basis for abstinence, possibly correlated with lack of social support or economic stress. In order to try to isolate a subgroup of women for whom the level of sexual activity is least susceptible to selection bias, analyses may be restricted to women who are thought to have equal baseline risk of preterm birth. In an attempt to reduce or eliminate selection bias, we would eliminate those women who were told to refrain from sexual activity by their physicians, based on perceived elevated risk and those who experienced symptoms associated with genital tract infection as the basis for remaining sexually inactive. We might eliminate those who are unmarried or not living with a partner. The goal is to find a subset of women for whom the allocation of sexual activity is as random as possible, i.e., to simulate as closely as possible a randomized trial in which the allocation of exposure is independent of baseline risk, accepting that some reasons for being unexposed are too closely tied to disease risk to be informative.

An illustration of a specific candidate source of selection bias is provided by studies of whether physical activity protects against depression. A key issue is whether those who are inactive due to disability, and are more likely to be depressed as a result of their disability, should be excluded from such studies. The potential gain in validity from excluding disabled participants was examined by Strawbridge et al. (2002) using data from the Alameda County Study, a prospective cohort study of nearly 7000 adults. The authors examined the 1947 adults who were over age 50 and living in 1999 and had all essential data for addressing physical activity and depression. Disability was defined as the inability to walk 0.25 miles, walk up 10 stairs without resting, stand from a stooping or kneeling position, or stand after sitting in a chair. Considering various potential confounding factors, those who were more physically active had a 25% lower risk of depression (Table 4.6). Excluding the 151 individuals who were disabled ac-

TABLE 4.6. Sequential Logistic Regression Models Showing Relations Between 1994 Physical Activity and Depression in 1994 and 1999, with Adjustments for Other Risk Factors Among 1947 Men and Women, Alameda County Study, California, 1994–1999

MODEL AND 1994 COVARIATES	Prevalent 1994 Depression (cross-sectional analyses) with All Subjects Included (n = 1947)		Incident 1999 Depression (Longitudinal Analyses) with 1994 Depressed Subjects Excluded			
			Disabled Included (n = 1802)		Disabled Excluded (n = 1651)	
	OR*	95% CI†	OR	95% CI	OR	95% CI
1. Age, sex, and ethnicity	0.75	0.68, 0.84	0.75	0.66, 0.85	0.73	0.63, 0.85
2. Model 1 + education, financial strain, and neighborhood problems	0.78	0.70, 0.87	0.76	0.67, 0.87	0.75	0.65, 0.87
3. Model 2 + physical disability,† chronic conditions, BMI, smoking, and alcohol consumption	0.86	0.76, 0.96	0.82	0.72, 0.94	0.78	0.67, 0.91
4. Model 3 + no. of relatives, no. of friends, and satisfaction with relations	0.90	0.79, 1.01	0.83	0.73, 0.96	0.79	0.67, 0.92

*Odds ratios (OR) represent the approximate relative likelihood of being depressed associated with a one-point increase in the physical activity scale. Because the incidence rate for depression is relatively small (5.4%), the resulting odds ratios for the longitudinal analyses closely approximate relative risks.

†This variable is omitted from models in which physically disabled subjects were excluded.

CI, confidence interval; BMI, body mass index.

Strawbridge et al., 2002.

cording to the above criteria made no material difference in the results, with no tendency whatsoever to move closer to the null value. In this example, it appeared that omission of disabled persons was not necessary to enhance validity and only produced a small loss in precision. Nonetheless, the strategy of restricting to evaluate selection bias is well illustrated by this study, with regard to methods, implementation, and interpretation.

INTEGRATED ASSESSMENT OF POTENTIAL FOR SELECTION BIAS IN COHORT STUDIES

The evaluation of potential selection bias in cohort studies is much like the evaluation of confounding. We first specify known determinants of the health outcome of interest, since it is only selection in relation to such factors that can generate erroneous comparisons. Those markers may be broad (e.g., social class, geographic setting) or narrow (e.g., biological indices of risk, dietary constituents). The question of selection bias is whether, conditional on adjustment for known determinants of disease risk, the exposed and unexposed groups are comparable except for differing exposure status. Since we cannot repeat the experiment and assign the exposed population to a no exposure condition to measure their true baseline risk, we need to make statistical adjustments and ultimately make a judgment regarding the comparability of the groups. Accepting the exposed population as given, the challenge is to evaluate whether the unexposed population has done its job, i.e., generated disease rates that approximate those that would have been found in the exposed population had they lacked exposure.

A number of indirect tools can be applied to address the following questions:

1. Is the disease rate in the unexposed population similar to that in external populations, conditional on adjusting for known influences?
2. Do the patterns of disease risk within the unexposed population correspond to those expected from the literature?
3. For postulated mechanisms of selection bias, do the strata in which selection bias is least likely to be present show similar results to the total cohort? Is there a gradient of association across the gradient of hypothesized selection bias?
4. Are disease rates for conditions thought to be unrelated to the exposure similar for the exposed and unexposed groups?
5. Were there markers of disease risk introduced by selection bias that needed to be controlled? Is it likely that residual selection bias is present after making those adjustments?
6. Can the reasons for exposure be divided into those more and less vulnerable to selection bias? What is the pattern of results among those who are least likely to be affected by selection bias?

Though none of these is a definitive test for selection bias, all bear on the probability of selection bias of varying magnitudes. An array of favorable responses adds markedly to the evidence against selection bias, and responses suggestive of selection bias would warrant more refined analysis or even further data collection to examine the possibility. Again, the model of the healthy worker effect in occupational epidemiology illustrates the fundamental importance of selection bias but also how much progress can be made with concerted effort to elucidate and control the sources of bias. Most specific scenarios of selection bias can be postulated and tested using the above tools, either diminishing the credibility of the results through discovery that significant amounts of bias are likely to be present or strengthening the credibility by refuting these hypothesized sources of bias.

REFERENCES

Arrighi HM, Hertz-Picciotto I. The evolving concept of the healthy worker survivor effect. Epidemiology 1994;5:189–196.

Checkoway H, Pearce N, Crawford-Brown DJ. Research methods in occupational epidemiology. New York: Oxford University Press, 1989:78–91.

Choi BCK. Definition, sources, magnitude, effect modifiers, and strategies of reduction of the health worker effect. J Occup Med 1992;34:979–988.

Chow W-H, Linet MS, Liff JM, Greenberg RS. Cancers in children. In D Schottenfeld, JF Fraumeni Jr (eds), Cancer Epidemiology and Prevention, Second Edition. New York: Oxford University Press, 1996:1331–1369.

Dayan J, Creveuil C, Herlicoviez M, Herbel C, Baranger E, Savoye C, Thouin A. Role of anxiety and depression in the onset of spontaneous preterm labor. Am J Epidemiol 2002;155:293–301.

Elwood M, Elwood H, Little J. Diet. In JM Elwood, J Little, and JH Elwood (eds), Epidemiology and Control of Neural Tube Defects. New York: Oxford University Press, 1992:521–602.

French JI, McGregor JA. Bacterial vaginosis: history, epidemiology, microbiology, sequelae, diagnosis, and treatment. In Borschardt KA, Noble MA (eds), Sexually transmitted diseases: Epidemiology, pathology, diagnosis, and treatment. Boca Raton, Florida: CRC Press, 1997:3–39.

Greenland S. Randomization, statistics, and causal inference. Epidemiology 1990;1:421–429.

Greenland S, Robins JM. Confounding and misclassification. Am J Epidemiol 1985;122:495–506.

Greenland S, Robins JM. Identifiability, exchangeability, and epidemiologic confounding. Int J Epidemiol 1986;15:413–419.

Little J, Elwood H. Socio-economic status and occupation. In JM Elwood, J Little, and JH Elwood (eds), Epidemiology and Control of Neural Tube Defects. New York: Oxford University Press, 1992a:456–520.

Little J, Elwood M. Ethnic origin and migration. In JM Elwood, J Little, and JH Elwood (eds), Epidemiology and Control of Neural Tube Defects. New York: Oxford University Press, 1992b:146–167.

Matthews KA, Kuller LH, Wing RR, Meilahn EN, Plantinga P. Prior to use of estrogen replacement therapy, are users healthier than nonusers? Am J Epidemiol 1996;143: 971–978.

Miettinen OS, The "case-control" study: valid selection of subjects. J Chron Dis 1985;38:543–548.

Morgenstern H, Thomas D. Principles of study design in environmental epidemiology. Environ Health Perspect 1993;101 (Suppl 4):23–38.

Pope CA III, Burnett RT, Thun MT, Calle EE, Krewski D, Ito K, Thurston GD. Lung cancer, cardiopulmonary mortality, and long-term exposure to fine particulate air pollution. JAMA 2002; 287: 1132–1141.

Punnett L. Adjusting for the healthy worker selection effect in cross-sectional studies. Int J Epidemiol 1996;25:1068–1076.

Read JS, Klebanoff MA. Sexual intercourse during pregnancy and preterm delivery: Effects of vaginal microorganisms. Am J Obstet Gynecol 1993;168:514–519.

Ries LAG, Hankey BF, Harras A, Devesa SS. Cancer incidence, mortality, and patient survival in the United States. In D Schottenfeld, JF Fraumeni Jr (eds), Cancer Epidemiology and Prevention, Second Edition. New York: Oxford University Press, 1996:168–191.

Rostrepo M, Muñoz N, Day NE, Parra JE, de Romero L, Nguyen-Dinh X. Prevalence of adverse reproductive outcomes in a population occupationally exposed to pesticides in Colombia. Scand J Work Environ Health 1990;16:232–238.

Rothman KJ. Modern Epidemiology. Boston: Little, Brown and Co., 1986.

Rothman KJ, Greenland S. Modern epidemiology, Second edition. Philadelphia: Lippincott-Raven Publishers, 1998.

Savitz DA, Barón AE. Estimating and correcting for confounder misclassification. Am J Epidemiol 1989;129:1062–1071.

Sayle AE, Savitz DA, Thorp JM Jr, Hertz-Picciotto I, Wilcox AJ. Sexual activity during late pregnancy and risk of preterm delivery. Obstet Gynecol 2001;97:283–289.

Stampfer MJ, Colditz GA, Willett WC, Manson JE, Rosner B, Speizer FE, Hennekens CH. Postmenopausal estrogen therapy and cardiovascular disease. N Engl J Med 1991;325:756–762.

Steenland K, Stayner L. The importance of employment status in occupational cohort mortality studies. Epidemiology 1991;2:418–423.

Strawbridge WJ, Deleger S, Roberts RE, Kaplan GA. Physical activity reduces the risk of subsequent depression for older adults. Am J Epidemiol 2002;156:328–334.

Writing Group for the Women's Health Initiative Investigators. Risks and benefits of estrogen plus progestin in healthy postmenopausal women. Principal results from the Women's Health Initiative randomized controlled trial. JAMA 2002;288:321–333.

5

SELECTION BIAS IN CASE–CONTROL STUDIES

For many years, there was the misperception that case–control studies were fundamentally inferior to cohort designs, suffering from backward logic (health outcome leading to exposure rather than exposure to health outcome). As the conceptual basis for the design is more fully understood (Miettinen, 1985), it has become clear that the only unique threat to validity is the susceptibility to selection bias. The logistics of selecting and enrolling cases and controls are often fundamentally different from each other, making the concern with selection bias justifiably prominent.

CONTROL SELECTION

Subject Selection in Case–Control and Cohort Studies

A case–control study involves the comparison of groups, namely cases and controls, in order to estimate the association between exposure and disease. By choosing persons with the adverse health outcome of interest (cases) and a properly constituted sample from the source population (controls), we assess exposure prevalence in the two groups in order to estimate of the association between exposure and disease. A cohort study also has the same goal, estimating the association between exposure and disease, and also does so by comparing two groups, i.e., the exposed and the unexposed. Unfortunately, there is a temptation to select cases and controls in a manner that mimics the selection of exposed and unexposed subjects in a cohort study. The role of an unexposed group in a cohort study however, and a control group in a case–control study are entirely different. In a cohort study, the goal is to select an unexposed group that has identical baseline risk of disease as the exposed group other than any effect of the exposure itself. If that goal is met, then the disease experience of the unexposed group provides a valid estimate of the disease risk the exposed persons would have had if they had not been exposed (counterfactual comparison). Cohort studies attempt to mimic a randomized trial or experiment in which the exposure of interest is manipulated to ensure, to the maximum extent possible, that the exposed and unexposed are identical in all respects other than the exposure of interest.

In a case–control study, by contrast, given a set of cases with the disease, the goal is to select controls who approximate the exposure prevalence in the study base, that is, the population experience that generated the cases. The key comparison to assess whether the control group is a good one is not between the cases and the controls, but between the controls and the study base they are intended to approximate. The available cases define the scope of the study base, namely the population experience that gave rise to that particular set of cases. Once defined clearly, the challenge for control selection is unbiased sampling from that study base. If this is done properly, then the case–control study will give results as valid as those that would have been obtained from a cohort study of the same population subject to sampling error. It should be noted, however, that biases inherent in that underlying cohort, such as selection bias associated with exposure allocation, would be replicated in the case–control study sampled from that cohort.

Consider two studies of the same issue, agricultural pesticide exposure and the development of Parkinson's disease. In the cohort study, we identify a large population of pesticide users to monitor the incidence of Parkinson's disease and an unexposed cohort that is free of such exposure. We would then compare the incidence of Parkinson's disease in the two groups. In the case–control study, assume we have a roster of Parkinson's disease cases from a large referral center and select controls for comparison from the same geographic region as the cases, in order to assess the prevalence of exposure to agricultural pesticides in each group and thereby estimate the association. The methodologic challenge in the cohort study is to identify an unexposed cohort that is as similar as possible to the exposed group in all other factors that influence the risk of developing Parkinson's disease, such as demographic characteristics, tobacco use, and family disease history. Bias arises to the extent that our unexposed group does not generate a valid estimate of the disease risk the pesticide-exposed persons would have had absent that exposure.

Bias arises in case–control studies not because the cases and controls differ on characteristics other than exposure but because the selected controls do not accurately reflect exposure prevalence in the study base. In our efforts to choose appropriate controls for the referred Parkinson's disease cases, we need to first ask what defines the study base that generated those cases—what is the geographic scope, socioeconomic, and behavioral characteristics of the source population for these cases, which health care providers refer patients to this center, etc. Once we fully understand the source of those cases, we seek to sample without bias from that study base. The critical comparison that defines whether we have succeeded in obtaining a valid control group is not the comparison of controls to Parkinson's disease cases but the comparison of controls to the study base that generated those cases. Only if the cases are effectively a random sample from the study base, that is, only if it is a foregone conclusion that there are no predictors of disease, would the goal of making controls as similar as possible to cases be appropriate.

Properly selected controls have the same exposure prevalence, within the range of sampling error, as the study base. Selection bias distinctive to case–control studies arises when the cases and controls are not coherent relative to one another (Miettinen, 1985), i.e., the groups do not come from the same study base. Thus, the falsely seductive analogy that "exposed and unexposed should be alike in all respects except disease" in cohort studies and therefore "cases and controls should be alike in all respects except disease" is simply incorrect.

Selection of Controls from the Study Base

A key concept in case–control studies that guides control selection is the study base (Miettinen, 1985), defined simply as the person–time experience that gives rise to the cases. Conceptually, the study base is populated by the people at risk of becoming identified as cases in the study if they got the disease during the time period in which cases are identified. Note that this is more than just being at risk of developing the disease in that membership in the study base also requires that if the disease should develop, the individual would end up as part of the case group for that study. The question of "Who would have become a case in this study?" often has a complex, multifaceted answer. Beyond the biological changes involved with disease development, it may involve behavioral response to symptoms or seeking medical care from certain physicians or hospitals, if those are components of becoming recognized, enrolled cases in the study. If the constitution of the study base can be unambiguously defined in both theoretical and operational terms, then sampling controls is reduced to a probability sampling protocol. In fact, one of the major virtues of case–control studies nested within well-defined cohorts is precisely that clarity: all members of the study base are enrolled in the cohort, and sampling from that roster is straightforward in principle and in practice.

In many case–control studies, however, the very definition of the study base is complex. In some instances, the study base is defined a priori, e.g., all persons enrolled in a given health care plan for a defined period of time, or all persons who reside in a given geographic area over some time period, and the challenge is to accurately identify all cases of disease that arise from that study base (Miettinen, 1985). Given that the investigator has chosen the study base, the conceptual definition is clear, though practical aspects of sampling from that base in an unbiased manner may still pose a challenge. Random sampling from a geographically defined population is often not easy, at least in settings in which population rosters are lacking.

In other instances, a roster of cases is available, for example, from a given medical practice or hospital, and even the conceptual definition of the study base is unclear. The investigator must consider the entire set of attributes that are prerequisites to being enrolled as a case. The conceptual definition of the study base producing cases may include whether symptoms come to attention, whether people seek a diagnosis for those symptoms, whether they have access to medical care, and who they choose as their health care provider (Savitz & Pearce, 1988). Thus, the assessment of whether a particular mechanism of control selection has generated an unbiased sample from the study base (Miettinen, 1985) requires careful evaluation and informed judgment.

Obtaining perfectly coherent case and control groups from the same study base guarantees that there will be no additional selection bias introduced in the case–control sampling beyond whatever selection bias may be inherent in the underlying cohort. The failure to do so, however, does not automatically produce selection bias; it just introduces the possibility. In a cohort study, the ultimate purpose of the unexposed group is to estimate the disease risk of the exposed group absent exposure. In a case–control study, the purpose of the controls is to generate an accurate estimate of the exposure prevalence in the study base that gave rise to the cases. Given this goal, by good fortune or careful planning, a control group that is not coherent with the cases may nevertheless generate a valid estimate of exposure prevalence in the study base that gave rise to the cases. If, for example, the exposure of interest in a case–control study of melanoma among women were natural hair color (associated with skin pigmentation and response to sunlight), and we knew that hair color was not related to gender, we might well accept the exposure prevalence estimates among male controls in a geographically defined study base as a valid estimate for female cases. In no sense could we argue that the controls constitute a random sample from the study base that produced the cases, which must be exclusively female, yet the exposure prevalence of the controls would be a valid estimate of the exposure prevalence in that study base under the assumptions noted above.

A second consideration is that a control group can be well suited to address one exposure and yet be biased for assessing others. If controls are sampled in a valid manner from the proper study base, then they will generate accurate estimates of prevalence for all possible exposures in the study base, and thus case–control comparisons of exposure prevalence will generate valid measures of association. However, with deviations from the ideally constituted controls, the potential for selection bias needs to be considered on an exposure-by-exposure basis. In the above example of a case–control study of melanoma, males would not serve well as controls for female cases in efforts to address the prevalence of sunscreen use or diet, let alone reproductive history and oral contraceptive use. The question of whether the controls have generated a good estimate of exposure prevalence in the study base, and thus a valid measure of the exposure–disease association of concern, must be considered for each exposure of interest.

Among the most challenging exposures to evaluate are those that are associated with social factors or discretionary individual behaviors, e.g., diet, exercise, tobacco use. These characteristics are often susceptible to selection bias in that they may well be related to inclination to seek medical care, source of medical care, and willingness to voluntarily participate in studies. In contrast, if exposure were determined solely by genetic factors, e.g., blood type or hair color, or those not based on conscious decisions, e.g., public water source, eating at a restaurant discovered to employ a carrier of hepatitis, then selection bias is less likely. Therefore, it is much easier to choose controls for studies of some exposures, such as blood type, than others, such as psychological stress or diet.

In asking whether a particular method of control selection constitutes an unbiased method of sampling from the study base, corrections can be made for intentionally unbalanced sampling, e.g., stratified sampling by demographic attributes or cluster sampling. Consideration of confounding may justify manipulation of the sampling of controls to better approximate the distribution of the confounding factor among cases. Such manipulation of control selection is a form of intentional selection bias (Rothman, 1986), which is then removed through statistical adjustment. When it is known that stratification and adjustment for the confounding factor will be required to obtain valid results, then there may be some benefit from manipulating the distribution of the confounding factor among the controls. If that stratified sampling makes the distribution of the confounding factor among controls more similar to the distribution among cases, then the stratified analysis will be more statistically efficient and thus generate more precise results than if the distribution were markedly different among cases and controls.

For example, we may be interested in the question of whether coffee consumption is associated with the risk of developing bladder cancer. We know that tobacco use is a major determinant of bladder cancer and also that coffee consumption and smoking tend to be positively associated. Thus, we can anticipate that in our analysis of the association between coffee consumption and bladder cancer, we will need to make adjustments for a confounding effect of cigarette smoking. If we take no action at the time of control selection, we will have many more cases who are smokers than controls (given that tobacco use is a strong risk factor for bladder cancer). We lose precision by creating strata of smoking in which there is gross imbalance of cases and controls, i.e., many controls who are nonsmokers relative to the number of cases and few controls who are heavy smokers relative to the number of cases. In anticipation of this problem, we may well choose to distort our control sampling to oversample smokers, i.e., intentionally shift the balance using probability sampling among strata of smokers and nonsmokers to make the smoking distribution of controls more similar to that of the cases. We will still need to adjust for smoking, as we would have without stratified sampling, but now when we do adjust we will have a better balance of cases and controls across the smoking strata, and a more statistically precise result for the estimated measure of association.

Given the ability to account for stratified sampling from the study base, we do not need a mechanism to achieve a simple random sample that represents exposure prevalence but only a mechanism to achieve a defined probability sample from the study base. Even when the uneven sampling in relation to measured attributes is unintentional, we can correct for it in data analysis. For example, if a door-to-door sampling procedure inadvertently oversamples older women, we can readily adjust for age and gender distribution in the analysis. The key question then is whether the exposure prevalence reflects that in the study base within those strata known to be unbalanced. In the example with overrepresentation of elderly women, we need only assurance that the exposure prevalence among older women in the study base has been sampled accurately and that the exposure prevalence among young women and men of all ages in the study base has also been sampled accurately, not necessarily that the proportion of women and men in the study base has been sampled accurately (unless gender is the exposure of interest). Conversely, selecting a sample that is representative with regard to social and demographic factors does not guarantee that it reflects accurately exposure prevalence and thus would generate an unbiased estimate of the association between exposure and disease. Exposed persons may be oversampled (or undersampled) inadvertently in each of the age-sex strata even if the distribution by age and sex is perfectly representative of the study base. For example, participants in studies generally are less likely to be users of tobacco than are nonparticipants. This might well be true in all age and gender strata so that a control sample that is perfectly balanced across age and gender could well underestimate tobacco use in all those strata and yield a biased measure of association between tobacco use and disease.

Coherence of Cases and Controls

Focusing on coherence between cases and controls emphasizes that it is not *one* of the groups that is at fault if they cannot be integrated to yield valid measures of the association between exposure and disease, but rather their composition *relative to one another*. Thus, there is no such thing as poorly constituted cases or poorly constituted controls, only groups that are incoherent with one another. In practice, once one group, cases or controls, has been operationally defined, then the desired attributes of the other is defined and the challenge is a practical one of meeting that conceptual goal. Miettinen (1985) coined the terms *primary study base* and *secondary study base*. With a primary study base, the definition of the population-time experience that produces the cases is explicitly demarcated by calendar periods and geographic boundaries. In such instances, the challenge is to fully ascertain the cases that arise from within that study base and to accurately sample controls from that study base. A secondary base corresponds to a given set of cases identified more by convenience, such as those that appear and are diagnosed at a given hospital, posing the challenge of identifying a means of properly sampling controls from the ill-defined study base.

In reality, there is a continuum of clarity in the definition of study bases, with the goal being the identification of a study base that lends itself to selection of coherent cases and controls. A choice can be made in the scope of the study base itself that will make coherent case and control selection more or less difficult. It may be more useful to focus on the identification of a coherent base for identifying both cases and controls than to first focus on making case or control selection alone as easy as possible and then worrying about how to select the other group. The ability to formally define the geographic and temporal scope of a study base is less critical than the practical ability to identify all the cases that are produced in a study base and to have some way to properly sample controls from it.

Coherence may sometimes be achieved by restricting the constitution of one of the groups to make the task easier. For example, in a study of pregnancy outcome based in prenatal care clinics, the case group may include women who began normal pregnancies and developed the disease of interest, e.g., pregnancy-induced hypertension, as well as women who began prenatal care elsewhere and were referred to the study clinic because they developed medical problems, including the one of interest. The source of referrals is very difficult to identify with clarity, since it depends on financial incentives, patient and physician preferences, etc. Therefore, one option would be to simply exclude those referred from other prenatal care providers from the case group and thereby from the study base itself, and instead study non-referred cases and a sample of patients who enrolled in prenatal care at the study settings without necessarily being at high risk. Note that the problem is not in identifying referred cases, which is straightforward, but rather in sampling from the ill-defined pool of pregnant women who would, if they had developed health problems, have been referred to the study clinics. Restricting cases and controls to women who began their care in the study clinics improves the ability to ensure that they are coherent.

In this example, as in most case–control studies, the burden is placed on proper selection of controls given a roster of cases. Selection bias is defined not as having chosen a set of cases from an ill-defined, intractable study base but rather having the inability to identify and sample controls from that base. Given a set of cases, we ask whether the chosen controls accurately reflect the prevalence of exposure in the study base that generated them, regardless of how complex the definition of that study base may be. One of the primary reasons to conduct case–control studies is the rarity of disease, in that a full roster of cases plus a sample from the study base is more efficient than the consideration of the entire study base, as is done in cohort studies. Given the goal of including as many cases as possible for generating precise estimates, solutions such as the one proposed for referrals to prenatal care clinics that require omission of sizable numbers of cases are likely to be unattractive. Typically, all possible cases are sought, and the search is made for suitable controls.

The more idiosyncratic the control sampling method and the more it deviates from a formal, random sample from the study base, the more scrutiny it requires. Sometimes, we have a clearly defined, enumerated study base, as in case–control studies fully nested within a defined cohort. When cases of disease arise in a population enrolled in a health maintenance organization, there is often a data set that specifies when each individual joins and leaves the program. Those are precisely the individuals who would have been identified as cases if they had developed the condition of interest (aside from those persons who for some reason forego the benefits of the plan and seek their care elsewhere). Medical care coverage affords the opportunity to comprehensively define the population at risk and thus sample from it. One of the primary strengths of epidemiologic studies in health maintenance organizations is the availability of a roster of persons who receive care, and are thus clearly at risk of becoming identified as cases.

As we move away from clear, enumerated sampling frames, the problems of control selection become more severe. Even in studies conducted within a defined geographic area, there is the challenge of identifying all cases of disease that occur in the area. Doing so is easier for some conditions than for others. Several diseases are fully enumerated by registries in defined geographic areas, most notably cancer and birth defects. Vital records provide a complete roster of births, and thus certain associated birth outcomes, and deaths, including cause of death. For most conditions of interest, however, there is not a geographically based register in place. Chronic diseases such as diabetes, myocardial infarction, or osteoporosis require essentially developing one's own register to fully ascertain cases in a geographically defined population, tabulating information from all medical care providers, developing a systematic approach to defining cases, etc. Beyond the potential difficulties in identifying all cases from a given region in most countries, probability sampling from geographically defined populations is extremely difficult and becoming more difficult over time. As privacy restrictions increase, accessibility of such data sources as drivers' license rosters is becoming more limited. Furthermore, public wariness manifested by increased proportions of unlisted telephone numbers and use of telephone answering machines to screen calls has made telephone based sampling more fallible. At their best, the available tools such as random-digit dialing telephone sampling, neighborhood canvassing, or use of drivers' license rosters are far from perfect, even before contending with the problems of non-response that follow. Conceptually, a geographically defined study base is attractive, but it may not be so on logistical grounds.

Sampling from the study base that generates patients for a particular hospital or medical practice raises even more profound concerns. The case group is chosen for convenience and constitutes the benchmark for coherent control sampling, but the mechanisms for identifying and sampling from the study base are daunting. Without being able to fully articulate the subtleties of medical care access, preference, and care-seeking behavior, diseased controls are often chosen on the assumption that they experience precisely the same selection forces as the cases of interest. To argue that choosing patients hospitalized for non-malignant gastrointestinal disease, for example, constitutes a random sample from the population that produced the cases of osteoporotic hip fracture may be unpersuasive on both theoretical and empirical grounds. Such strategies are rarely built on careful logic and there is no way to evaluate directly whether they have succeeded or failed, even though by good fortune they may yield valid results. Their potential value would be enhanced if it could be demonstrated that the other diseases are not related to the exposure of interest and that the sources of cases are truly identical.

Selection in still more conceptually convoluted ways, such as friend controls, is also not amenable to direct assurance that they represent the appropriate study base. We need to ask whether friend controls would have been enrolled as cases in the study had they developed the condition of interest and whether they constitute a random sample of such persons. Viewed from a perspective of sampling, it is not obvious that such methods will yield a representative sample with respect to exposure. When the procedure seems like an odd way of sampling the study base, attention should be focused on the ultimate question of whether the controls are odd in the only way that actually matters—Do they reflect the exposure prevalence in the study base that produced the cases? That question is synonymous with "Is selection bias present?"

EVALUATION OF SELECTION BIAS IN CASE–CONTROL STUDIES

Temporal Coherence of Cases and Controls

A critical initial exercise is to enumerate, in conceptual terms, the specific requirements for enrollment as a case in the study versus the requirements for enrollment as a control. Some of the relevant attributes are easily and routinely considered, such as age range for eligibility and geographic scope of residence, but others may be more subtle and difficult to assess.

Calendar time is an often-neglected component in the definition of the study base, particularly when cases were diagnosed over some period of time in the past. Case registries for diseases such as cancer are a convenient resource for mounting case–control studies, but obtaining an adequate number of cases often necessitates including not just cases diagnosed subsequent to the initiation of the study, but also some who were diagnosed and registered in the past. Because the cases occurred over some period of historical calendar time, the study base from which controls are recruited should accommodate the temporal aspects of case eligibility if the exposure prevalence may change over time. At the extreme, if we had enrolled cases of colon cancer aged 45–74 diagnosed in metropolitan Atlanta, Georgia during 1992–1995, the roster of Atlanta residents aged 45–74 in 1990 or 1998 would not be coherent with the cases due to the changes that occurred in the dynamic cohort of residents. The questions must be asked, "Were all members of the study base eligible for control selection *at the time of case occurrence*, considering time-varying factors such as residence, age, and health status? Would the roster of potential controls available at the instant of case occurrence correspond to those from which controls were actually sampled?" In the ideal study, we would have enrolled cases as they occurred, in the period 1992–1995. As each case occurred, controls would be randomly sampled from the roster of the persons in the community. Note that the roster would be different in 1990, 1992, and 1995 due to changes in age, in- and out-migration, and death. Only if the prevalence of exposure is invariant, and thus the prevalence in 1990, 1992, 1995 and every year in between is the same, can we safely assess exposure among controls over a different period of time than for cases and thus employ a non-coherent study base.

Several studies addressing the potential association of elevated levels of magnetic fields from electric power lines in relation to childhood cancer selected controls, at least in part, some years after the cancer cases had been diagnosed (Savitz et al., 1988; London et al., 1991; Preston-Martin et al., 1996). Given the rarity of childhood leukemia or brain cancer, accrual of a sufficient number of cases through prospective monitoring of the population is challenging. This requires either conducting the study in a very large population from which cases arise, as was done in a study in large segments of the Midwest and eastern United States (Linet et al., 1997) and in the United Kingdom (United Kingdom Childhood Cancer Study Investigators, 1999), or by sustaining an active study to accrue cases over many years. It is much more efficient in time and expense to extend the case accrual period into the past using historical cancer registry data rather than solely into the future.

For example, in the study conducted in Denver, data collection began in 1984, yet cases diagnosed as early as 1976 were eligible (Savitz et al., 1988). Given a case that occurred several years before data collection for the study began, for example in 1976 or 1977, how do we properly select controls from the study base of the past that no longer exists?

Imagine the fate of the roster of eligible controls for a case occurring eight years before the start of the study. Over the intervening years, the population of the geographic area has changed, some otherwise eligible children have died, and those children of similar age as the case are now much older. Age is easily back-calculated to determine who, based on current age, would have been eligible at some point in the past. Past residence is a much more serious concern. Of all the potentially eligible controls at the time of case occurrence, a small number of children have died, but many may have moved out of the geographic area and many new children have probably moved into the geographic area. One source of ineligibility for control selection is rather easily addressed, namely whether the potential control resided in the study area at the time in the past when the case occurred. We can simply ask this present-day resident where they were living at the relevant time in the past. The otherwise eligible potential control who has left the geographic area, however, cannot readily be identified. We simply have no convenient way of tracking and including those who moved elsewhere but would have been eligible for sampling if we had been conducting our study at the optimal time in the past. Thus, our ideal roster of controls is inaccessible in the absence of true historical population registers, such as those that can be reconstructed in Sweden (Feychting & Ahlbom, 1993).

In the Denver study of magnetic fields and cancer, we chose to restrict the controls to those who resided in the area at the time of case diagnosis and continued to reside there at the time the study was initiated (Savitz et al., 1988; Savitz & Kaune, 1993a). There have been concerns raised over the consequences of our inability to fully sample from the study base and the resulting exclusion of residentially mobile controls (Jones et al., 1993). The magnitude of bias from this restriction is difficult to assess directly. A suggested solution to this problem is to restrict the cases comparably to those who remained residentially stable following their diagnosis. The logic of restricting on postdiagnosis experience, however, is questionable and it is quite possible that the reasons for moving would differ among families who suffered from having a child diagnosed with cancer compared to other families.

The optimal solution to the temporal incoherence of cases and controls is to eliminate it. If there were rosters from times in the past, we could effectively sample from the study base. As noted, records in Sweden allow reconstruction of neighborhoods as they were configured in the past. Records from schools, health care plans, birth records, town records, telephone directories, drivers' license rosters, or voter registration lists are examples of data resources that allow stepping back to the time of interest. Each has imperfections and potential sources of selection bias, and the challenge of locating persons who are identified through such historical rosters is apparent. Any archival information that allows for selection from the desired historical population roster is worthy of serious consideration. The only alternative is to mount studies in large enough populations to permit control selection to be concurrent with case diagnosis.

Selection bias from non-concurrent case and control selection can arise when trying to define a suitable sampling frame for cases whose disease began prior to the initiation of data collection for the study. Often, cases diagnosed in the past are combined with those newly diagnosed as the study progresses, leading to subsets of concurrent (for newly diagnosed cases) and non-concurrent (for past cases) controls. Even within the stratum of non-concurrent, the more remote in time, the more susceptible to selection bias, whatever the exact mechanism that produces it. Controls selected for marginally non-concurrent cases, e.g., those in the past year, are less susceptible to this bias than controls selected for cases diagnosed in the more remote past, e.g., five years ago. Critiques of studies of residential magnetic fields associated with power lines near homes and childhood leukemia had appropriately raised concerns about the influence of selection bias due to this phenomenon (Poole & Trichopoulos, 1991; Jones et al., 1993) in a study in Denver, Colorado (Savitz et al., 1988). Specifically, the study data collection began in 1983, with cases diagnosed over the period 1976–1983. The most direct test to address all conceivable problems of non-concurrence is to stratify cases by *degree* of non-concurrence using the year of diagnosis, i.e., 1976–1979 (more non-concurrent) and 1980–1983 (less non-concurrent), to assess the patterns of association in those groups. In this instance, the magnitude of association was stronger, not weaker, for the most recently diagnosed cases (Table 5.1), suggesting this form of selection bias was unlikely to have biased the odds ratio upwards (Savitz & Kaune, 1993b).

Consider Discretionary Health Care of Cases and Controls

In addition to experiencing the biological process of disease occurrence, in many studies the identified cases of disease either recognized a manifestation of the biological problem and sought treatment for it, or had incidental contact with the health care system that led to a diagnosis. In some instances, the investigators engage in systematic case-finding and eliminate the discretionary component of being diagnosed, but often the cases in case–control studies are identified through a health care provider. The questions to be asked for characterizing the study base, and thereby evaluating the suitability of controls, must include the implicit steps between developing the disease of interest and coming to be identified as a case in the study.

Identifying suitable hospital controls or ill controls for cases selected from a health care provider poses a particular challenge. The major motivation in selecting such ill controls is the convenience of access, often from the same source

TABLE 5.1. Sratum-Specific Results for High Wire Code Versus Low Wire Code: Denver, Colorado, 1976–1983, Interviewed Subjects

	Total Cancers		Leukemia		Brain Cancer	
PARAMETER	OR	CI	OR	CI	OR	CI
Age at diagnosis						
0–4 years	1.9	0.9–4.2	3.9	1.4–10.6	1.0	0.2–5.3
5–9 years	1.8	0.3–10.2	2.3	0.3–19.0	2.3	0.3–19.0
10–14 years	2.9	1.0–8.5	4.1	0.9–19.0	6.2	1.0–38.2
Gender						
Male	1.6	0.8–3.3	2.4	1.0–6.0	1.7	0.5–6.2
Female	3.3	1.2–9.1	7.0	1.9–26.3	2.4	0.5–11.2
Father's education						
< 16 years	1.8	0.9–3.8	4.2	1.6–11.1	2.3	0.8–7.0
≥ 6 years	2.3	0.8–6.2	2.5	0.7–8.9	—	
Per capita income						
< $7000/year	2.1	1.0–4.4	3.6	1.5–8.9	1.7	0.6–5.2
≥$7000/year	1.8	1.1–3.1	2.8	0.7–11.4	1.8	0.2–18.5
Year of diagnosis						
Before 1980	1.3	0.5–3.5	1.8	0.5–6.3	0.9	0.2–5.0
1980 or later	3.7	1.4–9.7	7.1	2.3–22.1	3.8	1.5–9.9
Residential stability						
Unstable	2.9	1.3–6.6	4.7	1.8–12.5	1.7	0.4–7.1
Stable	1.5	0.6–3.6	2.7	0.8–9.4	2.1	0.5–8.5
Residence type						
Single family	2.1	1.1–4.1	3.9	1.7–8.9	2.0	0.6–6.2
Other	2.0	0.4–11.2	2.8	0.3–28.3	1.4	0.1–13.6

OR, odds ratio; CI, confidence interval.
Savitz & Kaune, 1993.

as the cases. Another consideration is the tradeoff between potential selection bias (from choosing ill controls) and non-response (often a greater problem among controls selected from the community than from the hospital). Our focus here is on the concern with selection bias, with non-response addressed in detail in Chapter 6. Assume, for example, that a set of cases, e.g., women with osteoporotic hip fracture, have been identified at a large medical center and we are interested in determining whether there is an increased risk associated with low levels of calcium intake during adulthood. The hypothetical source of controls consists of those women who would, had they developed osteoporotic hip fracture, have come to the hospital at which case ascertainment is occurring. How do we operationally define this requirement that they "would go to that hospital" if they experienced a hip fracture?

First, we must focus on exactly how and why the cases ended up going to that particular hospital, beyond the fact of their health condition. Location of residence or workplace is often influential. If there are a small number of cases who came to that hospital for peculiar reasons, for example, they were visiting friends who live in the area when their hip fracture occurred, we may prefer to exclude them since the roster of such visitors would be virtually impossible to identify for control selection purposes. The identity of the woman's regular physician, or whether she even has a regular physician, may influence the specific hospital she would go to when hip fracture occurs. Financial aspects of their health care, such as insurance plan or Medicare/Medicaid eligibility, could influence the patient's likely source of care.

All the steps that resulted in the identification of these cases contribute to the definition of the study base, and therefore are elements to be considered in constituting the sampling frame for selection of controls. If the geographic coverage of the hospital is well defined, then only persons who reside in that area are part of the study base. In fact, if the medical care system were based solely on geography, then residence would unambiguously determine source of medical care. In the United States and many other settings, however, geography alone does not determine the health care provider. The choice of physician, insurance coverage, and physician and patient preferences are often relevant considerations in the selection of a hospital. If medical practices constituted the network for patient referral, then the study base would consist of patients seen within those practices, since they would have come to the study hospital in case of a hip fracture. If particular insurance plans direct patients to that hospital, then to be eligible as a control, the woman should be insured through such a plan. One reason that health maintenance organizations are particularly attractive for epidemiologic research, as noted above, is that the source population is unambiguously defined by enrollment in the plan. In the current, largely disorganized system of medical care in the United States, anticipating who would go to a given health care facility for a particular condition is a complex and only partially predictable process dependent on physician inclination, whether alternative facilities are available, finances, and subjective considerations of physician and patient preferences.

In light of this complexity, the traditional approach is to try to identify other health conditions that have a *comparable* source population (Miettinen, 1985), even without being able to articulate just what is required to be a member of that source population. Thus, we may speculate that women who come to the hospital for acute gastrointestinal conditions (gallstones, appendicitis) effectively represent a random sample from the study base, at least with respect to the exposure of interest. The conditions that define the source of controls must be unrelated to calcium intake, of course, for this strategy to be valid. Inability to operationally define the study base and thereby circumscribe the roster of potential controls constitutes a major disadvantage in evaluating the suitability of the chosen controls. Some degree of luck is required for the sampling mechanism of choosing persons with other diseases to yield an effectively random sample from the study base, and there is no direct way to determine if one has succeeded. It is clearly not a conceptually appropriate control group in terms of identifying and sampling from a well-defined roster, and will yield a valid measure of association only under the assumption that it nonetheless yields an accurate estimate of the prevalence of the exposure of interest in the study base.

Choosing controls based on having other, specific health conditions presumes that the exposure of interest has no direct or indirect positive or negative relation to the controls' diseases. The classic concern is that the exposures are as yet undiscovered risk factors for the control disease, as occurred in choosing patients with chronic bronchitis as controls in an early study of lung cancer and cigarette smoking (Doll & Hill, 1950). At that time, it was believed that smoking was unlikely to be related to bronchitis, so that choosing bronchitis patients would give a good estimate of smoking prevalence in the source population. Given the epidemiologists' well-founded belief that disease does not occur randomly, it is difficult to argue with confidence that a given exposure has no relation, direct or indirect, positive or negative, with a given disease. When we choose the presence of a disease as the basis for sampling controls, and the exposure of interest is related through any means, not necessarily causal, to the disease for which controls are sampled, the estimate of exposure prevalence in the study base will be distorted.

There are also more subtle ways in which persons with illness may have exposures that are not representative of those in the appropriate study base, especially when health behaviors or other aspects of lifestyle are involved. Continuing with the interest in calcium intake and osteoporotic hip fracture, assume the goal is to identify hospitalized patients whose past diet is representative of the study base of patients with hip fracture and we have chosen patients with benign gynecologic conditions. Assume that these hospitalized patients are truly members of the study base, i.e., if they had experienced a hip fracture, they would have become cases in the study. Thus, the only question is whether the sampling mechanism of other diseases is suitable.

First, diet is likely to have an etiologic relationship with a wide range of conditions, some of which have not yet been discovered. It is difficult to argue that *any* health condition is certain to be free of dietary influences. Second, early or preclinical illness is likely to alter diet subtly so that even in the absence of a causal relationship with the other diseases, reported diet may be distorted. Even when respondents are asked to report on diet at times in the more remote past, they tend to be influenced by recent diet (Wu et al., 1988), and may well report diet that has been altered by early or subclinical disease. Third, even if past diet were truly representative of the study base, the reporting of it may be affected by the presence of an unrelated illness. The psychological impact of the illness may well cause patients to misreport diet. (The point concerns information bias or misclassification rather than selection bias, and is discussed in more detail in Chapter 8.) An argument for the use of ill controls is that their reporting tendencies will be more comparable to the cases and thus yield more valid measures of association. The benefits of creating such offsetting biases are uncertain and difficult to evaluate empirically.

The proposed solutions to the problem of varying degree of medical surveillance can themselves introduce bias. In the 1970s and 1980s, there was a major controversy about the question of whether exogenous estrogen use caused endometrial cancer or simply brought existing cancers to diagnosis by producing vaginal bleeding, a symptom which led to medical care that in turn led to diagnosis. There was no question that an association was present, but its etiologic significance was debated intensely.

In order to address a concern with detection of such cancers, specifically whether the increased medical surveillance associated with receipt of estrogen therapy resulted in identification of otherwise subclinical disease, some investigators had proposed using as controls women who had undergone dilatation and curettage (D&C) (Horwitz & Feinstein, 1978). In that study, there was little association between estrogen use and endometrial cancer, in contrast to virtually all the previous studies. Hulka et al. (1980) conducted a case–control study in which they included alternate control groups to address specific hypothesized biases. Under the scenario that estrogen use increases bleeding and thereby brings latent cancer to light, an appropriate control group would consist of women who experienced bleeding for other reasons and thus were subjected to the same diagnostic scrutiny. Compared to results for more conventionally constituted hospital or community controls (Table 5.2), those controls who underwent D&C showed markedly reduced odds ratios. According to the proponents of the detection bias argument, these reduced measures of association reflect the benefit of removing bias due to enhanced surveillance among the estrogen users. In addition, the constitution of a control group based on having undergone a specific gynecologic procedure has compromised all other principles of control selection, namely the generation of a sample that represents the exposure prevalence in the study base that generated the cases. The proposed solution to examining a case group that reflects both a medical condition and health care that resulted in diagnosis was to generate a control group with an equally convoluted path to identification as a non-case. As demonstrated convincingly by Hulka et al. (1980) and others subsequently, the proposed solution generates an aberrantly reduced measure of association through inflating the prevalence of estrogen use among controls.

Compare Exposure Prevalence in Controls to an External Population

Analogous to the manner in which disease rates in the unexposed cohort may be compared to disease rates in external populations as one means of assessing

TABLE 5.2. Effect of Duration of Estrogen Use on Relative Risks, Using Three Control Groups Among White Women: Case-Control Study of Endometrial Cancer and Exogenous Estrogen, North Carolina, 1970–1976

DURATION OF USE	NO. OF CASES	D&C			Controls — Gynecology			Controls — Community		
		NO.	RR	95% CI	NO.	RR	95% CI	NO.	RR	95% CI
None used	125	136			118			172		
< 6 months	8	13	0.7	(0.3, 1.8)	12	0.7	(0.3, 1.8)	20	0.8	(0.3, 1.9)
6 months–< 3.5 years	9	14	0.7	(0.3, 1.7)	9	0.9	(0.3, 2.6)	21	0.7	(0.3, 1.6)
3.5 years–< 6.5 years	9	16	0.8	(0.3, 1.8)	1 ⎫	3.8	(1.2, 12.1)	7	1.7	(0.7, 4.7)
6.5 years–< 9.5 years	9	11	1.2	(0.5, 3.1)	2 ⎬			5	2.5	(0.8, 7.4)
≥ 9.5 years	19	10	2.0	(0.8, 4.7)	2	5.1	(1.4, 18.5)	4	5.5	(1.9, 16.2)
No data on duration	7	8			9					

*Age-adjusted with four age groups: < 50, 50–59, 60–69, and 70+ years.

D&C = dilatation and curettage; CI, confidence interval; RR, relative risk.

Hulka et al., 1980.

whether they fall within an expected range, with appropriate caution, exposure prevalence among controls can sometimes be beneficially compared to the exposure prevalence in external populations. Because typically we have less extensive information concerning exposure prevalence than disease patterns in external populations, however, the opportunity to apply this strategy in case–control studies is more limited than the corresponding approach in cohort studies.

Controls are selected in a case–control study to provide an estimate of exposure prevalence in the study base; for example, the proportion of women using estrogen replacement therapy or the proportion of men aged 50–59 who eats five or more servings of beef per week. If data from population surveys on prevalence of use of estrogen replacement therapy were available, for example, stratified as needed by age, social class, and other important influences on patterns of use, then a comparison could be made between exposure prevalence in the study controls and exposure prevalence in the general population. Data are most widely available for exposures of general interest, such as reproductive history, use of medications, tobacco and alcohol use, diet, and certain social and economic factors. Even when such data are available, however, the exact method of measuring and reporting them may differ from the methods used in the case–control study and thereby diminish the informativeness of the comparison. If perfectly suitable data were already available from an appropriate population, then there would be no need to identify and collect information from controls at all. At best, data from somewhat similar populations on roughly comparable exposures can yield comparisons with the study controls that can identify gross aberrations. If supplemental estrogen use from sociodemographically similar populations to those in the study ranges from 10% to 20%, and the controls in our study report 3% use or 53% use, we would have reason to look carefully at the manner in which the controls were chosen (as well as our methods for ascertaining supplemental estrogen use). If we measured exposure in the reported range or close to it, however, we would have some added confidence that the controls are more likely to be appropriately constituted and the exposure was properly assessed.

Continuing with the example of estrogen use and endometrial cancer introduced previously, Hulka et al. (1980) examined the question of whether selecting controls based on having had a D&C would produce an erroneous estimate of the prevalence of estrogen use in the population. They examined three control selection strategies, one consisting of community controls (the "gold standard" for this purpose), the second consisting of women with other gynecological conditions, and the third consisting of women who had undergone D&Cs. As anticipated, relative to the community controls, the D&C controls had an inflated prevalence of estrogen use, reflecting selection bias (Table 5.3). Approximately 35% of white women and 24% of African-American women had used estrogens in the D&C group as compared to 27% and 8% of white and African-American

TABLE 5.3. Percent of Cases and Controls Reporting Any Estrogen Use, by Race: Case-Control Study of Endometrial Cancer and Exogenous Estrogen, North Carolina, 1970–1976

	Cases			Controls								
				D&C			Gynecology			Community		
		Estrogen			Estrogen			Estrogen			Estrogen	
RACE	TOTAL NO.	NO.	%	TOTAL NO.	NO.	%	TOTAL NO.	NO.	%	TOTAL NO.	NO.	%
White	186	61	32.8	208	72	34.6	153	35	22.9	236	64	27.1
African-American	70	7	10.0	108	26	24.1	71	9	12.7	85	7	8.2

D&C, dilatation and curettage.

Hulka et al., 1980.

women, respectively, in the community controls. It appears that the distortion is especially pronounced for African-American women.

If comparisons of exposure prevalence are to be made between study controls and an external population, it will usually be necessary to make adjustments for known determinants of exposure. At a minimum, differences in such attributes as age, sex, race, and social class would have to be considered, as well as calendar time, if exposure prevalence has changed. For supplemental estrogens, there may well be differences related to geographic region, health care coverage, and reproductive history. The comparison is then made between the external population and the controls within strata that are more likely to show comparable exposure patterns, strengthening the value of the comparison. Some surveys such as the National Health and Nutrition Examination Survey and other large, national, probability samples conducted by the National Center for Health Statistics allow for isolation of subgroups most comparable to the study population of interest because of their size and diversity. To estimate supplemental estrogen use among Hispanic women aged 60–64 in the southwestern United States would be quite feasible, for example.

If the exposure prevalences are roughly similar between study controls and the external population, modest comfort may be taken that extreme selection bias is less likely to be present. If the observed prevalence in the study controls is grossly discrepant from that in the external population, one of two conclusions may be drawn. The study base may simply be substantially different from the sample that generated the external prevalence measure, and thus the disparity is not indicative of a problem within the study. There may be such profound regional and socioeconomic differences in exposure prevalence as to render national data uninformative, for example. The potential for large disparities needs to be evaluated using what is known about the determinants of exposure and interpreted according to the level of confidence that the external population should be similar to the study population. Powerful, but previously unrecognized, determinants of exposure may be present.

If there is no explanation for the disparity based on known determinants of exposure, then the constitution of the control group may be called into question and the argument for selection bias becomes more tenable. Information would need to be gathered on whether the controls appear to overstate or understate the exposure prevalence in the study base and on the amount of over- or underestimation that would therefore be expected in the measure of association. The exposure prevalence in the external population could be substituted for the exposure prevalence observed in the controls and odds ratios based on external and internal controls compared to characterize the importance of the disparity. In addition to selection bias, the potential for information bias would need to be entertained given that the methods by which exposure is ascertained could markedly influence the reported exposure level. In fact, the problems in ascertainment could come from either the controls in the study or from the external population survey to which they are compared. Like many "red flags," the disparity in exposure prevalence is a trouble sign but not a definitive indicator that trouble is present or just what has caused the trouble.

Determine Whether Exposure Prevalence Varies as Expected Among the Controls

An aberration in the manner in which controls are selected may manifest itself as an unusual pattern of exposure among subsets of controls if the faulty selection does not apply equally to all segments of the study base. Often we know from previous research that exposure prevalence varies by subgroup, e.g., men tend to drink more alcohol than women, White smokers tend to smoke more heavily than African-American smokers, leisure-time physical activity is greater among persons of higher socioeconomic status. If some erroneous method of selection has been applied that is similarly problematic for all subgroups of controls, defined by gender, race, age, etc., then the pattern of exposure prevalence across those markers of exposure may be as expected. If, however, the problems in selection are more extreme for some groups than others, or simply affect subgroups differentially, we will observe patterns of exposure comparing subsets of controls that deviate from those that would normally be expected.

To evaluate this possibility, the pattern of exposure among controls must be examined to determine whether it conforms to expectations based on external knowledge of patterns among subgroups. For this exercise to be helpful, there must be some basis for such expectations, ideally empirical evidence of exposure patterns from previous surveys. Even reasonably justified intuitive expectations may be helpful as a benchmark, however, recognizing that deviations between our expectations and the data may be a result of our intuition being incorrect. Health-related behaviors such as diet, alcohol and tobacco use, physical activity, and preventive health behaviors, are frequently considered in population surveys. The predictors of such attributes or behaviors often include social and demographic characteristics such as age, race, education, occupation, or location of residence. Confirming the presence of expected patterns among the controls lends support to the contention that the controls have been properly constituted, as well as some evidence that the exposure was accurately measured.

For example, if we chose controls for a study of physical activity and myocardial infarction among women through driver's license rosters, our sampling frame might be quite suitable for younger women, but could be increasingly ineffective with advancing age. As people age, and particularly as they age and become more physically impaired, they may be less inclined to maintain a drivers' license. If the older age groups were increasingly different from the source population in that age range, we might see an aberrant pattern in which physical activity levels did not decline with advancing age among the controls and perhaps even rose with advancing age. This would run counter to the expected patterns of declining physical activity with advancing age, suggesting that we had obtained a sample that was deviant among older age groups.

An empirical application of this strategy comes from a study of serum lycopene (an antioxidant form of carotenoid found in fruits and vegetables) in relation to the risk of prostate cancer (Vogt et al., 2002). A multicenter case–control study was conducted in the late 1980s in Atlanta, Detroit, and 10 counties in New Jersey. Controls were chosen through random-digit dialing for men under age 65 and through the Health Care Financing Administration records for men age 65 and older. Among a much larger pool of participants, 209 cases and 228 controls had blood specimens analyzed for lycopenes. Serum lycopene was inversely associated with risk of prostate cancer and found to be lower among African-American controls as compared to white controls (Table 5.4). To corroborate the plausibility of lower levels among African Americans (who experience a markedly higher risk of prostate cancer generally), the authors examined pertinent data from the National Health and Nutrition Examination Survey. In fact, there is strong confirmatory evidence that African Americans in the United States do have lower lycopene levels than whites across the age spectrum (Fig. 5.1). Other methodological concerns aside, this pattern provides evidence in support of having enrolled reasonably representative African-American and white men into the case–control study.

Internal comparisons could, of course, reveal the patterns that would be expected based on prior information, but still have stratum-specific and overall exposure prevalences that are disparate from that in the study base. If we recruited our controls for the study of physical activity and myocardial infarction by random digit dialing, and had a resulting preference for women who stayed at home across the age spectrum, we might well over-sample physically inactive women with some fraction of such women unable to maintain employment due to limited physical ability. The patterns by age might still be exactly as expected, but with a selectively inactive sample within each stratum and therefore a biased sample overall. Nonetheless, for at least some hypothesized mechanisms of selection bias, we would expect the extent of it to vary across strata of other exposure and disease predictors, and for those candidate pathways, examination of exposure prevalence across subgroups may be useful.

Examine Markers of Potential Selection Bias in Relation to Measures of Association

Based on the postulated mechanism for the occurrence of selection bias, predictions can be made regarding segments of the study base in which the problem would be more or less substantial, even if it pervades all groups to some degree.

TABLE 5.4. Median Serum Carotenoid Concentrations (10th–90th Percentile) for African-American Cases and Controls, and White Cases and Controls, from a U.S. Multicenter Case-Control Study of Prostate Cancer, 1986–1989

| | African-American | | | | Whites | | | |
| | Cases | | Controls | | Cases | | Controls | |
SERUM CAROTENOIDS ($\mu G/DL$)	MEDIAN	10TH–90TH PERCENTILE	MEDIAN	10TH–90TH PERCENTILE	MEDIAN	10TH–90TH PERCENTILE	MEDIAN	10TH–90TH PERCENTILE
α-Carotene	3.2	0.8–6.8	3.1	0.8–6.0	3.6	1.1–9.0	3.5	1.0–8.2
β-Carotene	17.6	6.0–40.8	16.5	6.6–36.8	15.6	5.8–37.9	13.8	5.1–32.8
β-Cryptoxanthin	7.7	3.5–19.1	7.5	3.9–16.0	6.8	3.5–15.7	6.6	3.0–14.5
Lutein/zeaxanthin	25.3	12.1–44.9	21.2	11.1–41.2	18.9	9.3–34.6	18.3	9.7–31.8
Lycopene	14.5	3.7–32.3	15.4	4.8–32.0	16.9	6.5–31.9	18.7	6.3–35.9
Total carotenoids	75.4	37.8–128.7	66.8	35.3–117.3	64.6	33.9–120.4	63.5	33.5–115.6

Vogt et al., 2002.

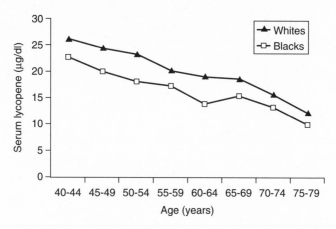

F<small>IGURE</small> 5.1. Median serum lycopene concentrations by age and race among males from the Third National Health and Nutrition Examination Survey, 1988–1994 (Vogt et al., 2002).

To address this possibility, we can evaluate measures of association between exposure and disease within strata that are expected to suffer from greater and lesser degrees of the selection bias.

In the earlier example in which controls for a study of physical activity and myocardial infarction were to be recruited from a drivers' license roster, we might expect that the sampling frame would be quite good for younger women, say under age 60, and become increasingly non-representative for older women. We may even have external data to indicate the proportion of women in each age stratum who have a driver's license. In the subset of the study population that is thought to be relatively free of selection bias, for example women under age 60, we would expect the odds ratio to be free from that source of bias. With higher and higher age strata, we would expect increasing amounts of selection bias to be present, so that the measures of association would be biased downward to increasing degrees (uncharacteristically active control women in the older age strata).

Referring to the Denver childhood cancer study examining magnetic field exposure (Savitz et al., 1988; Savitz & Kaune, 1993a), a major concern was with selection bias related to socioeconomic status. Despite reasonably consistent evidence from cancer registries that childhood leukemia is more common in higher social classes, nearly all case–control studies find the opposite pattern, i.e., higher risk in lower social classes. The presumed mechanism for this is underrepresentation of lower social class controls. Case response is generally better across the socioeconomic spectrum, whereas control response is thought to be poorer among persons of lower education and income. In order to examine the potential for such bias and to isolate the strata in which such bias is less severe, results were stratified by father's education and per capita income in the family (Table 5.1). The expected pattern of results would be to observe less bias in the upper education and income groups. In this case, there is some tendency for the measures of association to be less elevated among upper socioeconomic status participants overall, but subject to the imprecision in stratified analyses, the odds ratios are not markedly different across strata.

One of the challenges in interpreting the results of this aspect of potential selection bias is the inability to distinguish between measures of association that truly differ across subgroups (effect measure modification) and varying measures of association across strata that result from differential selection bias across strata. In the above examples, if physical activity truly had a different effect on risk of myocardial infarction among younger and older women, the exact same pattern might be seen as the one that would result from selection bias that affects younger and older women differently. Similarly, in the example of residential magnetic fields and childhood cancer, if there were some reason that the pattern of risk truly differed by socioeconomic status, the effect of selection bias could not be isolated from a genuine modification of the measure of association across strata of education or income. If there were changes in the prevalence of other conditions necessary for the causal process to operate or changes in the nature of the exposure across socioeconomic groups, the exact same pattern of results could be found. As is often the case, outside evidence and insights need to be applied in assessing the implications of apparent effect measure modification.

Adjust Measures of Association for Known Sources of Non-Comparability

When we can identify and measure the process by which selection bias is thought to operate, we can adjust for those determinants just as we adjust for confounders. Some forms of selection bias can be viewed as unintentional stratified sampling, exactly comparable to intentional stratified sampling as discussed earlier under Selection of Controls from the Study Base if the selection acts to sample randomly within the strata. Thus, if the method of sampling from the study base has generated an excess (or deficit) of men, or younger people, or those who reside in one county rather than another, we can readily stratify and adjust for those attributes in the analysis. The question then is whether there is selection bias *within* the strata, i.e., whether among young men sampled from a given county the exposure prevalence is reflective of young men in that county.

In the conventional application of sampling principles, the question of selection bias is equivalent to a question of whether the exposure prevalence is correctly estimated within strata. In the above example using a drivers' license registry to sample women for a case–control study of physical activity and myocardial infarction, the sampling is distinctly non-random across age strata.

Intentionally stratified sampling, as is done in frequency matching, uses algorithms for selection that are intended to generate unbiased samples within the strata. Whether the imbalance is intentional or unintentional, the strata in the chosen controls are not weighted as they are in the study base, and proper analyses must take this imbalance into account and make necessary adjustments by reweighting the strata. When we choose to sample unevenly across strata, we are careful about implementing a random algorithm and monitoring its effectiveness. In contrast, when we unintentionally sample unevenly across strata, there is no such planning and control, and thus biased sampling is more likely. Some amount of good fortune is required for the biased sampling to function as an effective mechanism of stratified sampling. To the extent that the selection bias is even partially acting like stratified sampling, however, confounding by the stratification factors may be introduced, and removed at least partially through adjustment (Rothman, 1986).

Consider a case–control study of the role of cocaine use in relation to migraine headache, built on a case register from a regional referral hospital that specializes in the treatment of migraine headaches. If we select controls by random-digit dialing from the same geographic area as the cases, we will have to contend with the potential biases arising from differential tendency to seek medical care and particularly, medical care from this institution. Socioeconomic status is likely to be one such influence on the opportunity and ability to access care at this referral center, so that we recognize and accept that there will not be a natural balance between the social class distribution of selected controls and the true (but unknown) study base for these cases seen at this health care facility. Furthermore, social class is one predictor of cocaine use, with greater prevalence among lower social class persons. Adjusting for socioeconomic status will be beneficial to the extent that this one source of non-comparability, imbalance across social class, is ameliorated. In order for the adjustment to be fully effective, the prevalence of cocaine use among selected controls within social class strata would have to accurately reflect the prevalence of cocaine use in that segment of the study base.

The extent to which a community sample selected by random digit dialing differs from the results of a privately conducted census was examined empirically for Otsego County in New York State (Olson et al., 1992). Given that so many case–control studies rely on random digit dialing as a method of control selection, any systematic tendency to overrepresent some groups and underrepresent others introduces potential bias and suggests that adjustment be made for markers of participation. Overall, the sample selected by random digit dialing and the census yielded very similar distributions. There was a tendency however, for the random digit dialing controls to have participated to a greater extent in certain medical screening tests (Table 5.5), suggesting greater health consciousness or more access to health care. If we were conducting a case–control study of post-

Table 5.5. Distribution of Sample Chosen by Random Digit Dialing and Census Population Aged 40–74 Years According to Whether Respondents Had Certain Screening Tests, Otsego County, New York, 1989

SCREENING TEST	Random Digit Dialing Sample		Census Population	
	NO.	%	NO.	%
Had blood pressure checked in past 2 years				
Yes	306	89.7	13,403	86.1
No	30	8.8	1503	9.7
No response	5	1.5	657	4.2
Total	341	100.0	15,563	100.0
Had cholesterol checked in past 2 years*				
Yes	230	67.4	8699	55.9
No	102	29.9	5855	37.6
No response	9	2.6	1009	6.5
Total	341	99.9	15,563	100.0
Ever had stool test or rectal examination for colon cancer				
Yes	174	51.0	7215	46.4
No	155	45.5	7238	46.5
No response	12	3.5	1110	7.1
Total	341	100.0	15,563	100.0
Among women only				
Ever had Papanicolaou test for cervical cancer				
Yes	157	89.2	6890	84.9
No	15	8.5	738	9.1
No response	4	2.3	492	6.1
Total	176	100.0	8120	100.1
Ever had mammogram for breast cancer				
Yes	110	62.5	4475	55.1
No	61	34.7	3104	38.2
No response	5	28	541	6.7
Total	176	100.0	8120	100.0

[a] $\chi^2 = 12.72$, df $= 1$; $p < 0.001$ (based on those responding).

menopausal estrogen use and osteoporosis, there might be no causal relation between screening history and that outcome. If there were an association between screening and use of estrogens, however, which is plausible, then the distortion due to random digit dialing would require adjustment in the analysis. The control sampling mechanism would have generated an association with disease status because of the overrepresentation of women who tend to have more health screening (and may well have a higher prevalence of estrogen use as well).

The impact of factors that cannot be captured directly or completely can still be addressed to some extent. We rarely have a measure of the precise indicator of the source of selection bias, e.g., proclivity to seek medical care or health consciousness or willingness to participate in telephone surveys. We may have markers however, that are at least associated to some extent with those attributes, for example, insurance coverage, frequency of routine physical examinations, and level of education. In the same manner that adjustment for an imperfectly measured confounder adjusts only partially, adjustment for these imperfect markers would adjust partially for the selection bias. Not only might adjustment for such factors yield a less biased measure of association, but the comparison of unadjusted and adjusted measures of association would help to determine the direction of bias and estimate how large the residual effect is likely to be, analogous to the examination of residual confounding (Savitz & Barón, 1992). If adjustment for the proxy indicator shifted the measure of association in a given direction, then we can safely expect that a refined measure of that attribute would have shifted the measure of association even further in the same direction, and if adjusting for the marker has a large impact on the measure of association, more complete adjustment is likely to move the estimate farther still.

Confirm Known Exposure–Disease Associations

A direct approach to examining not just the suitability of controls but rather the coherence between cases and controls is to determine whether known or strongly suspected exposure–disease associations are corroborated in a given study. Typically, case–control studies include information on a spectrum of potential risk factors, and known influences on disease are incorporated as potential confounders of the association(s) of primary interest in the study. To the extent that some of these are firmly established, there is potential value in conducting preliminary analyses to determine whether we can confirm the obvious. When we do so, there is some assurance that our subject selection mechanisms have not gone seriously awry. When we fail to confirm known associations, the question must be raised more seriously as to whether (and how) our study methods may have generated deviant study groups.

For example, in a Swedish study of the role of dietary retinol intake on risk of hip fracture, Melhus et al. (1998) were addressing a relatively unexplored issue so that their results for the primary hypothesis could not be used to demonstrate the efficacy of their approach to the research. There are a number of well-established risk factors for hip fracture however, that could be considered for this purpose. Before focusing on dietary retinol, the pattern of other known risk factors was characterized by analyzing the 247 hip fracture cases and 873 controls (Table 5.6). Well-established associations with lean body mass index, physical

TABLE 5.6. Odds Ratios for Covariates in the Hip Fracture Study, Swedish Mammography Cohort, 1987–1995

VARIABLE	CASE–PATIENTS	CONTROLS	ODDS RATIO (95% CI)
	n		
Body mass index			
< 23.0 kg/m^2	93	206	1.0 (reference)
23.0–25.2 kg/m^2	50	206	0.44 (0.28–0.69)
25.3–27.9 kg/m^2	50	210	0.49 (0.31–0.78)
> 27.9 kg/m^2	39	207	0.37 (0.23–0.61)
Daily energy intake			
< 1183 kcal	56	218	1.0 (reference)
1183–1437 kcal	69	219	1.49 (0.96–2.29)
1438–1695 kcal	54	218	1.20 (0.76–1.91)
> 1695 kcal	68	219	1.27 (0.82–1.98)
Physical activity			
Quartile 1 (lowest activity)	76	185	1.0 (reference)
Quartile 2	57	151	1.05 (0.66–1.67)
Quartile 3	68	324	0.58 (0.38–0.88)
Quartile 4 (highest activity)	40	175	0.59 (0.36–0.97)
Former athletic activity			
Never	233	845	1.0 (reference)
Ever	14	29	1.60 (0.72–3.55)
Menopausal age			
< 49 years	77	268	1.0 (reference)
49–50 years	107	305	1.35 (0.92–1.99)
51–52 years	26	129	0.71 (0.41–1.21)
> 52 years	37	172	0.78 (0.48–1.27)
Menopausal status			
Premenopausal	29	124	1.0 (reference)
Postmenopausal	218	750	1.10 (0.66–1.81)
Smoking status			
Never smoker	161	653	1.0 (reference)
Former smoker	42	128	1.40 (0.90–2.18)
Current smoker	44	93	1.87 (1.18–2.98)

(continued)

TABLE 5.6. Odds Ratios for Covariates in the Hip Fracture Study, Swedish Mammography Cohort, 1987–1995 (*continued*)

VARIABLE	CASE–PATIENTS	CONTROLS	ODDS RATIO (95% CI)
	n		
Hormone replacement therapy			
Never user	229	741	1.0 (reference)
Former user	15	80	0.58 (0.32–1.08)
Current user	3	53	0.11 (0.02–0.49)
Oral contraceptives			
Never user	232	812	1.0 (reference)
Ever user	15	62	0.73 (0.35–1.56)
Oral cortisone			
Never user	227	815	1.0 (reference)
Ever user	17	53	1.18 (0.65–2.14)
Diabetes mellitus			
No diabetes	219	835	1.0 (reference)
Oral treatment of diabetes	17	30	2.45 (1.24–4.86)
Insulin treatment of diabetes	11	9	5.10 (1.87–13.9)
Previous osteoporotic fracture			
Never	165	709	1.0 (reference)
Ever	82	165	2.29 (1.61–3.25)

CI, confidence interval.
Melhus et al., 1998.

inactivity, and use of hormone replacement therapy were verified, providing a general indication that the selection of subjects was successful and thereby increasing confidence that the patterns of association for uncertain risk factors is more likely to be valid as well.

Conventional wisdom can be incorrect, of course, with supposedly known associations subject to error in previous studies. Furthermore, the prevalence of important cofactors may vary across populations, so that an exposure that operates as a risk factor in one population may truly not operate in that manner in another. As discussed above, the potential for selection bias will vary across risk factors, with a given study able to generate valid measures of association for one exposure yet incapable of doing so for others. Even if valid for confirming known associations, the study may not be valid for addressing the association of primary interest. Finally, there is the ever-present random error to consider, a particular concern in attempting to corroborate well-accepted associations that are modest in magnitude. Failure to confirm an association between a history of heavy cigarette smoking and lung cancer would raise serious doubts about the validity of other measures of association with lung cancer identified in a case–control study, whereas many of the established risk factors for diseases such as breast cancer are so modest in magnitude that random error alone could well yield a spurious absence of measurable association. For example, although a positive association between alcohol intake and breast cancer is generally accepted (Longnecker, 1994), the magnitude is modest. Thus, studies that fail to find it, a non-trivial proportion of all studies (Singletary & Gapstur, 2001), are not by any means rendered invalid as a result. Like the other strategies, the examination of known and strongly suspected associations helps to direct the effort to scrutinize potential selection bias without providing conclusions in isolation from other considerations.

INTEGRATED ASSESSMENT OF POTENTIAL FOR SELECTION BIAS IN CASE–CONTROL STUDIES

The initial step in evaluation of selection bias is to articulate in very specific terms what is required for the cases to be enrolled as cases in the study. The eligibility criteria start with the structural requirements based on age, gender, and geography, but often go well beyond these attributes to include medical care determinants, behaviors, and even attitudes. With the cases well defined, the study base will also be conceptually well defined as the population experience that generated those cases. Such a conceptual understanding however, is only one step toward translation into a sampling frame for the controls. Without undue worry regarding feasibility, initially at least, the study base should be fully described.

   The chosen controls need to be evaluated against the ideal controls, a random sample from the study base that generated the cases. Now, we must contend with the practical constraints that interfere with identifying and sampling the study base. We encounter unmeasurable notions of what individuals would have done had they developed the disease and inaccessible members of the study base that should have been included in the ideal sampling frame. Errors of inclusion, in which controls were selected who were not part of the study base, and errors of exclusion, in which segments of the study base were not represented, should be described, ideally in quantitative terms: What is the nature and magnitude of deviation from the ideal? Can we exclude those who are truly not members of the study base? Can we estimate the number and likely effect of excluding those who should have been included but could not be?

   This evaluation needs to occur with a focus on a particular exposure, including the nature of the exposure, how it is distributed in the population, and what

impact imperfect selection mechanisms are likely to have on estimating its prevalence. Consideration of the deviations from the ideal method of sampling from
the study base should focus on the impact on exposure prevalence. Are the erroneously included or excluded segments of the study base likely to have an exposure prevalence that differs from the properly constituted study base? If so, in
which direction and by how much?

Evaluation of control selection strategies that are not closely linked to a defined study base, such as selection of hospital controls, must go directly to the
evaluation of whether the exposure prevalence that has been generated is likely
to be similar to that which would have been obtained by sampling the appropriately defined study base. In other words, the mechanism of control selection is
so far removed from sampling the study base that we can only consider whether
it is likely to have yielded a valid result, not whether the mechanism was a good
one. A distinct disadvantage of such an approach is the difficulty in addressing
this question with empirical evidence.

Sometimes, the prevalence of exposure can be compared to suitable external
populations to determine whether the chosen controls are roughly similar to others who have been appropriately constituted and measured. The pattern of exposure distribution among the controls may be compared to known or expected
patterns to determine whether there is likely to have been a differential selection
bias among the controls. If there are segments of the study base that are likely
to have been sampled more effectively than others, measures of association should
be generated with stratification on those potential markers of the degree of selection bias. The more valid result comes from the stratum in which selection
bias is least likely to have occurred. The influence of adjustment for markers,
both direct and indirect, of selection bias should be evaluated to determine the
direction and amount of influence of adjustment. Where there is an imperfect
proxy measure of the basis for selection bias rather than the exact measure of interest, the influence of the unmeasured factor on the results should be estimated
and the bias controlled in the same manner as confounding. The ability to repli-
cate known and strongly suspected exposure–disease associations should be attempted and failures to do so considered in more detail. All these tools are suitable for control selection mechanisms that attempt to choose directly from the
study base as well as for those mechanisms that do not. The more that the method
of control selection deviates from sampling the study base, however, the greater
the need for evidence that the result is valid.

Whereas a perfectly coherent set of controls for a given set of cases assures
freedom from selection bias, a non-coherent control group does not guarantee
that bias will occur. That depends entirely on the exposure of interest and whether
that exposure is related to the source of the lack of coherence. In the example
regarding residential mobility and magnetic field exposure from power lines,
there would be no selection bias if residential mobility were not associated with

nearby electrical wiring and residential magnetic fields. If the source of non-coherence were unrelated to the exposure, then restricting the sampling to those potential controls who did not change residences over the period between case diagnosis and study conduct would introduce no bias. Sampling in an unbalanced way from those who are residentially stable relative to those who are residentially mobile is only a problem if residential mobility is related to the exposure of interest. A group that is not coherent based on having omitted residentially unstable members could still generate the correct estimate of exposure prevalence in the study base and thus the correct measure of association. Using as a benchmark the ideal source of controls, critical evaluation must focus on the extent to which the less than ideal control group has generated a valid result. The question that must be asked is whether omitting parts of the study base or including experience outside the study base has distorted the estimate of exposure prevalence.

REFERENCES

Doll R, Hill AB. Smoking and carcinoma of the lung: preliminary report. Br Med J 1950;739–748.

Feychting M, Ahlbom A. Magnetic fields and cancer in children residing near Swedish high-voltage power lines. Am J Epidemiol 1993;138:467–481.

Horwitz RI, Feinstein AR. Alternative analytic methods for case-control studies of estrogens and endometrial cancer. N Engl J Med 1978;299:1089–1094.

Hulka BS, Grimson RC, Greenberg RG, Kaufman DG, Fowler WC Jr, Hogue CJR, Berger GS, Pulliam CC. "Alternative" controls in a case-control study of endometrial cancer and exogenous estrogen. Am J Epidemiol 1980;112:376–387.

Jones TL, Shigh CH, Thurston DH, Ware BJ, Cole P. Selection bias from differential residential mobility as an explanation for associations of wire codes with childhood cancer. J Clin Epidemiol 1993;46:545–548.

Linet MS, Hatch EE, Kleinerman RA, Robison LL, Kaune WT, Friedman DR, Severson RK, Haines CM, Hartsock CT, Niwa S, Wacholder S, Tarone RE. Residential exposure to magnetic fields and acute lymphoblastic leukemia in children. N Engl J Med 1997;337:1–7.

London SJ, Thomas DC, Bowman JD, Sobel E, Cheng T-C, Peters JM. Exposure to residential electric and magnetic fields and risk of childhood leukemia. Am J Epidemiol 1991;134:923–937.

Longnecker M. Alcoholic beverage consumption in relation to risk of breast cancer: meta-analysis and review. Cancer Causes Control 1994;5:73–82.

Melhus H, Michaelsson K, Kindmark A, Bergström R, Holmberg L, Mallmin H, Wolk A, Ljunghall S. Excessive dietary intake of Vitamin A is associated with reduced bone mineral density and increased risk for hip fracture. Ann Intern Med 1998;129:770–778.

Miettinen OS, The "case-control" study: valid selection of subjects. J Chron Dis 1985;38:543–548.

Olson SH, Kelsey JL, Pearson TA, Levin B. Evaluation of random digit dialing as a method of control selection in case-control studies. Am J Epidemiol 1992;135:210–222.

Poole C, Trichopoulos D. Extremely-low frequency electric and magnetic fields and cancer. Cancer Causes Control 1991;2:267–276.

Preston-Martin S, Navidi W, Thomas D, Lee P-J, Bowman J, Pogoda J. Los Angeles study of residential magnetic fields and childhood brain tumors. Am J Epidemiol 1996;143: 105–119.

Rothman KJ. Modern Epidemiology. Boston: Little, Brown and Co., 1986.

Savitz DA, Barón AE. Estimating and correcting for confounder misclassification. Am J Epidemiol 1989;129:1062–1071.

Savitz DA, Kaune WT. Childhood cancer in relation to a modified residential wire code. Environ Health Perspect 1993a;101:76–80.

Savitz DA, Kaune WT. Response: potential bias in Denver childhood cancer study. Environ Health Perspect 1993b;101:369–370.

Savitz DA, Pearce NE. Control selection with incomplete case ascertainment. Am J Epidemiol 1988;127:1109–1117.

Savitz DA, Wachtel H, Barnes FA, John EM, Tvrdik JG. Case-control study of childhood cancer and exposure to 60-Hz magnetic fields. Am J Epidemiol 1988;128:21–38.

Singletary KW, Gapstur SM. Alcohol and breast cancer. Review of epidemiologic and experimental evidence and potential mechanisms. JAMA 2001;286:2143–2151.

United Kingdom Childhood Cancer Study Investigators. Exposure to power-frequency magnetic fields and the risk of childhood cancer. Lancet 1999;354:1925–1931.

Vogt TM, Mayne ST, Graubard BI, Swanson CA, Sowell AL, Schoenberg JB, Swanson GM, Greenberg RS, Hoover RN, Hayes RB, Ziegler RG. Serum lycopene, other serum carotenoids, and risk of prostate cancer in US Blacks and Whites. Am J Epidemiol 2002; 155:1023–1032.

Wu ML, Whittemore AS, Jung DL. Error in reported dietary intakes. II. Long-term recall. Am J Epidemiol 1988;128:137–145.

6

BIAS DUE TO LOSS OF STUDY PARTICIPANTS

CONCEPTUAL FRAMEWORK FOR EXAMINING BIAS DUE TO LOSS OF STUDY PARTICIPANTS

The previous chapters addressed the mechanism by which subjects were selected and the distinctive biases that may result from the methods of selection in cohort and case–control studies. The focus in those chapters was on the manner in which the groups were constituted, and whether, if implemented as designed, the selection process would yield a valid measure of association. With a poor choice for the non-exposed group in a cohort study, even flawless execution of that selection method would yield biased results. Similarly, if the control group defined for a case–control study fails to reflect the prevalence of the exposure of interest in the study base, then selection bias is present regardless of how successfully we identify and recruit subjects from that poorly chosen sampling frame. The concern in previous chapters was in the *definition* of the study groups, not in the *implementation* of the selection method. In this chapter, we focus on the potential for bias that arises in the implementation of the selection process, focusing on the problems resulting from the inability of researchers to enroll and follow the individuals who were chosen for the study. Even with a perfectly valid plan that meets all the conceptual goals for a valid study, systematic loss from the defined study groups is such a common source of bias that it warrants extended discussion.

Many of these problems with attrition are unique to studying free-living human populations. Controlled laboratory experiments do not have to contend with rodents moving and leaving no forwarding address, or bacteria that refuse to permit the investigator to impose the potentially noxious exposure. If the organism and experimental conditions are properly chosen and implemented, with the investigator in complete control, there is little room for the selective loss of subjects to yield an erroneous result. On occasion, an outbreak of infection will disrupt laboratory experiments or failures to follow the protocol will occur due to human or machine error. However, the experimental control of the investigator is rather complete.

Contrast that tight experimental control with the typical situation in observational epidemiology and to a large extent, in experimental studies in human populations. The investigator designates a study group of interest, for example, all men diagnosed with ulcerative colitis in a given geographic area or a randomly selected sample of children who receive medical care through a health maintenance organization. Even with the good fortune of starting with complete rosters of eligible participants, a rare situation in practice, there are multiple opportunities for losses in going from those desired to those who actually contribute data to the final analysis. The disparity between the persons of interest and those who are successfully enrolled in the study and provide the desired data poses a significant threat to validity.

Complete documentation of study methods in epidemiology includes a complete and honest accounting of eligible subjects and the numbers lost for various reasons, culminating in the tally of those who were included in the final analyses. This accounting is vital to quantifying the potential for biased results through evaluation of the disparity between those sought for the study and those actually in the study. Multiple processes contribute to those losses, with the reason for the losses critical to evaluating the potential impact on the validity of the study results. These losses are not failings of the investigators or research staff, but an inherent and undesirable feature of studying human populations.

All other considerations equal, the smaller the volume of loss, the less susceptible the study is to erroneous results of a given magnitude. Also, the more random the losses are, the less damage they do to the validity of results. A perfectly random pattern of loss only reduces precision and can, if the sampling frame is large enough, be compensated by increasing the sampling fraction. For example, if a computer error deleted every tenth subject from a randomly ordered list, there would be no impact on validity, and increasing the sampling fraction by 10% would result in no loss in precision either. In sharp contrast, loss of 10% of eligible subjects because they could not be contacted by telephone is a distinctly non-random process, not compensated by increasing the sampling fraction by 10%.

The key question is whether those who remain in the study after losses are systematically different in their key attributes (risk of disease in cohort studies, prevalence of exposure in case–control studies) compared to those in the initial sampling frame. Some mechanisms of loss are likely to be very close to random. For example, in studies that recruit from patients in a clinic setting, sometimes there are insufficient resources to recruit during all clinic hours so that otherwise eligible patients are lost because of lack of staff coverage at particular times of day or certain days of the week. Even for such ostensibly random sources of loss, however, questions may be raised about whether subjects who come to a clinic at inconvenient times (weekends, nights) are different than those who come at times that staff are more readily available (weekdays).

In a recent study in which pregnant women were recruited in a prenatal care setting, those lost due to missed opportunity to recruit were somewhat different than women who were contacted, more often young and less educated (Savitz et al., 1999). We hypothesized that one of the reasons for our inability to contact women in the clinic was that they had changed names or rescheduled visits on short notice, events quite plausibly related (though indirectly) to risk of adverse pregnancy outcome as a result of a less favorable demographic profile. In fact, those women who we were unable to contact in the clinic had a slightly higher risk of preterm birth as compared to women we could speak to and attempt to recruit for the study.

Mechanisms of loss that are based on the decisions or lifestyle of potential participants, such as refusal, absence of access to a telephone, screening calls with an answering machine, not being home during the day, or changing residences are more obviously non-random in ways that could well affect the study's result. Socioeconomic and demographic characteristics, behavioral tendencies, exposures of interest, and disease risk are often intertwined. This same complex set of factors is likely to extend to the determinants of the ability to be located, the inclination to agree to be enrolled, and the decision to drop out once enrolled. With a little imagination, the many correlates of "difficult to contact" or "unwilling to contribute time to research" make such losses non-random with regard to the exposures and health outcomes of interest to epidemiologists.

Table 6.1 illustrates some of the processes by which subjects may be lost across the phases of a study, and suggests some of the underlying mechanisms that may be operative. Not all of these phases apply to every study, nor is the list exhaustive. Limited data are available to empirically assess which reasons for losses are more tolerable, i.e., closer to random losses, than others. Even when data on the nature of such losses are available from other studies, the patterns of reasons for loss and the implications for study validity are likely to vary across populations, time periods, and for different exposures and diseases of interest, making it difficult to generalize. These processes are in large part cultural, sociological, and psychological, so that universal predictors that apply to all humans are un-

TABLE **6.1.** Mechanisms of Subject Loss and Potential Implications

Insufficient staff coverage in clinical setting

• Employment affects timing of medical care
• Social support or economic resources affects timing of medical care

Physician refusal of access to subject

• Perceived vulnerability of patient
• Perceived hostility (lawsuit potential) of patient
• Physician attitude toward patient autonomy

Unable to locate subject

• Limited economic resources leaves few leads (credit bureau, employer, telephone)
• Extensive economic resources permit privacy (unlisted numbers, answering machines, isolation from neighbors)
• Greater geographic mobility due to desire to move, economic need, or job opportunities

Subject refusal

• Hostility towards research based on bad experience or limited understanding
• Poor health precludes provision of data
• Protective of privacy due to engagement in embarrassing or illegal behaviors
• Overburdened with work or family responsibilities and thus lacking in time
• Self-confidence to refuse requests from authorities

Missing data

• Refusal to provide information that is unusual, embarrassing, or illegal
• Exhaustion due to poor health that precludes completion of survey
• Poor communication skills or low educational attainment

likely to exist. Nonetheless, repeated documentation of the magnitude and pattern of losses is extremely helpful to investigators who plan and evaluate studies. Decisions must be made regarding where to target resources and informed decisions are needed for allocating those resources optimally. If losses due to changing residence are typically more or less important as a potential source of bias than losses due to respondent refusal, then our energy (and funds) for conducting a study and scrutinizing its results can be allocated accordingly.

The ultimate impact of the losses is a function of the magnitude of loss and how aberrant those lost are with regard to their health or exposure status. Although we focus here on losses and the reasons for loss, the study will actually be analyzing those *not* lost. The concern with potential for bias focuses on how those available compare to the full complement of those of interest. Obviously, if those lost are notably deviant, those available will differ from the original pool of participants. The quantitatively greatest sources of loss tend to be the most worthy of attention in assessing the potential for bias. Most often, participant refusal is the dominant reason for loss, and its familiarity and inevitability should not be misinterpreted as an indication that it is benign. The magnitude of deviation between those lost and those enrolled is ideally evaluated empirically, but since this requires information that is often unavailable, indirect evidence may be brought to bear on the issue. After enumerating and quantifying the many sources of loss, priorities can be defined regarding which problems deserve scrutiny, validation substudies, or sensitivity analyses.

Like other forms of selection bias, if the losses are related to measured attributes, like age and educational level, but random within strata of those attributes, then adjustment for the measured factors will eliminate bias just as it eliminates confounding. That is, if refusals are more common among less educated eligible subjects, but random within strata defined by education, then after adjustment for education, the bias due to non-participation will be reduced. Questions must be asked regarding whether the measured attributes (e.g., educational level) adequately approximate the attributes of ultimate interest (e.g., proclivity to participate in studies) in order to fully adjust for the potential bias. Even though adjustment can ameliorate the bias, it is very unlikely to fully eliminate it.

The specific exposures and diseases under investigation must be scrutinized carefully in order to assess the potential for bias. The abstract question of whether those available in the analysis are or are not representative of the desired study population has little meaning without consideration of the particular characteristics of concern. The guiding question is whether the omission of some eligible participants affects the disease rate in a cohort study or the exposure prevalence in a case–control study. In studying a disease that is closely associated with a number of health behaviors, such as lung cancer or coronary heart disease, subjects lost due to refusal to participate are likely to introduce distortion due to deviant smoking and dietary habits, for example, relative to those who enroll. It has been found repeatedly across diverse modes of data collection that smokers tend to refuse study participation more frequently than do nonsmokers (Criqui et al., 1978; Macera et al., 1990; Psaty et al., 1994). In contrast, for diseases less closely related to such behaviors, e.g., prostate cancer, the distortion due to refusals may well be less, or perhaps we simply lack sufficient information at present to make an informed judgment for such diseases. Analogously, when assessing the impact of losses due to physician refusal to permit patient contact in a case–control study, we might have little concern if the exposure of interest were a genetic variant, not likely to be directly related to physician judgment, whereas if the exposure were the level of psychological stress, physician refusals could have disastrous consequences if the cases perceived to have the highest stress levels were systematically eliminated.

Several years ago, the patterns of loss that would and would not produce bias were clearly specified (Greenland, 1977; Greenland & Criqui, 1981). In a cohort study, loss of subjects from the exposed and unexposed groups that are not differential by disease status do not result in bias, even if losses are unequal for the exposed and unexposed groups. Furthermore, even losses that are selective for persons with (or without) the disease of interest do not introduce bias in ratio measures of association, so long as those disease-selective losses are quantitatively the same in the exposed and unexposed groups. In case–control studies, losses that distort the exposure prevalence among cases and controls are tolerable so long as the losses are comparably selective for the two groups. Even if exposed (or unexposed) subjects are preferentially lost, so long as the magnitude of that preferential loss is comparable in cases and controls, bias in the odds ratio will not result.

Only when the losses are differential by exposure *and* disease status is there selection bias. That is, in cohort studies, the key question is whether there is a preferential loss of diseased subjects that differs for the exposed and unexposed. If each group loses 10% of diseased and 5% of non-diseased, there is no bias, but if the exposed lose 10% of diseased and 10% of non-diseased and the unexposed lose 5% of diseased and 10% of non-diseased, bias will result. Similarly, if losses of subjects from a case–control study are related to exposure and of different magnitude for cases and controls, for example, 10% of exposed subjects and 10% of non-exposed subjects are lost from the control group whereas 5% of exposed subjects and 10% of non-exposed subjects are lost from the cases. The harmful pattern can be summarized as occurring when response status acts as an effect–modifier of the exposure–disease association. Under such circumstances, the magnitude of the exposure–disease relation differs among those who participate in the study and those who do not.

EVALUATION OF BIAS DUE TO LOSS OF STUDY PARTICIPANTS

The ultimate solution to the problem of response bias is to eliminate it altogether or at least minimize the magnitude of non-response from all sources. Before discussing the approaches to assessing or minimizing the impact of non-response, the compelling preference for addressing it directly through increasing response should be noted. Non-response can rarely be avoided entirely, but efforts to reduce it deserve great attention in study design and implementation. All other approaches to evaluating its impact or attempting to make corrections are indirect and subject to substantial uncertainty. Given that non-response is inevitable, however, careful examination of the magnitude and patterns can be helpful in indicating how much bias is likely to be present and the direction of that bias.

Characterize Nonparticipants

A straightforward approach to assessing the potential impact of non-response on measures of association is to characterize a sample of nonrespondents with regard to key attributes of exposure and disease, as well as other important predictors of disease. A sample of subjects lost for each major reason (refused, not traceable, etc.) is subjected to the intense effort required to obtain the desired information, anticipating at least partial success in obtaining information on some of the potential participants who had been initially considered lost. This approach is predicated on the assumption that there is a gradation of effort that can be expended to obtain participation and a corresponding gradation of difficulty in recruiting potential respondents. Every study balances available resources with the expected yield, and some limit must be placed on the amount of effort that can be devoted to reaching and obtaining the participation of all eligible subjects. In general, expanding the effort to locate or recruit nonparticipants will yield some additional participants and data obtained from those recovered participants is informative.

Subject refusal probably remains the predominant reason for losses in most epidemiologic studies. Even after intensive efforts to persuade subjects to participate in interviews or specimen collection have failed, uniquely talented, motivated interviewers can usually persuade a sizable proportion of subjects who had initially refused to change their minds (refusal converters). Locating subjects is even more clearly tied to resources expended. Commercial tracking companies typically have an explicit policy—the more money you are willing to spend to locate a given person, the more intensive the effort, and the more likely it is that they will be able to locate that person. Thus, after a reasonable, affordable level of effort has been expended to locate subjects, a subset of formerly untraceable subjects can be subjected to more intensive tracking methods and located to generate the desired data. The product of these refusal conversions or intensive tracking efforts is information on formerly nonparticipating subjects who can help us make some inferences about the otherwise eligible subjects who remain nonparticipants.

Assuming that at least some of the former nonrespondents can be enrolled, the goal is to characterize the exposure or health outcome of primary interest. In a cohort study, the occurrence or non-occurrence of disease is central. After normal follow-up procedures, some fraction of the original cohort is likely to remain lost to follow-up. To evaluate the impact of that loss, a fraction of those lost to follow-up would be located through more intensive means in order to determine their disease outcomes. With that information in hand, formal corrections can be made if one assumes that those former nonrespondents who were found represent their counterparts who remain nonrespondents. For example, if the disease incidence among the 10 subjects who were formerly lost to follow-up but located through intensive effort were 20%, one might assume that of the total 100 subjects lost to follow-up, 20 of them developed disease as well. Such a calculation assumes that those who were converted from lost to found represent those who were permanently lost, which is subject to uncertainty. When the recovered subjects constitute a complete roster of a randomly chosen subset, confidence in generalizing to all those remaining lost is much greater than when those who are recovered are simply the most easily recovered from the pool of those initially lost and are thus likely to differ systematically from those who remain lost. Incorporating the data on those subjects who were found directly reduces the non-response, whereas extrapolating from that subset that could be found to the entire roster of those lost is more akin to a sensitivity analysis. ("What if those lost had the disease experience of those we could find?") Nevertheless, the alternative assumption that nonrespondents are identical to respondents is lacking in any empirical support and thus far more tenuous.

Beyond the reduction in non-response that results from these intensive follow-up efforts, and the subsequent ability to estimate the association of interest without such losses, this strategy can provide additional insight into the underlying reasons for non-participation. In some cases, direct inquiry built into the follow-up process can reveal the ways in which those who were included differ from those who initially were not. In the case of subject refusal, information on social and demographic attributes, occupation, medical history, etc. will help to describe the patterns and potential bias, but also to better understand why they refused in the first place. Former refusals can be queried directly regarding their reason for having been reluctant to participate in the study. To the extent that honest answers can be generated, there is the opportunity to examine whether study methods could be refined to improve response or at least add to the understanding of the process that resulted in their having been lost.

Similarly, eligible subjects who were initially untraceable and then located can be evaluated to reveal why they were untraceable or at least to characterize the types of persons who fall into that category. Perhaps they were less likely to use credit cards or more likely to be self-employed. Such general descriptors of the lost individuals and informed speculation about the underlying process help the investigator and reviewer to judge the potential for biased measures of association among the participants who were included. Also, information may be generated to indicate cost-effective approaches to reducing the magnitude of non-response in the ongoing study or at least in future ones.

In comparing those who were lost to those who participated, investigators often focus on broad demographic attributes of the two groups because those are most readily available. Unwarranted comfort may be taken when the demographic profile of those lost is similar to those who were enrolled. Such a pattern is used to infer that those lost are effectively a random sample of those enrolled, and thus, on average, participants would generate measures of association equivalent to those from all eligible subjects. Data sources on nonrespondents, such as public records or city directories typically provide some information on gender, age, and sometimes occupation or educational level. Such descriptors do provide some insight into the process by which subjects were lost, and provide limited data to address the hypothesis that the loss process has generated a random sample from those eligible. The reassurance that can be provided by sociodemographic similarity of respondents and nonrespondents is not directly relevant to assessing potential for bias, however, which depends on the specific exposure and disease under study. The ultimate question is not whether they are socially and demographically similar, but rather whether, conditional on those social and demographic factors that are readily measured and adjusted as needed, the losses result in distortion of disease rates or exposure prevalence.

In a cohort study, what we would really like to know is whether disease incidence is similar among nonparticipants and participants *within* cells defined by social and demographic factors. Do those women aged 40–49 with 12 years of education who did not enroll in the study have the same disease risk as women aged 40–49 with 12 years of education who did enroll? Determination of whether the proportion who are women aged 40–49 with 12 years of education differs between participants and nonparticipants does not help a great deal in making this assessment. Whether or not the sociodemographic profile is similar, within gender, age, and education cells, disease risk may be consistently greater among nonparticipants. A small sample with the information of ultimate interest on exposure or health outcome may be of greater value in assessing bias than assessing demographic data on a larger proportion of non–participants.

A thorough analysis of several sources of potential bias in a large case–control study of magnetic fields and childhood leukemia provides a useful illustration of examining nonrespondents (Hatch et al., 2000). One of the major methodologic concerns in the original analysis was the potential for non-response to have distorted study findings pertaining to two indices of magnetic field exposure, wire codes that estimate magnetic fields in the home and measurements of magnetic fields in the home. Information on complete nonrespondents was unavailable, of course, but they did have two indicators of partial participation—subjects who refused to permit indoor magnetic field measurements but could be characterized by measurements at the front door, and subjects who did and did not agree to participate in the interview phase of the study. By comparing complete and partial participants, patterns were identified that help to assess the broader concern with non-response (Table 6.2).

The profile that emerges is that those who provided only part of the desired data (i.e., front door measurement only, those without interview) tended to be of lower social class based on not residing in a single family home, lower income, and less education, as well as showing some indication of higher levels of magnetic field exposure indices. Interestingly, these patterns were reported to hold for both cases and controls, but to be stronger among controls. That is, the socioeconomic gradient of partial response (and thus, perhaps, non-response) was stronger among controls, introducing the potential for biased measures of association to the extent that socioeconomic status could not be fully adjusted.

TABLE 6.2. Selected Characteristics of Subjects with Indoor Magnetic Field Measurements vs. Subjects with Front Door Magnetic Field Measurements Only and of Wire Coded Subjects with and without In-Person Interview, National Cancer Institute Childhood Leukemia Study

CHARACTERISTIC	SUBJECTS WITH INDOOR MEASUREMENTS ($N = 1101$)	SUBJECTS WITH FRONT DOOR MEASUREMENTS ONLY ($N = 147$)	WIRE CODED SUBJECTS WITH INTERVIEW ($N = 1052$)	WIRE CODED SUBJECTS WITHOUT INTERVIEW ($N = 107$)
Living in single family home	83	58	78	70
With income < $20,000	12	23	14	29
Mothers with ≤ high school education	38	46	40	55
Rented residence	18	40	22	35
Unmarried mothers	10	25	13	22
Urban	22	23	25	30
> 0.2 μT	12.7	15.6		
VHCC	6.3	8.8	6.7	8.4
Controls	47	67	48	76

VHCC, Very High Current Configuration wire code
Hatch et al., 2000.

Consider Gradient of Difficulty in Recruitment

Although participation is ultimately dichotomous, i.e., individual subjects are or are not located and they do or do not agree to participate in the study, there are several ways in which a spectrum or gradient of difficulty in recruitment can be examined. The rationale for examining such a gradient is to understand the patterns going from those who were readily enrolled to those who were less readily enrolled and then extrapolate to those who did not participate at all. This strategy is built on the assumption that the many reasons for failure to participate in the study act probabilistically, and that those who fall at one end of the continuum of participation predictors are extremely likely to enroll and those at the other end of the continuum are almost certain not to enroll, with all potential participants falling somewhere along that spectrum. Under this scenario, those individuals who have some of the non-participation profile but are still recruited can tell us something about those who have the more extreme version of the non-participation profile and do not participate. For example, potential participants who moved but were located or who were located only with intensive effort may give hints about those who moved and could not be found. Similarly, we might expect that those who were reluctant to participate but were ultimately persuaded to do so would fall in between the eager participants and those who chose not to participate at all. Estimation of a quantitative dose-response function of nonparticipation and formal extrapolation to nonrespondents would be the ultimate goal, but a qualitative assessment may be all that is feasible.

In mail surveys, the design typically calls for a series of steps to enhance response (Dillman, 1978), each step yielding more respondents and depleting the pool of refusals. Some respond directly to the initial questionnaire, some respond only to reminder postcards, others respond only to repeat mailing of the questionnaire, continuing to those who must be interviewed by telephone because they ignore all mailed material. It can be difficult in practice to determine exactly which action precipitated a response, but through careful coding of questionnaires, monitoring mailing and receipt dates, and some inferences based on those dates, a gradient of willingness to cooperate can be defined among the participants. Those who promptly returned the questionnaire without a reminder are at one end of that spectrum, and those who responded only after the most extreme efforts, e.g., telephone calls, are at the other end of the spectrum.

The characteristics of those who responded at each stage can be examined, both to describe them in broad social and demographic terms, but more importantly to determine their statuses with regard to the variables of primary interest and the estimated measure of effect for that subgroup. In a cohort study in which disease is ascertained by questionnaire, the proportion affected by the disease, stratified by the effort required to elicit a response, would indicate whether the ultimate nonrespondents were likely to have higher or lower disease rates than the respondents. Stratifying by exposure might address the critical question of whether exposed nonrespondents are likely to have a different health outcome than unexposed nonrespondents. Similarly, in a case–control study, the exposure prevalence can be assessed across strata of cooperativeness, separately for cases and controls, to extrapolate and assess whether the ability to include the remaining nonrespondents would be likely to change the pattern of results. In a sensitivity analysis, the nonrespondents could be assumed to have the traits of reluctant respondents, or a more extreme version of the reluctant respondent profile, and an assessment made of the expected results for the full study population. In contrast to making arbitrary and implausible extreme assumptions (e.g., all those missing are exposed cases), the evaluation of reluctant respondents provides a basis for much more credible estimates.

In a community survey in Montreal, Siematycki and Cambell (1984) examined participant characteristics for those who responded at the first stage of the survey that was conducted by mail, compared to the cumulation of first- and second-stage responders, with second-stage participants only responding with further contact, including a home interview if needed. As shown in Table 6.3, few

TABLE 6.3. Selected Characteristics and Responses of Early Respondents Compared with All Respondents in a Mail Strategy in Montreal

	FIRST STAGE RESPONDENTS: MAIL (N = 1065) % ± SE	ALL RESPONDENTS: MAIL, TELEPHONE, HOME (N = 1258) % ± SE
Sociodemographic characteristics		
Female	52.6 ± 1.5	52.1 ± 1.4
Age distribution: 17–35	36.9 ± 1.5	36.4 ± 1.4
36–55	34.1 ± 1.5	34.6 ± 1.3
56+	28.4 ± 1.4	27.8 ± 1.3
11 or more years of schooling	59.1 ± 1.5	58.1 ± 1.4
Live in a household with children	39.1 ± 1.5	38.7 ± 1.4
Reported morbidity and health care		
Has chronic condition	16.2 ± 1.1	15.7 ± 1.0
Was unable to carry out usual activities in past month due to illness	18.0 ± 1.2	18.4 ± 1.1
Reported 3 or more symptoms in checklist of 14	37.9 ± 1.5	38.1 ± 1.4
Saw physician in past 2 weeks	25.4 ± 1.3	24.6 ± 1.2
Saw dentist in past 2 weeks	9.3 ± 0.9	9.1 ± 0.8
Took prescribed medication in past 2 weeks	25.7 ± 1.3	25.8 ± 1.2
Ever smoked cigarettes	69.0 ± 1.4	69.1 ± 1.3
Current cigarette smoker	48.5 ± 1.5	49.4 ± 1.4

SE, standard error.

Siemiatycki & Campbell, 1984.

differences were noted between results based on the first stage alone versus the first and second stages combined. Note however, that this presentation of results does not isolate the second-stage respondents, who in fact had a lower level of education and were more likely to be current smokers, but not to a sufficient extent to influence the cumulative sample.

By isolating those responding in each of the stages, there is an opportunity to extrapolate to those who did not participate at all. In studies that are large enough, measures of association can be calculated for subgroups defined by the stage at which they responded. In a study using a mailed questionnaire, for example, the relative risk for those responding to the first questionnaire, the reminder postcard, the second questionnaire, and the telephone interview can be calculated to identify a gradient and estimate what the relative risk would be in those who did not participate at all. Through this approach, it is possible to assess directly whether inclusion of all eligible participants is likely to generate a relative risk that is larger or smaller than that found for the participants alone, and even to provide some quantitative basis for how much different it would be. If the gradient of relative risks moving from easy to difficult response were 1.2, 1.4, 1.4, and 1.7, one might guess that the relative risk for those who did not participate would be approximately 1.8–2.0, and therefore conduct a sensitivity analysis under that assumed value. Although this is subject to uncertainty, the alternative is to assume nonrespondents are identical to respondents, and the data make that assumption even less tenable.

Telephone and in-person interviews have a comparable spectrum of difficulty, though it may be less easily measured as compared to mailed questionnaires. Interviewed respondents vary greatly in their initial enthusiasm for the study, with some requiring intensive efforts to persuade them to become involved and others much more readily agreeable. The amount of persuasion that is required is worth noting to facilitate extrapolation to those who could not be persuaded even with intensive effort. The number of telephone calls required to reach a respondent is another dimension of difficulty in recruitment, reflective of accessibility or cooperativeness. Those who require many calls may give some insights into those who would have required an infinite number of calls (i.e., those who were never reached). Subjects who ultimately participate after one or more missed appointments may be reflective of those who repeatedly miss appointments and ultimately become nonrespondents for that reason. Because refusal to participate has multiple etiologies, including lack of belief in the value of research, insufficient time, and inability to be located, there is some danger in seeking a single dose-response function for recruitability. It may be more informative to separate out the degrees of reluctance for each causal pathway and extrapolate for each specific reason they could not be enrolled,

The other major source of loss is due to the inability to locate presumably eligible subjects. Efforts to locate individuals can be documented and placed into ordinal categories of required effort. For example, some subjects are readily found through the available address or telephone number, or they are listed in the telephone directory at the expected address. Others can be traced through a forwarding address or are found in directories at their new address. Further down the list, some are found by contacting neighbors or by calling former employers. Studies generally follow a well-defined sequential algorithm based on the nature of the population and the impressions of the investigators regarding the most efficient approach. Whatever series of steps is followed, the documentation of what was ultimately required to locate the subject should be noted and examined so that the pattern of results can be extrapolated to those never found. Here the gradient of traceability may be more obvious than for refusals, since those who move multiple times or are lost would be expected to be similar to those who move and are found, only more so.

An important caveat with this strategy is that ultimate nonrespondents may be qualitatively different than reluctant respondents. That is, there may be a discontinuity in which easy and reluctant respondents are similar to one another and intransigent nonrespondents are altogether different from either group. There is no easy way to detect this, in that the most uncooperative subjects or those most difficult to locate will remain nonparticipants regardless of the amount of effort that is expended. To the extent that this is true, the sensitivity analysis that assumes otherwise will be misleading, and this untestable possibility should temper the degree to which extrapolation to nonrespondents is viewed as a solution rather than an exploration of the problem.

Stratify Study Base by Markers of Participation

If subgroups can be identified in which participation is more complete and thus less susceptible to bias, then stratification on those markers of participation can be informative for several purposes. The stratum in which participation is more favorable provides more valid estimates of the association of interest, less vulnerable to bias from non-response. Moreover, if there is a gradient of nonparticipation across strata, then examining the pattern of measures of association across strata of diminishing participation may reveal the pattern of selection bias, if any, that has been produced. Like any causal hypothesis, if it is postulated that nonparticipation causes an upward or downward bias in the measure of effect, then estimates of the measure of effect across levels of non-participation will be highly informative regarding that hypothesis.

For example, if geographic location were a marker of the likelihood of participation in a multicenter study, the measure of association could be stratified by geographic area to identify the presumably more valid estimate in certain geographic areas with a high response proportion, and provide effect estimates across areas of increasing vulnerability to selection bias. If, in fact, the estimates of association were similar across strata that are known to vary in the proportion participating, then the potential for selection bias due to non-response in the study can be inferred to be less likely to be present at all. If response proportions differed across geographic area in a multicenter study, yet the measures of association were similar across those sites, then bias due to non-response would be less likely to be a problem overall, including in the areas with lower participation proportions. Such data would be counter to the hypothesis that selection bias has distorted the study results. If, on the other hand, results differed in relation to the degree of response, such evidence would be consistent with the presence of selection bias and the strata in which selection bias was minimal could be assumed to generate the most valid results.

A limitation in this exercise is that selection bias due to non-response is rarely if ever the only possible basis for subgroups to differ or not differ from one another. The extent of other biases may differ across those same strata or there may be true effect measure modification across subgroups. If no gradient in effect estimates is found across subgroups with varying completeness of response, other biases may be compensating for the bias due to non-response to hide its effect. Analogously, and perhaps even more plausibly, observation of a gradient in relation to the marker of participation may be indicative of true effect-modification by the marker of response proportion rather than a product of selection bias. Markers of participation, such as socioeconomic factors, ethnicity, and geographic location, may well be true modifiers of the effect of exposure, and simultaneously influence the participation proportion. These competing explanations cannot readily be separated empirically and require informed judgment based on knowledge of the specific exposure and disease under investigation.

Impute Information for Nonparticipants

Several of the strategies already considered, including generating estimates for a subset of nonparticipants and extrapolating from reluctant respondents to non-respondents, can be extended to more formal strategies for imputation of responses for nonparticipants. That is, explicit guesses are made regarding what the responses of nonrespondents would have been, and those imputed responses are used in the analysis. Such imputation can be viewed as another form of sensitivity analysis, in that it does not eliminate concern with non-response but makes reasonable assumptions about the missing data.

As an example of research in which selective response and missing data could markedly distort findings, a number of mail surveys were conducted in the 1970s and 1980s to address the hypothesis that exposure of pregnant workers to anesthetic gases might be associated with increased risk of spontaneous abortion (Tannenbaum & Goldberg, 1985). Operating room staff and health-care workers lacking such exposure were surveyed by mail and reported their reproductive experiences. Given the growing awareness of a potential association between anesthetic gases and adverse pregnancy outcome, it is quite plausible that response would be exaggerated for exposed cases, i.e., women who worked in such settings and had a spontaneous abortion, with the work setting and the experience motivating response to the survey. To the extent that such a phenomenon occurred, we would find a much stronger association among respondents than among all eligible participants. Faced with such results, we could either accept them with caveats or attempt to address the potentially critical concern of non-response with imputation of data for nonrespondents.

Many epidemiologists have a great reluctance to use imputed data, based on very legitimate concerns. At the extreme, imputation can be misused to gloss over the fact that the data are truly missing. That is, imputed data are not as good as actual data, and confidence in the validity of the results should be reduced due to the missing data, yet imputation can make it tempting to act as though the non-response problem has been solved. In many national surveys distributed by the National Center for Health Statistics, for example, the data are complete but with an imputation "flag." It is actually more convenient to use the full data set, including imputed values, than to regenerate a data set in which imputed values are treated as missing. Missing data should not be hidden or disguised, because non-response needs to be known to make an accurate assessment of the study's susceptibility to bias. Even when presented honestly as a sensitivity analysis, ("What would the results be if we made the following assumptions about nonparticipants?") it is intuitively unappealing to many to impute not just social or demographic factors but exposure or disease status. Imputation seems to violate our ingrained demands for real data, objectively described.

On the other hand, once we determine that there are eligible subjects who have not been enrolled, we are faced with a range of imperfect alternative approaches. Inevitably subjects are lost, and the proportions are typically in the range of 20%–30% in even the most meticulously conducted studies, with losses of 40%–50% not uncommon. Given that the losses have occurred, we can (1) ignore the losses altogether; (2) describe the losses by analyzing patterns among those who provided data, using a variety of tools and logic described in previous sections to speculate about the impact of those losses on the study results; or (3) impute data for nonparticipants, analyzing the combined set of subjects with real and imputed data, and discussing the strengths and limitations of the imputation.

When the analysis is restricted to those subjects who provided data, we are assuming that they are a random sample from the pool of eligibles and that results are valid, though somewhat less precise, as a result of those losses. As discussed above, that is a highly questionable assumption, with self-selection in particular unlikely to be random. To the extent that participants are a non-random sample with respect to key attributes of exposure or disease or both, the measures of association may be distorted (Rothman & Greenland, 1998).

Imputation makes a different set of assumptions, with a variety of techniques available but all are built on the strategy of using known attributes to impute unknown attributes. Regression techniques use information from all subjects with complete data to develop predictive equations for each of the missing measures. Those predictive models are then applied to those with some data available to predict values for missing items, and those predicted values are substituted for the missing ones. Another approach is to identify a set of subjects with complete data who are similar to the lost subject with respect to known attributes and use a randomly selected individual subject's profile to substitute for the missing one.

In any event, the guess is an informed one, though not subject to verification. The underlying assumption of imputation is that attributes can be predicted for those who are nonparticipants based on information from participants. To the extent that this is in error, then the data generated by imputation will be incorrect and the results using the imputed data will be biased.

Given the two options, accepting missing information as missing and imputing missing information, each with positive and negative aspects, perhaps the optimal approach is to do the imputation but retain the ability to examine results for subjects with measured data and the combined population with measured plus imputed data separately. In that way, the evaluator of the evidence, including the investigators who generated it, can consider the plausibility of the assumptions and make an informed judgment about which results are likely to be more valid. Similar results under the two approaches provides evidence that bias due to nonparticipation is less likely, whereas different results for complete and imputed subjects suggests that the losses may have introduced distortion and, subject to the level of confidence in the imputation process, that the more valid result is obtained through imputation.

An evaluation of the ability to impute data and assess its impact on study results is provided by Baris et al. (1999). They considered a study of magnetic fields and childhood leukemia conducted by the National Cancer Institute in which some of the children had lived in two or more homes. The "gold standard" measure of exposure in such instances was considered to be the time-weighted average of measurements in the two residences, but they were interested in comparing more cost-efficient approaches to determine whether information would be lost by failing to obtain measurements in both homes. To examine this, they presented results based on various approaches to imputing the value of the unmeasured home using available information on one measured home chosen as the longest-occupied or currently occupied (at the time of the study).

Using the exposure indices presented in Table 6.4, the gold standard measurements yielded odds ratios and 95% confidence intervals across the three groups above 0.065 microTesla (μT), a measure of magnetic flux density, as follows: 0.97 (0.52–1.81), 1.14 (0.63–2.08), and 1.81 (0.81–4.02), with a p-value for trend of 0.2. Whether overall means for study subjects were used for imputation (results on left) or case and control group-specific means were used (results on right), there was severe attenuation of the pattern from using imputed results. What had been a weak gradient, with some indication of higher risk in the highest exposure stratum, disappeared upon using imputed data for the second home. Even with a reasonable correlation of fields across homes, the loss of information to characterize exposure–disease associations was substantial in this instance.

TABLE 6.4. Odd Ratios (95% CI) from Different Imputation Strategies Categorized According to Initial Cut Off Points of Magnetic Field Exposure, National Cancer Institute Childhood Leukemia Study

Relative Risk for Acute Lymphoblastic Leukemia Calculated With:

Control Mean Imputation*

EXPOSURE CATEGORIES	TWA Based on Longer Lived in Homes Plus Imputed Values for Shorter Lived in Homes				TWA Based on Current Lived in Homes Plus Imputed Values for Former Lived in Homes			
	MEAN (μT)	CASES	OR	95% CI	MEAN (μT)	CASES	OR	95% CI
< 0.065 μT	0.056	26	1.00	—	0.058	22	1.00	—
≥ 0.065–< 0.099 μT	0.080	61	0.99	0.51 to 1.95	0.083	74	0.74	0.36 to 1.55
> 1.00–< 0.199 μT	0.134	45	1.14	0.56 to 2.32	0.124	46	0.85	0.39 to 1.86
≥ 0.200 μT	0.330	17	1.00	0.41 to 2.45	0.278	7	0.68	0.20 to 2.33
			$P_{trend} = 0.8$				$P_{trend} = 0.8$	

Status Specific Mean Imputation†

EXPOSURE CATEGORIES	TWA Based on Longer Lived in Homes Plus Imputed Values for Shorter Lived in Homes				TWA Based on Current Lived in Homes Plus Imputed Values for Former Lived in Homes			
	MEAN (μT)	CASES	OR	95% CI	MEAN (μT)	CASES	OR	95% CI
< 0.065 μT	0.056	23	1.00	—	0.058	21	1.00	—
≥ 0.065–< 0.099 μT	0.081	63	1.17	0.59 to 2.31	0.083	74	0.78	0.37 to 1.63
> 1.00–< 0.199 μT	0.134	46	1.31	0.64 to 2.72	0.124	47	0.91	0.41 to 2.00
≥ 0.200 μT	0.331	17	1.13	0.46 to 2.80	0.279	7	0.71	0.21 to 2.47
			$P_{trend} = 0.6$				$P_{trend} = 0.6$	

*Shorter lived in homes were imputed from observed mean of longer lived in control homes; former lived in homes were imputed from observed mean of current lived in control homes.

†Shorter lived in homes were imputed from case mean of longer lived in homes (if case) or from control mean of longer lived in homes (if control); former lived in homes were imputed from case mean of current lived in homes (if case) or from control mean of current lived in homes (if control).

CI, confidence interval; OR, odds ratio; TWA, time = weighted average

Baris et al., 1999.

INTEGRATED ASSESSMENT OF POTENTIAL FOR BIAS DUE TO LOSS OF STUDY PARTICIPANTS

Among the threats to the validity of epidemiologic studies, none is more ubiquitous or severe than the problem of non-participation. By choosing to study free-living humans, epidemiologists face an unavoidable loss due to the characteristics distinguishing those who are eligible and those who provide all the desired information. The loss of desired participants is rarely random with respect to the attributes of interest, and thus the participants will often be non-representative on key attributes and have serious potential to generate biased measures of association.

The only unambiguous solution, free of assumptions, is to eliminate nonresponse. Before embarking on indirect, fallible approaches to assessing or controlling effects of nonparticipation, every effort should be made to eliminate or at least minimize the magnitude of the problem. At the point of choosing a study population, attention should be given to seeking study settings in which the losses will be minimized. There is often some tension between studying highly selective, cooperative groups, perhaps distinctive for being of higher social class or belonging to some motivated group (e.g., nurses), and the ultimate interest in applying findings to more diverse populations. Unless the study questions demand inclusion of a range of persons who differ in availability and willingness to participate, starting with a series of valid studies in highly selected populations may be the preferred strategy.

To evaluate the impact of nonparticipation, the specific pathways of subject loss need to be isolated, perhaps even more finely than is typically done in epidemiologic studies. Refusal due to distrust of medical researchers may have different implications than refusal due to lack of available time, for example. We are concerned with systematic (non-random) losses and whether those losses are related to the exposure and disease of concern. The more specificity with which the mechanism of loss can be stated, the greater our opportunity to consider empirically or theoretically the effect such losses will have on the study results. Those losses most likely to be related to the occurrence of disease in a cohort study or the prevalence of exposure in a case–control study deserve the greatest scrutiny. The potential for distortion plus the magnitude of loss combine to determine the importance of the phenomenon.

Within each of the pathways of loss, there are several parallel approaches to assessing the impact on study results: Intensive effort can usually rescue some proportion of those lost. This allows a comparison of the characteristics of those successfully enrolled despite initial failure to those enrolled more readily. In turn, if those who were rescued can be assumed to have traits in common with the nonparticipants, the impact of non-response can be estimated. If there is a gradient associated with the mechanism of loss, e.g., degree of reluctance or difficulty of tracing, the pattern of results across that spectrum can be analyzed to project to those who remained lost. Characteristics of those with lesser doses of the tendency to be lost can be compared to those with greater amounts of that same tendency and then extrapolated to the most extreme subset (who remain lost). Subsets of the study base in which the loss was less severe can be examined and compared to subsets in which there was greater loss, both to assess the pattern in measures of association across that spectrum as well as to generate results for subsets in which non-response bias is unlikely to be a major problem. Finally, methods of imputation should be considered, with appropriate caveats, to estimate what the results would have been without losses.

Many of these techniques depend on the foresight of the investigators in acquiring and presenting relevant data. Without presenting the needed information on study attrition, the reviewer may be left with much more generic speculation about non-response and its impact. Published papers typically give some clues at least regarding the reasons for loss and some characteristics of those not participating. With those clues regarding the sources and magnitude of non-participation, the key questions can at least be formulated and partial answers provided. Non-participation represents a challenge in which greater effort is likely to yield reduced risk of bias and revealing more information is certain to help the user of information from the study to draw more valid inferences.

REFERENCES

Baris D, Linet MS, Tarone RE, Kleinerman RA, Hatch EE, Kaune WT, Robison LL, Lubin J, Wacholder S. Residential exposure to magnetic fields: an empirical assessment of alternative measurement strategies. Occup Environ Med 1999;56:562–566.

Criqui M, Barrett-Connor E, Austin M. Differences between respondents and non-respondents in a population-based cardiovascular disease study. Am J Epidemiol 1978;108:367–372.

Dillman DA. Mail and telephone surveys. The total design method. New York: John Wiley & Sons, 1978.

Greenland S. Response and follow-up bias in cohort studies. Am J Epidemiol 1977;106:184–187.

Greenland S, Criqui MH. Are case-control studies more vulnerable to response bias? Am J Epidemiol 1981;114:175–177.

Hatch EE, Kleinerman RA, Linet MS, Tarone RE, Kaune WT, Auvinen A, Baris D, Robison LL, Wacholder S. Do confounding or selection factors of residential wiring codes and magnetic fields distort findings of electromagnetic field studies? Epidemiology 2000;11:189–198.

Macera CA, Jackson KL, Davis DR, Kronenfeld JJ, Blair SN. Patterns of non-response to a mail survey. J Clin Epidemiol 1990;43:1427–1430.

Psaty BM, Cheadle A, Koepsell TD, Diehr P, Wickizer T, Curry S, VonKorff M, Perrin EB, Pearson DC, Wagner EH. Race- and ethnicity-specific characteristics of participants lost to follow-up in a telephone cohort. Am J Epidemiol 1994;140:161–171.

Rothman KJ, Greenland S. Modern epidemiology, Second edition. Philadelphia: Lippincott-Raven Publishers, 1998.

Savitz DA, Dole N, Williams J, Thorp JM, McDonald T, Carter AC, Eucker B. Determinants of participation in an epidemiologic study of preterm delivery. Paediatr Peri-
nat Epidemiol 1999;13:114–125.

Siemiatycki J, Campbell S. Nonresponse bias and early versus all responders in mail and
telephone surveys. Am J Epidemiol 1984;120:291–301.

Tannenbaum TN, Goldberg RJ. Exposure to anesthetic gases and reproductive outcomes.
A review of the epidemiologic literature. J Occup Med 1985;27:659–668.

7

CONFOUNDING

DEFINITION AND THEORETICAL BACKGROUND

Confounding is one of the fundamental methodological concerns in epidemiology. Although rarely as explicitly examined in other disciplines, and sometimes identified with different terminology, confounding is also a theme in other branches of science. Wherever one is concerned with identifying causal associations, whether through observational or experimental studies, a key focus of study design and analysis is to address the potential effects of confounding.

The concept of confounding can be expressed in a number of different ways. One simple definition refers to confounding as the mixing of effects, in which there is "distortion of the effect estimate of an exposure on an outcome, caused by the presence of an extraneous factor" (Last, 2001). A more conceptually complete view is the counterfactual definition of confounding (Greenland & Robins, 1986). The ideal comparison group for the exposed group is the exposed group itself but under the condition of not having been exposed, an experience that did not, in fact, occur (thus it is counterfactual). If we could observe this experience (which we cannot), we would be able to compare the disease occurrence under the situation in which exposure has occurred to the counterfactual one in which everything else is the same except exposure was not present. Instead, we choose some other group, sometimes one that has been randomized not to receive exposure, to provide an estimate of what the experience of the exposed group would have been absent the exposure. Ignoring various forms of selection and measurement error and random processes, the reason that comparing the exposed to the unexposed group would fail to accurately measure the causal effect of exposure is confounding. That is, the unexposed group may have other influences on disease, due to both measurable factors and unknown influences, which make its disease experience an inaccurate reflection of what the exposed subjects themselves would have experienced had they not been exposed. Other disease determinants have rendered the comparison of disease risk across exposure levels an inaccurate reflection of the causal impact of exposure. This has been referred to as *non-exchangeability* in that the exposed and unexposed are not exchangeable, aside from any effect of the exposure itself.

There is an important distinction to be made between the concept of confounding as defined above and the definition of a confounder or confounding variable. A confounding variable is a marker of the basis for non-comparability. It provides at least a partial explanation for the underlying differences in disease risk comparing the exposed and unexposed aside from the exposure itself. If we wish to assess the influence of coffee drinking on the risk of bladder cancer, we should be concerned that coffee drinkers and abstainers may not have comparable baseline risk of disease independent of any effects of coffee itself, i.e., confounding is likely to be present. One important source of such non-comparability would be attributable to the fact that persons who habitually drink different amounts of coffee also tend to differ in cigarette smoking habits, and cigarette smoking is a known cause of bladder cancer. Thus, we are concerned with cigarette smoking as a confounder or marker of the non-comparability among persons who consume different amounts of coffee. Put in other terms, we would like for the disease experience of the non-coffee drinkers in our study to accurately reflect the disease experience that the coffee drinkers themselves *would* have had if they had not been coffee drinkers. If smoking habits differ between the two groups, however, then the consequences of coffee drinking will be mixed with those of cigarette smoking and give an inaccurate representation of the effect of coffee drinking as a result.

Because the concept of confounding based on the counterfactual model relies on unobservable conditions, epidemiologists usually concentrate on the more practical approach of searching for specific confounders that may affect the comparison of exposed and unexposed, and make extensive efforts to control for confounding. Although this effort is often fully justified and can help markedly to remove bias, we should not lose appreciation for the underlying conceptual goal. Exchangeability of exposed and unexposed is the ideal and the search for markers of non-exchangeability is undertaken to better approximate that ideal. Statistical adjustment for confounding variables is simply a means toward that end.

The inability to identify plausible candidate confounding variables, for example, or extensive efforts to control for known and suspected confounding variables by no means guarantees the absence of confounding. Doing one's best is laudable, but circumstances outside the control of the investigator often make some degree of confounding inescapable. In observational studies in which exposure cannot be assigned randomly, the attainment of exchangeability is a very high aspiration. When randomization of exposure is feasible, the opportunity to force the exposed and unexposed groups to be exchangeable is greatly enhanced. The randomization process itself is precisely for the purpose of making sure that the groups are exchangeable. If exposure is assigned randomly, those persons (or rats or cell cultures) that receive the exposure should be exchangeable with those that do not receive the exposure. Regardless of how extensive the measurement and control of extraneous determinants of disease may be in observational studies, producing groups that are functionally randomized is a nearly unattainable goal.

Consider efforts to truly isolate the effects of specific dietary practices, occupational exposures, or sexual behavior. The challenges are apparent in that these exposures are not incurred in any sense randomly. The choice of diet, job, or sexual partner is integrally tied to many other dimensions of a person's life, at least some of which are also likely to affect the risk of disease. We obviously cannot ethically or feasibly randomize such experiences, however, and thus must accept the scientifically second-best approach of trying to understand and control for the influences of other associated factors. We must reflect carefully on other known determinants of the health outcomes of interest that are likely to be associated with the exposure of primary interest and make statistical adjustment for those markers, simulating to the extent possible a situation in which the exposures themselves had been randomly allocated. Accepting that the ideal is not attainable in no way detracts from the incremental value of feasible approaches to improve the degree of comparability of exposed and unexposed.

Statistical methods of adjusting for confounding variables are exercises in which we estimate the results that would have been obtained had the exposure groups been balanced for those other disease determinants even though, in fact, they were not. For the extraneous disease determinant or confounder, which is associated with the exposure of interest, we estimate the influence of exposure on disease after statistically removing any effect of the extraneous exposures. The most straightforward approach is to stratify on the potential confounding factor, creating subgroups in which the extraneous factor is not related to exposure. In the above illustration, in which our interest was in isolating the effect of coffee drinking on bladder cancer from that of cigarette smoking, we can stratify on smoking status and estimate the coffee–bladder cancer association separately among nonsmokers, among light smokers, and among heavy smokers. Within each of those groups, cigarette smoking would not distort the association because smoking is no longer related to coffee drinking. We can, if desired, then pool the estimate of the association across levels of smoking to generate a summary estimate that addresses coffee drinking and bladder cancer under the scenario in which smoking is not associated with coffee drinking.

Stratification by smoking simulates a population in which smoking is not associated with coffee drinking. It is hypothetical, not the actual experience of the population, because in the real population coffee drinking and cigarette smoking *are* associated. The product of the stratification is the removal of the effects of the specific confounding factor, to the extent it was accurately measured and analyzed properly. We can say that the association of coffee drinking and bladder cancer has been adjusted for cigarette smoking, or that cigarette smoking no longer confounds the association. That is not to say that all confounding has been removed so that coffee drinking is now effectively randomly allocated, but rather one of the likely sources of non-exchangeability of coffee drinkers and nondrinkers has been addressed. To the extent we have been successful, we have moved closer to the situation in which coffee drinking was incurred randomly.

Viewing confounding as non-exchangeability serves as a reminder that the direction and magnitude of confounding depend on the specific determinants of disease and how they are distributed with respect to the exposure. The disease risk of the unexposed may be greater or less than the hypothetical disease risk the exposed would have experienced had they not been exposed. If the disease risk of the unexposed exceeds that of the exposed group absent exposure, i.e., the unexposed have a higher risk than the exposed would have had if not exposed, then the bias in the risk ratio is downwards, towards a smaller value. An exposure that truly increases disease will appear to pose less of a hazard and an exposure that protects against disease will appear to have a greater benefit. If the disease risk of the unexposed is less than that of the exposed group absent exposure, i.e., the unexposed are of lower risk than desired for the counterfactual comparison, then an exposure that increases risk of disease will have a spuriously elevated risk ratio and one that protects against disease will show less of a benefit than it otherwise would.

Thus, confounding variables can act as positive confounders, raising the measure of effect above what it would otherwise be, or they can be negative confounders, falsely lowering the measure of effect. The null value does not serve as an anchor or reference point in assessing confounding. Following from this, efforts to recognize and control confounding should not be limited to a focus on challenging positive associations. There is no logical reason to postulate confounding solely for positive associations, asking what factors may have spuriously created it. Confounding is just as plausibly present when we observe no association, having masked a truly positive or negative association. At the extreme, we might even observe an inverse association due to confounding of a positive association or vice versa.

A final point about confounding concerns the role of randomization in removing confounding. By assigning exposure randomly in a sufficiently large study, the potential for confounding can be minimized to any desired extent. Known confounding factors are likely to be balanced across exposure groups, though they can be measured and adjusted if the randomization does not achieve perfect balance. More importantly, unknown influences on disease are increasingly likely to be balanced as well as study size increases. That is, without being able to even identify what those determinants are, one can achieve a balance of pre-existing risk such that the remaining differences between exposed and unexposed are due to the exposure, or with measurable probability, due to random error arising from the exposure allocation process (Greenland, 1990). In contrast to the arbitrary and largely uninterpretable use of statements about probability and random error in observational studies, the statistical methods to generate p-values are directly interpretable as "the probability of having obtained as or more extreme values under the null hypothesis" with random assignment of exposure. In the latter condition, random error corresponds to the failure of the randomization process, for reasons of chance, to yield a balanced baseline risk across exposure groups. It is quantifiable and can be minimized by increasing the study size, unlike confounding in observational studies, which is not necessarily ameliorated as study size increases.

QUANTIFICATION OF POTENTIAL CONFOUNDING

The conceptual underpinnings of confounding concern counterfactual comparisons and exchangeability, but the focus in conducting and analyzing studies is on how much distortion confounding has produced in the measure of effect with what probability. We would like to know what the unconfounded measure is, and therefore wish to estimate how deviant the observed measure of effect is likely to be relative to that unconfounded value. Equivalently, the goal is to estimate the magnitude of confounding. If we obtain a risk ratio of 1.5 relating coffee drinking to the risk of bladder cancer, and have not made adjustments for cigarette smoking or are concerned that we have not fully adjusted for cigarette smoking, we would like to be able to estimate how much of an impact the confounding might have relative to the unknown unconfounded measure of interest. How probable is it that the unconfounded measure of the risk ratio is truly 1.4 or 1.0 or 0.7? In the context of randomized exposure assignment, the probability of obtaining an aberrant allocation of subjects can be considered equivalent to the probability of confounding of a given magnitude, and the formal tools of statistical inference have direct applicability (Greenland, 1990). In contrast, in observational studies in which exposure is not randomly allocated, this assessment is based on informed speculation, quantitative if possible, but hypothetical in nature.

To move forward in understanding, controlling, and estimating the magnitude of uncontrolled confounding, specific sources of the confounding must be hypothesized. There is little benefit to noting that exposed and unexposed groups *may* differ in baseline disease risk for unspecified reasons. While this is always true, it is of no value given that without further specification the statement just constitutes an inherent feature of observational studies and to some extent, a feature of studies in which exposure *is* randomized. Instead, the basis for the confounding must be hypothesized in measurable terms to be useful in the interpretation of potential causal associations.

The magnitude of confounding due to an extraneous variable is a function of two underlying associations, namely that of the confounding variable with exposure and the confounding variable with disease. A full algebraic description of both of these associations predicts the direction and magnitude of confounding that the extraneous variable will produce. If both associations are fully known and quantified, the confounding can be measured and removed, which is the purpose of stratified or regression analyses, in which the confounder–exposure association is eliminated.

In general, the magnitude of both the confounder–exposure and confounder–disease associations must be considered to assess the extent of confounding, not just one alone. At the extremes, however, meaningful inferences can be made based on knowledge regarding one of those associations. If there is either no confounder–exposure or no confounder–disease association present, that is, the potential confounding variable is not related to disease or it is not related to exposure, the magnitude of the other association is irrelevant: no confounding could possibly be present. If speculating about confounding factors in the smoking–lung cancer association, one might initially (and naively) ask about match carrying as a potential confounder given that it is such a strong correlate of tobacco smoking. We would find that carrying matches has no independent relation to lung cancer, however, and in the absence of an association with lung cancer, it cannot possibly be a confounder of the association between smoking and lung cancer. Similarly, there are clearly genetic factors that predispose to the development of lung cancer, but if it could be demonstrated that the distribution of those genetic factors were completely unrelated to cigarette smoking, a hypothesis to be tested empirically and not one to be casually dismissed as implausible, then the genetic factor could not confound the smoking–lung cancer association.

The other extreme case in which either the confounder–exposure or confounder–disease association yields definitive information regardless of the other is when the potential confounding variable is completely associated with exposure or disease. Regardless of the magnitude of the other association, when there is complete overlap of the confounder with exposure or disease, there is no opportunity to isolate the component of the association due to the exposure of interest from the association due to the confounding factor. In the above example, imagine that coffee drinkers were always smokers, and that the only non-coffee drinkers were never smokers. We would be unable to extricate the effect of coffee drinking from that of smoking and vice versa, even though in theory the observed association with disease may be wholly due to one or the other or partially due to both. One exposure might well confound the other but there would be no opportunity to measure or control that confounding. Similarly, if some condition is completely predictive of disease, such as exposure to asbestos and the development of asbestosis, then we cannot in practice isolate that exposure from others. We cannot answer the question, "Independent of asbestos exposure, what is the effect of cigarette smoking on the development of asbestosis?" The confounder–disease association is complete, so that we would be able to study only the combination and perhaps consider factors that modify the association.

In practice, such extreme situations of no association and complete association are rare. Potential confounding variables will more typically have some degree of association with both the exposure and the disease and the strength of those associations, taken together, determines the amount of confounding that is present. In examining the two underlying associations, the stronger association puts an upper bound on the amount of confounding that could be present and the weaker association puts a lower bound on the amount of confounding that is plausible. If one association is notably less well understood than the other, some inferences may still be possible based on estimates for the one that is known.

In practice, much of the attention focuses on the confounder–disease association, given that this association is often better understood than the confounder–exposure association. Epidemiologists typically focus on the full spectrum of potential causes of disease and less intensively on the ways in which exposures relate to one another. The strength of the confounder–disease association places an upper bound on the amount of confounding that could be present, which will reach that maximum value when the exposure and confounder are completely associated. That is, if we know that the risk ratio for the confounder and disease is 2.0, then the most distortion that the confounder could produce is a doubling of the risk. If we have no knowledge at all about the confounder–exposure association, we might infer that an observed risk ratio for exposure of 1.5 could be explained by confounding (i.e., the true risk ratio could be 1.0 with distortion due to confounding accounting for the observed increase), a risk ratio of 2.0 is unlikely to be fully explained (requiring a complete association between confounder and exposure), and a risk ratio of 2.5 could not possibly be elevated solely due to confounding.

As reflected by its dependence on two underlying associations between the potential confounding variable and disease and between the potential confounding variable and exposure, the algebraic phenomenon of confounding is *indirect* relative to the exposure and disease of interest. In contrast to misclassification or selection bias, which directly distorts the exposure or disease indicators and their association by shifting the number of observations in the cells that define the measure of effect, confounding is a step removed from exposure and disease. In order for confounding to be substantial, *both* the underlying associations, not just one of them, must be rather strong. Such situations can and do arise, but given the paucity of strong known determinants for many diseases, illustrations of strong confounding that produces spurious risk ratios on the order of 2.0 or more are not common.

The amount of confounding is expressed in terms of its quantitative impact on the exposure–disease association of interest. This confounding can be in either direction, so it is most convenient to express it in terms of the extent to which it distorts the unconfounded measure of association, regardless of whether that unconfounded value is the null, positive, or negative. Note that the importance of confounding is strictly a function of how much distortion it introduces, with no relevance whatsoever to whether the magnitude of change in the confounded compared to the unconfounded measure is statistically significant. Similarly, there is no reason to subject the confounder–exposure or confounder–disease associations to statistical tests given that statistical testing does not help in any way to evaluate whether confounding could occur, whether it has occurred, or how much of it is likely to be present. The sole question is with the magnitude, not precision, of the underlying associations.

The more relevant parameter to quantify confounding is the magnitude of deviation between the measure of association between exposure and disease with confounding present versus the same measure of association with confounding removed. We often use the null value of the association as a convenient benchmark of interest but not the only one: Given an observed association of a specified magnitude in which confounding may be present, how plausible is it that the true (unconfounded) association is the null value? We might also ask: "Given an observed null measure of association in which confounding may be present, how likely is it that the unconfounded association takes on some other specific value?" Based on previous literature or clinical or public health importance, we might also ask: "How likely it is that the unconfounded association is as great as 2.0 or as small as 1.5?"

The amount of confounding can also be expressed in terms of the *confounding risk ratio*, which is the measure of distortion it introduces. This would be the risk ratio which, when multiplied by the true (unconfounded) risk ratio would yield the observed risk ratio, i.e., RR (confounding) $\times$ RR (true) = RR (observed). If the true risk ratio were the null value of 1.0, then the observed risk ratio would be solely an indication of confounding whether above the null or below the null value. A truly positive risk ratio could be brought down to the null value or beyond, and a truly inverse risk ratio (<1.0) could be spuriously elevated to or beyond the null value. Quantitative speculation about the magnitude of confounding consists of generating estimates of RR (confounding) and the associated probabilities that those values occur.

EVALUATION OF CONFOUNDING

The assessment and control of confounding should be recognized as an effort to mitigate non-comparability through statistical adjustment for indirect markers, not as a complete solution to the problem of non-comparability of disease risk among the exposed and unexposed. When we speculate that confounding may be present, and we define the variables that are thought to serve as markers for that confounding, we are entertaining a hypothesis. The hypothesis in this case is that underlying disease risks differ between exposed and unexposed groups because a particular characteristic that is predictive of disease is associated with exposure status. When statistical adjustments are made for this hypothesized marker of confounding, we generate results that will be more valid only if the initial hypothesis was correct. If our initial hypothesis about the presence of confounding or the role of the specific variable in producing that confounding was incorrect, or the measure of the confounder is faulty, then the adjusted estimate may well be no more valid or even less valid than the unadjusted measure. Unfortunately, we have no direct way of assessing which hypothesis is correct in that the truth is unknown. Therefore, rather than viewing adjusted estimates as correct or even necessarily better than the unadjusted estimates, the plausibility of the confounding hypothesis and approach to addressing it need to be critically examined. The statistical evidence comparing unadjusted and adjusted measures of effect will not reveal the underlying phenomenon or provide information on which estimate is more valid.

Despite the somewhat speculative nature of postulating and adjusting for confounding, this approach has the virtue of providing a means of quantifying the extent of possible confounding empirically. That is, we can say that if the confounding is present, and if the confounding variable captures the phenomenon to at least some extent, then the statistically adjusted measure is closer to the correct value than the unadjusted measure. In order for a hypothesis regarding confounding to have practical value in the interpretation of epidemiologic evidence, there must be an opportunity to evaluate its implications through some form of adjustment. Some hypotheses regarding confounding are so generic as to be untestable and therefore of little value. For example, the suggestions that exposed and unexposed are inherently non-comparable or that some unknown confounding factor may be present are untestable and therefore of no value in assessing the potential for confounding to have affected the study results.

More constructive hypotheses pose specific scenarios by which confounding arises, even if those are not necessarily amenable to measurement and control. If a medication is given solely for a specific disease, and some adverse health conditions are associated with the use of that drug, confounding by indication may be present. That is, the underlying disease for which the drug was given may be responsible for the adverse health consequences that are mistakenly attributed to the drug. Even though the hypothesis is clear and the means for addressing it is clear in principle, evaluation of the hypothesized confounding requires the availability of persons who have the disease and do not receive the drug and persons who receive the drug who do not have the disease. Such persons may not actually exist. All persons with the disease may be given the drug, and only those with the disease are given the drug. If that is the case, then the evaluation of confounding by indication must be through approaches other than empirical evaluation of the data, for example, consideration of biologic mechanisms or historical evidence on the sequelae of the disease before the drug of concern became available. Even when there is not a straightforward empirical test of the hypothesized confounding by indication, the development of the scenario is useful in the scrutiny and interpretation of the results of a study of potential effects of the drug of interest.

Another challenge to addressing confounding occurs when the hypothesized confounding arises through a construct that is very difficult to measure and thus evaluate or control. If we wish to evaluate the effect of social contacts on maintenance of functional ability in the elderly, we may have concern that the underlying motivation to sustain both social and physical functioning confounds the relationship. That is, rather than social contacts directly benefiting functional ability, both are reflective of the underlying inspiration required to expend effort socially and to be self-sufficient in activities of daily living. While worthy of examination, the postulated confounding factor of motivation is very difficult to measure and isolate from the exposure and disease of concern. The scenario of confounding is worthy of consideration, but tests of the hypothesized confounding are subject to great uncertainty and unlikely to yield definitive evidence simply because the construct is so challenging to measure.

Assess Consequences of Inaccurate Confounder Measurement

The markers of confounding that are available inevitably fall short, to varying degrees, of the ideal, just as exposure measures generally do not capture precisely the construct that they were intended to measure. In seeking to measure and control for confounding factors, we look for handles on the basis for noncomparability of the unexposed and exposed groups, a challenging mission that is almost guaranteed to be less than totally successful. The groups to be compared are not naturally comparable, in which case there would be no confounding, nor has randomized exposure assignment been employed to address the problem without needing to fully understand its origins. Our goal is to measure and control for the attributes that will make these non-comparable groups as comparable as possible. Viewed in this manner, effectiveness is not measured as a dichotomy, in which we succeed in eliminating confounding completely or fail to have any beneficial impact, but should be viewed as a continuum in which we mitigate confounding to varying degrees.

The conceptual challenge is to identify those characteristics of exposed and unexposed subjects, other than exposure, which confer differing disease risks. The underlying basis for the confounding may be such elusive constructs as socioeconomic status or tendency to seek medical care. Undoubtedly, information is lost as we operationalize these constructs into measures such as level of education or engaging in preventive health behaviors. Just as for exposures of interest, something is often lost in moving from the ideal to operational measures, and although it is often difficult to quantify that loss, it is an important contributor to incomplete control of confounding. Misclassification at the level of conceptualizing and operationalizing the construct of interest dilutes the ability to control confounding through statistical adjustment.

The more familiar problems concern accuracy of measurement of the potential confounding variable and the way in which the variable is treated in the analysis, e.g., categorized versus continuous, number of categories used. Errors arise in all the ways considered in the discussion of exposure measurement (Chapter 8): clerical errors, misrepresentation on self-report, faulty instrumentation, etc. In addition, for a given confounding variable, there is an optimal way of measuring it and constructing it to maximize its association with disease, thus enhancing the extent to which confounding is controlled. If we are concerned about a confounding effect of cigarette smoking in studying exposure to air pollution and lung cancer, then we can measure tobacco smoking in a number of ways, including "ever smoked," "years of smoking," "cigarettes per day," or "pack–years of smoking." In choosing among these measures, the guiding principle is to choose the one that best predicts risk of developing lung cancer, typically "pack–years of smoking." By choosing the one most strongly related to the health outcome, adjustment would be most complete, far better than if we relied on a crude dichotomy such as "ever versus never smoked."

There are different ways the confounding variable can be handled in the statistical analysis phase, and the same goal applies: define the measure to maximize its association with disease. A measure like "pack–years of smoking" could be treated as continuous measure and included in a logistic regression model in which the relationship with disease is presumed to be log-linear. Alternatively, it could be categorized into two or more levels, with many potential cutpoints, or modeled using more flexible approaches such as spline regression (Greenland, 1995). All these options apply to assessing the exposure of primary interest as well, but for the confounding variable, the goal is to remove its effect, not necessarily to fully understand its effect.

Regardless of the underlying reasons for imperfect measurement of the sources of confounding, the effect is the same: incomplete control for the confounding that arises from the specific phenomenon it is intended to address. That is, whatever the amount of confounding that was originally present, only a fraction will be removed through the adjustment efforts and the size of that fraction is dependent on the quality of assessment (Greenland & Robins, 1985; Savitz & Barón, 1989). If a perfectly measured confounder completely adjusts for the distortion, and a fully misclassified measure is of no benefit, adjustment for an imperfectly measured confounder falls somewhere in between. The more the measure used for adjustment deviates from the ideal, the less of the confounding is eliminated. This dilution of confounder control can arise by poor selection of an operational measure, measurement error, or inappropriate choices for categorization in the analysis.

The magnitude of confounding present after attempts at adjustment depends on both the magnitude of confounding originally present and the fraction of that confounding that has been effectively controlled. Incomplete control of confounding due to imperfect assessment and measurement of the confounding variables is proportionate to the amount of confounding originally present. If the amount of original confounding was substantial, then whatever the fraction that was controlled, the amount that is not controlled, in absolute terms, may still be of great concern. On the other hand, if the amount of confounding originally present were small, which is often the case, then leaving some fraction of it uncontrolled would be of little concern in absolute terms.

Kaufman et al. (1997) provide a quantitative illustration of a common problem of inaccurate confounder measurement. There is often an interest in isolating the effects of race from the strongly associated socioeconomic factors that both differ by race and are strongly associated with many health outcomes. The goal is generally to isolate some biological differences between African Americans and whites from their socioeconomic context. The challenge, of course, is to effectively eliminate the influence of such a strong confounder despite its elusive nature, often reverting to simplistic approaches such as adjusting for education. In a simulation, Kaufman et al. (1997) illustrate four ways in which frequently applied methods of adjustment for socioeconomic status fall short of controlling confounding of racial differences. One simple one suffices to illustrate the point—residual confounding due to categorization.

Many health outcomes vary continuously by measures of socioeconomic status, so that when a dichotomous measure or even one that has several levels is used, there will be residual confounding within strata. This problem is exacerbated in the case of racial comparisons when the mean levels are markedly different in the two groups and no single cutpoint will do justice to the two disparate distributions. In a series of simulations, the slope of the effect of education on disease was varied from −0.10 to −1.00 (on a log scale) in a logistic regression model using a realistic estimate of the difference in years of education between African Americans and whites (Table 7.1). In each case, the crude difference showed excess risk among African Americans solely as a result of socioeconomic differences, and the mean adjusted relative risk was also elevated, despite adjusting for a dichotomous measure of education. Note that adjustment for a continuous measure of education would have eliminated the effect of race entirely in this simulation. In most cases, the adjusted measure of African American/white differences was positive, and attenuated but not eliminated by the attempt at adjustment for education.

Measures of confounding, unless completely lacking in value, also provide some insight regarding the nature of the confounding that is likely to be present and help to estimate the unconfounded measure of effect. Statistical adjustments for markers of confounding, while known not to fully capture all confounding that is present, provide information for extrapolation to what the true measure of effect might be if confounding could be fully eliminated. By noting the direction

TABLE 7.1. The Spurious Association of African American Race with "Disease" Owing to Categorization Bias in the Exposure Variable: Results for Simulations with 1000 African Americans, 1000 Whites*

β	MEAN CRUDE OR FOR AFRICAN AMERICAN RACE[†]	MEAN ADJUSTED OR FOR AFRICAN AMERICAN RACE[‡]	REPETITIONS WITH OR ≥ 1.0 (%)[§]
−0.10	1.07	1.03	60
−0.20	1.13	1.05	70
−0.30	1.19	1.07	74
−0.40	1.27	1.09	81
−0.50	1.33	1.11	86
−0.60	1.40	1.13	90
−0.70	1.47	1.16	92
−0.80	1.53	1.18	94
−0.90	1.59	1.19	96
−1.00	1.65	1.21	97

*"Disease" generated randomly as: $p(d) = \dfrac{e^{(\beta z)}}{1 + e^{(\beta z)}}$ 1000 repetitions at each β; $Z_{white} \sim N(0.30, 1)$ and $Z_{\text{African-American}} \sim N(-0.30, 1)$, representing "education."

[†]From the model: logit(disease) $= \alpha + \beta_1 race + \epsilon$, where race is coded 1 = African-American, 0 = white.

[‡]From the model: logit(disease) $= \alpha + \beta_1 education + \beta_2 race + \epsilon$, where education is dichotomized at $Z \geq 0$ and race is coded 1 = African-American, 0 = white.

[§]The percentage of replications with adjusted odds ratios for African-American ≥ 1.0.

OR, odds ratio.

Kaufman et al., 1997.

of movement resulting from statistical adjustment, the direction of the confounding can be discerned and it can be predicted that better measures would move the measure of effect farther in the direction that the imperfect proxy has suggested. If adjustment for the proxy moved the measure of effect upward, then more complete adjustment would be expected to move it further upward, and similarly if the adjustment for the proxy moved the measure of effect downward. If there were no change whatsoever resulting from the proxy measure, then either there is no confounding present from the phenomenon that the proxy is intended to reflect, or the proxy is so poorly reflective of the phenomenon of interest to make it useless as a marker.

Some inferences can also be made based on what adjustment for the proxy measure of confounding did *not* do. For a specific source of confounding, if adjustment for the proxy measure moves the effect estimate in one direction, it is very unlikely that a more optimal measure of that source of confounding would move the effect estimate in the opposite direction. If the crude risk ratio were 2.0 and the adjusted risk ratio using an imperfect confounder marker were 1.8, then fully adjusted values of *greater* than 2.0 are unlikely. Fully adjusted values of 1.7 or even 1.5 may be quite plausible, however, given that it would require only more movement in the direction suggested by the proxy.

Techniques are available to estimate how much confounding is likely to remain based on the magnitude of change in the measure of effect resulting from adjustment using the available (imperfect) measure of the confounder (Savitz & Barón, 1989). Comparison of the unadjusted and partially adjusted measures, combined with an estimate of the extent of confounder misclassification, conveys useful information to assess how much confounding is likely to remain. If there is substantial change in the measure of effect from controlling a marker of confounding, and the measure is likely to be far from optimal, the amount of remaining confounding is likely to be substantial. If the measure is already quite good, then little residual confounding will be present. If the measure is only fair but the change in the measure of effect from adjustment for the exposure of interest is modest, then the amount of confounding remaining after adjustment is likely to be small.

Quantitative speculation is also possible, with an array of assumptions required to do so (Savitz & Barón, 1989). Quantification of the magnitude of change in the measure of effect due to adjusting for the imperfectly captured confounding variable, combined with assumptions about the quality of the measure of the confounding factor relative to an ideal measure of the source of confounding, provide the basis for estimating the fully adjusted association that would have been obtained had the confounding variable been measured perfectly. In simple terms, if adjustment for an imperfect marker causes a substantial shift in the measure of effect, then the additional shift that would result from improved measurement of the confounding factor may be substantial. In the above illustration in which the unadjusted risk ratio was 2.0, consider two situations: in one, adjustment for a marker of confounding yields a risk ratio of 1.8, in the other instance, adjustment yields a risk ratio of 1.4. If asked to make an assessment of how likely it is that a fully adjusted risk ratio would be at or close to the null value, it is more plausible in the second than the first scenario. That is, an imperfectly measured confounder that yields an adjusted risk ratio of 1.4 compared to the crude value of 2.0 indicates a more substantial amount of confounding than if the adjustment had yielded an adjusted risk ratio of 1.8, assuming that the quality of measurement is roughly comparable.

An illustration of this concern arises in assessing a potentially beneficial impact of barrier contraception on the risk of pelvic inflammatory disease, which can result in subsequent infertility. A potential confounding effect of sexually transmitted disease history must be considered, given that choice of contraception may well be related to risk of acquiring a sexually transmitted infection, and such infections are strong determinants of the risk of pelvic inflammatory disease. Virtually all approaches to measuring sexually transmitted infection are incomplete, with self-report known to be somewhat inaccurate, but even biologic measures are subject to uncertainty because they can only reflect prevalence at a given point in time. Assume we have obtained self-reported information on sexually transmitted diseases to be evaluated as a potential confounder of the barrier contraception—pelvic inflammatory disease association. Further assume that the unadjusted measure of association shows an inverse association with a risk ratio of 0.5. If adjustment for self-reported sexually transmitted diseases increased the risk ratio to only 0.6, we might argue that even with a perfect measure of sexually transmitted diseases, the adjustment would be unlikely to go all the way to the null value and perhaps 0.7 or 0.8 is the more accurate measure of association. On the other hand, if the adjusted measure rose from 0.5 to 0.8, we might infer that a more complete adjustment could well yield a risk ratio at or very close to 1.0. Insight into the quality of the confounder measure (often known in qualitative if not quantitative terms), unadjusted measure, and partially adjusted measure (always available) helps to assess the extent of incompleteness in the control of confounding and generate an estimate of what the (unknown) fully adjusted measure would be.

The ideal marker of confounding is presumed not to be available, because if it were, it would be used in preference to any speculation about residual confounding from suboptimal measures. There is often the option of examining confounders of varying quality within the range available, however, which would allow for assessing the impact of adjustment using markers of varying quality. The impact of successive refinements in control of a particular source of confounding can be informative in estimating what impact full adjustment would have, as described for exposure measures more generally in Chapter 8. No adjustment at all corresponds to a useless marker of confounding, and as the marker gets better and better, more and more of the confounding is controlled, helping to extrapolate to what the gold standard measure would accomplish.

For this reason, the opportunity to scrutinize unadjusted and adjusted measures is critical to assessing the extent to which confounding has been controlled. Merely providing the results of a multivariate analysis, without being able to assess what effect the adjustment for confounding variables had, limits the reader's ability to fully consider the amount of residual confounding that is likely to be present. As noted above, an adjusted risk ratio of 1.4 has a different interpretation if the crude measure was 2.0 and control of confounding is likely to be incomplete than if the crude measure were 1.5, and important potential confounders have been well controlled and properly analyzed. Even if the adjusted measure is conceded to be the best available, some attention needs to be paid to the source and pattern of any confounding that has been removed.

Apply Knowledge of Confounding Based on Other Studies

Although a specific confounding variable may not have been measured or not measured well in a particular study, there may be other similar research that can help to assess the potential for confounding. Previous research may provide a basis for judging whether the required confounder–exposure and confounder–disease associations are likely to be present, and even suggest the direction and magnitude of confounding that is likely to result from those associations. Alternatively, previous studies of the same exposure–disease association may have obtained relevant data on potential confounding variables and generated estimates of the magnitude of change in the effect estimate resulting from controlling confounding factors. If, for example, in previous studies of the exposure–disease association of interest, careful measurement and adjustment for the potential confounding factor had no impact, then concern with the failure to measure and inability to adjust for that factor in a given study would be diminished.

Extrapolation of results from one study to another carries a risk as well. The underlying basis for the associations of interest must be considered in order to judge whether relations found in one study would apply in other studies. Some exposures are associated with one another for largely sociological or cultural reasons, and such relations could not necessarily be extrapolated from one study population to another. Foundry workers in the United States who are exposed to silica may tend to be heavy cigarette smokers but extrapolation of that observation to assess potential for confounding in a study of silica exposure and lung cancer among Korean foundry workers would be tenuous. There is no biological basis for the confounding observed in the United States, driven by the higher smoking prevalence among blue-collar workers, to apply elsewhere. In some developing countries, smoking may be concentrated among the higher social classes or unrelated to social class.

In other cases, the basis for potential confounding is much more likely to be universal, and thus be more readily extrapolated from one study to another. If we are interested in the effect of one dietary constituent found in fruits and vegetables, for example, beta carotene, and concerned about confounding from other micronutrients found in fruits and vegetables, for example, vitamin C, the potential for confounding would be more universal. That is, if the same food products tend to contain multiple constituents or if people who consume one type of fruit or vegetable tend to consume others, then the amount and direction of confounding observed in one study may be applied to other studies.

The information on confounder–disease associations will more often be generalizable from one study to another to the extent that it reflects a basic biological link given that such relations are more likely to apply broadly. Once an association has been firmly established in a set of studies, it is reasonable to assume that the association would be observed in other populations unless known effect-modifiers are operative to suggest the contrary. We can safely assume, for example, that cigarette smoking will be related to risk of lung cancer in all populations, so that in seeking to isolate other causes of lung cancer, confounding by tobacco use will be a concern.

If attempts to identify and control confounding fail to influence the measure of effect, despite a strong empirical basis for believing that confounding should be present, concerns arise about whether the study has successfully measured the confounding variable of interest. In the above example of silica exposure and lung cancer, if we attempted to measure cigarette smoking and found it to be unrelated to risk of lung cancer, and thus not a source of confounding, we should question whether cigarette smoking had truly been measured and controlled. The strategies for evaluating potential exposure misclassification (Chapter 8) apply directly to confounding factors, which are just exposures other than those of primary interest.

To illustrate, when Wertheimer and Leeper (1979) first reported an association between residential proximity to sources of magnetic field exposure and childhood cancer, one of the challenges to a causal interpretation of the association was the potential for confounding. Because they had relied on public records, there was no opportunity to interview the parents and assess a wide range of potential confounding factors such as parental tobacco use, medications taken during pregnancy, and child's diet. When a study of the same exposure–disease association in the same community was undertaken roughly a decade later (Savitz et al., 1988), it included extensive consideration of potential confounding factors, and found essentially no indications of confounding. Although it is theoretically possible that undetected confounding due to those factors was present in the earlier study, the later study makes that possibility far less likely. That does not negate the possibility that both studies suffer from confounding by as yet undiscovered risk factors for those cancers, but at least the usual suspects are less of a concern in the earlier study based on the results of the latter study.

Ye et al. (2002) provide a quantitative illustration of the examination of confounding using evidence from previous studies. In a cohort study of alcohol abuse and the risk of developing pancreatic cancer in the Swedish Inpatient Register, information on smoking, a known risk factor for pancreatic cancer, was not available. The investigators applied indirect methods using the observed association found for alcohol use (relative risk of 1.4). By assuming a relative risk for current smoking and pancreatic cancer of 2.0, 80% prevalence of smoking among alcoholics and 30% in the general population of Sweden, a true relative risk of 1.0 for alcohol use would rise to 1.4 solely from confounding by smoking. That is, "The observed excess risk in our alcoholics without complications may be almost totally attributable to the confounding effect of smoking." (Ye et al., 2002, p. 238). Although this may not be as persuasive as having measured smoking in their study and adjusting for it directly, the exercise provides valuable information to help interpret their findings with some appreciation of the potential for the role of confounding.

To make appropriate use of information on confounding in studies other than the one being evaluated, the phenomenon occurring in the other studies needs to be fully understood. The ability to extrapolate the relations between the confounder and both exposure and disease should be carefully considered before asserting that the presence or absence of confounding in one study has direct implications for another study. If the study settings are sociologically similar and the study structures are comparable, such extrapolation may well be helpful in making an informed judgment. Extrapolation is not a substitute for measurement and control of confounding in the study itself, but speculation informed by previous research can be far superior to speculation without such guidance.

Assessing Confounding When Risk Factors Are Unknown

One of the most challenging situations for speculation about confounding arises when the risk factors for disease are largely unknown. Absence of known risk factors can give a false sense of security that there is freedom from confounding, but the inability to specify *confounding variables* does not protect against *confounding*. Something, as yet unidentified, is clearly causing the disease to occur, and just because those influences are currently unknown does not guard against their ability to introduce confounding. Inability to address the issue does not imply the issue is unimportant.

The available options for evaluation and control of confounding are limited when causes, and thus potential confounding factors, are largely unknown. Broad markers of exposure that often predict health and disease can be assessed, such as age, geographic region, social class, and occupation. None are direct causes, in that they are only markers of underlying etiologic relations. Geography per se does not cause disease, though it may enhance the probability of exposure to an infectious agent, and low income does not cause disease, though it can affect availability of certain foods that prevent disease. Given that these are intentionally non-specific indicators of many potential exposures, and imperfectly reflective of any one exposure, underlying confounding by specific exposures will not be fully controlled. Nevertheless, some insight would be gained regarding the potential for substantial confounding to be present based on these broad proxy measures.

Hypothetical scenarios can be described, indicating the strength of association between the confounder, exposure, and disease required to yield various alternative measures of effect, in the same manner as described above for imperfectly measured confounders. That is, the general marker can be viewed as a proxy confounder measure, and various candidate gold standard measures might be considered to ask about how much confounding may yet remain. As discussed previously, if control for the non-specific marker has no impact whatsoever, none of the exposures it reflects are likely to have an impact, whereas if it does change the measure of effect, we would expect that a sharper focus on the pertinent exposure would yield a more sizable change in the effect measure.

The danger of failing to control for true confounding factors in the face of ignorance is a threat, but also there is a danger of controlling for anything that happens to be measured if such adjustment changes the association of interest. When little is known about the causes of a particular disease, unnecessary adjustment for a broad range of factors that are not truly confounders results in a loss of precision under the assumption that the relations found reflect only random processes (Day et al., 1980). Moreover, if only those factors that reduce the association of interest are selected for adjustment, there will be bias toward the null value even when all associations are the product of random error (Day et al., 1980). When a lengthy list of candidate factors is screened for confounding, without adequate attention to the plausibility of their having an association with the health outcome based on mechanistic considerations and findings of prior studies, there is a danger of finding associations by chance and producing an adjusted effect estimate that is more rather than less biased than the unadjusted one.

Dose-Response Gradients and Potential for Confounding

It is possible for confounding to spuriously generate or mask a dose-response gradient, not just to produce distortion of measures based on dichotomized exposure indicators. When the confounding factor is associated with disease, and it is also associated with the exposure of interest in a stepwise fashion, then the amount of confounding will differ across levels of exposure. Assuming that the confounding variable is positively associated with the exposure, then more confounding will be present at higher as compared to lower levels of exposure generating the appearance of a dose-response gradient between the exposure of interest and the health outcome. Instead of simply asking if the exposure is associated with the confounding factor, we need to ask whether they are associated in a dose-response pattern.

Depending on the reasons for the exposure–confounder association, confounding that exaggerates or masks dose-response gradients may require increasingly implausible scenarios. For example, in the case of silica exposure and lung cancer being confounded by cigarette smoking, a global comparison of foundry workers and the general population may suffer from positive confounding if cigarette smoking is not carefully controlled. On the other hand, assume we now have information on levels of silica exposure, based on job activity and years of employment. The hypothesis that those individuals who have accrued greater amounts of silica exposure are heavier smokers, accounting for age, seems less plausible. That is, the sociological basis for foundry workers being more likely to smoke does not extend to an expectation that more heavily exposed foundry workers would be more likely to smoke than less heavily exposed foundry workers. The association of smoking with exposure only applies to employment in the foundry versus other types of work, not to the specific work location and job tasks within the foundry.

On the other hand, if the confounding is more tightly linked to the exposure itself, such as foods sharing multiple constituents that could confound one another, then it is likely that those who accumulate higher levels of one nutrient will consistently accumulate higher levels of another across the exposure spectrum. It may be difficult to obtain high levels of beta-carotene from fruits and vegetables without also obtaining large amounts of fiber and various micronutrients. The very source of exposure guarantees that confounding will follow a dose-response gradient.

The substantive knowledge of the reason for the confounder–exposure association demands closer evaluation and understanding than it typically receives from epidemiologists. We have to ask why smoking is associated with foundry work, at least to the extent that such understanding helps us assess whether the relationship is likely to extend to subgroups of foundry workers who differ in silica exposure. Unlike the confounder–disease association, which is of direct interest to epidemiologists and thus for which there is likely to be a relevant scientific literature, the confounder–exposure association is not of direct interest to epidemiologists. An understanding of *why* exposures are associated and the pattern of that association, however, would help markedly in anticipating, eliminating, and evaluating confounding.

An example showing that in some instances, the confounding factor may be associated in a dose-response fashion with the exposure of interest, is offered by coffee consumption and cigarette smoking in relation to cancer. Unlike the hypothetical example of a workplace association with smoking, the correlation *among* lifestyle factors has the potential to be much stronger and dose dependent. Stensvold and Jacobsen (1994) conducted a large prospective cohort study in Norway focused on the potential association between coffee drinking and cancer incidence. Over 43,000 men and women were given a questionnaire (self-administered) that included amount of coffee consumed and number of cigarettes smoked per day in addition to a range of other factors. The incidence of cancer over the subsequent 10-year period was evaluated.

Recognizing the strong potential for confounding of the coffee–cancer association by cigarette smoking, the authors presented data on the relationship between coffee consumption and smoking (Table 7.2). For both men and women, the probability of smoking daily rose steadily across levels of coffee consumption, and among smokers, the number of cigarettes smoked per day rose steadily across levels of coffee consumption. Given this pattern, it is not surprising that without adjustment for cigarette smoking, a gradient was observed for coffee consumption and total cancers as well as for smoking-related cancers. Across the coffee dose groups presented in Table 7.2, the relative risks of total cancer among men were 1.0 (referent), 1.08, 1.05, and 1.24. After adjustment for cigarettes per day, age, and county of residence, the relative risks were 1.0 (referent), 1.04, 0.96, and 0.99. For lung cancer, the relative risks prior to adjustment for smoking were 1.0 (referent group including < 5 cups/day), 1.6, and 4.1, whereas after adjustment, the relative risks for the upper two groups were 1.4 and 2.4, attenuated but still clearly elevated. For lung cancer, this may be reflective of residual confounding or perhaps a true effect of coffee consumption.

INTEGRATED ASSESSMENT OF POTENTIAL CONFOUNDING

In order to evaluate the extent to which confounding may have biased the results of an epidemiologic study, the conceptual basis for confounding must first be examined. The question of exchangeability of exposed and unexposed needs to be posed for the specific research question under consideration: Do nonsmokers have the risk of lung cancer that smokers would have had if they had not smoked? Do women with low levels of calcium intake have the same risk of osteoporosis that women with high levels of calcium intake would have had if their intakes had been low? This question, posed in the grammatically awkward but technically correct counterfactual manner serves to focus interest on the phenomenon of confounding rather than available covariates, which are at best, a means of addressing and mitigating the lack of comparability of the groups. The goal is not to achieve statistical control of covariates or to consider the longest possible list of potential confounders but rather to reduce or eliminate confounding. In some instances, there is little or no confounding present, or the confounding is readily addressed

TABLE 7.2. Characteristics of the Study Population According to Their Consumption of Coffee, Norway

| | Coffee Consumption, Cups per Day | | | | | | | |
| | Men | | | | Women | | | |
	≤ 2	3–4	5–6	≥ 7	≤ 2	3–4	5–6	≥ 7
Number at risk	2855	5599	6528	6753	2648	7350	6820	4420
Age (years)	45.9	46.5	46.2	45.1	46.0	46.5	45.9	44.9
Menopause (% yes)					27	30	27	24
Body mass index (g/cm²)	2.54	2.55	2.55	2.54	2.46	2.50	2.50	2.50
Smoke daily (% yes)	23	33	47	66	17	23	38	57
No. of cigarettes per day (among cigarette smokers)	11.5	11.6	12.6	15.5	9.1	8.6	9.8	12.1
Total cholesterol (mmol/l)	5.95	6.20	6.29	6.47	6.01	6.19	6.27	6.37
Triglycerides (mmol/l)	2.17	2.21	2.13	2.07	1.50	1.47	1.48	1.47
Physical inactivity (% sedentary)	15	14	15	20	17	15	17	22
History of cardiovascular disease and/or diabetes (% yes)	11	11	10	8	11	10	9	8
Beer consumption in an ordinary week (% yes)	27	25	25	26	8	7	6	6
Wine/liquor consumption in an ordinary week (% yes)	26	28	27	32	11	10	12	13
Residence (% in Finnmark)	12	16	24	43	15	18	25	41

Stensvold & Jacobsen, 1994.

with one or two markers, and in other instances, even a comprehensive effort with many potential confounders measured and adjusted will fall far short. By focusing on the conceptual basis for confounding, attention to confounding is less likely to be mistaken for elimination of confounding.

With the question clearly in mind regarding exchangeability, and reason to believe that the exposed and unexposed groups are not exchangeable, the next step is to consider what attributes may serve as markers of the basis for non-exchangeability. That is, if there is reason for concern about confounding in comparing exposed and unexposed, what are the underlying reasons for that confounding? Are the groups likely to differ in behaviors that go along with the one under investigation? Might the groups tend to interpret symptoms differently and have differential access to medical care? To the extent that the source of the confounding can be identified, it can be addressed through statistical methods. Again, the question is not "What variables are available to examine for their effect on the exposure–disease association?" but rather "What are the disease determinants which may make the exposed and unexposed non-exchangeable?"

Having identified the factors that are thought to generate the confounding, we now have to take on the challenge of measuring those factors for purposes of statistical control. Some sources of confounding are more easily measured than others due to the clarity of the concept and accessibility of information. An assessment of the effectiveness with which the construct of interest has been captured is helpful in addressing the question of how effectively that source of confounding has been controlled. Referring back to the underlying phenomenon of confounding, the availability and quality of markers should be contrasted with the ideal set of markers one would like to have available to control this source of confounding. If we are concerned with confounding by social class, and have data only on education, and none on income, occupation, wealth, etc., then we must acknowledge and contend with the inherent shortcoming in our control for confounding by social class. The potential for incomplete control of confounding draws upon substantive knowledge of the phenomenon, but also can be assessed to some extent within the available data. The change in the measure of effect resulting from the adjustment process can help in estimating what the measure of effect would have been had adjustment been complete.

Once candidate confounders have been operationalized and measured, the impact of statistical adjustment on the exposure–disease association can be assessed. Note again how many considerations arise prior to this point in the evaluation, all emanating from the concept of non-exchangeability. Errors in reasoning or measurement between the concept and the covariate will diminish or negate the effectiveness of control of confounding. Making statistical adjustments for confounding is an exercise, a form of sensitivity analysis, in that new information is generated to help in understanding the data and evaluating the hypothesis of interest. In order for the adjusted measure of effect to be superior to the unadjusted measure, a chain of assumptions about the phenomenon of confounding is required. If the marker of confounding is very poorly measured, there may be little effect of adjustment, with little impact on whatever confounding effect was originally present. On the other hand, the adjustment may have an influence on the measure of effect, but the adjusted estimate is not more valid than the unadjusted estimate. Errors in logic or implementation will not be revealed through the adjustment process or through scrutiny of the results that are generated. The adjusted results must be used to help interpret the presence, direction, and amount of confounding, but they do not necessarily eliminate the problem.

Hypotheses regarding confounding are subject to criticism and evaluation, just as hypotheses of causality are. The evidence tending to support or refute the hypothesis of confounding is derived through the conventional tools applied to observational data. Regardless of how thorough and careful that evaluation may be, uncontrolled confounding remains a candidate hypothesis to explain an observed association or lack of association. It is important, however, to consider the continuum of evidence in support of the hypothesized confounding. All observational studies, by their very nature, are vulnerable to confounding, but invoking exposure correlates that are unrelated to disease or risk factors for disease that are not related to exposure provides no support for the presence of confounding. Those who would put forward the hypothesis that confounding has influenced study results need to develop the logical and empirical basis to suggest that it is present. The more quantitative and testable the hypothesis of confounding can be made, the more effectively it can be addressed and confirmed or refuted in subsequent research.

REFERENCES

Day NE, Byar DP, Green SB. Overadjustment in case-control studies. Am J Epidemiol 1980;112:696–706.
Greenland S. Randomization, statistics, and causal inference. Epidemiology 1990;1: 421–429.
Greenland S. Dose-response and trend analysis in epidemiology: alternatives to categorical analysis. Epidemiology 1995;6:356–365.
Greenland S, Robins JM. Confounding and misclassification. Am J Epidemiol 1985; 122:495–506.
Greenland S, Robins JM. Identifiability, exchangeability, and epidemiologic confounding. Int J Epidemiol 1986;15:413–419.
Kaufman JS, Cooper RS, McGee DL. Socioeconomic status and health in blacks and whites: the problem of residual confounding and the resiliency of race. Epidemiology 1997;8:621–628.
Last JM. A Dictionary of Epidemiology, Fourth Edition. New York: Oxford University Press, 2001:37–38.

Savitz DA, Barón AE. Estimating and correcting for confounder misclassification. Am J Epidemiol 1989;129:1062–1071.

Savitz DA, Wachtel H, Barnes FA, John EM, Tvrdik JG. Case-control study of childhood cancer and exposure to 60-Hz magnetic fields. Am J Epidemiol 1988;128:21–38.

Stensvold I, Jacobsen BK. Coffee and cancer: a prospective study of 43,000 Norwegian men and women. Cancer Causes Control 1994;5:401–408.

Wertheimer N, Leeper E. Electrical wiring configurations and childhood cancer. Am J Epidemiol 1979;198:273–284.

Ye W, Lagergren J, Weiderpass E, Nyrén O, Adami H-O, Ekbom A. Alcohol abuse and the risk of pancreatic cancer. Gut 2002;51:236–239.

8

MEASUREMENT AND CLASSIFICATION
OF EXPOSURE

Many of the concepts and much of the algebra of misclassification are applicable to assessing and interpreting errors in exposure and disease misclassification. Differences arise based on the structure of epidemiologic studies, which are designed to assess the impact of exposure on the development of disease and not the reverse. Also, the sources of error and the ways in which disease and exposure are assessed tend to be quite different, and thus the mechanisms by which errors arise are different as well. Health care access, a determinant of diagnosis of disease, does not correspond directly to exposure assessment, for example. Health and disease, not exposure, are the focal points of epidemiology, so that measurement of exposure is driven by its relevance to health. The degree of interest in an exposure rises or falls as the possibility of having an influence on health evolves, whereas the disease is an event with which we are inherently concerned, whether or not a particular exposure is or is not found to affect it. Once an exposure has been clearly linked to disease, e.g., tobacco or asbestos, then it becomes a legitimate target of epidemiologic inquiry even in isolation from studies of its health impact.

The range of exposures of interest is as broad, perhaps even broader, than the spectrum of health outcomes. Exposure, as defined here, includes exogenous agents such as drugs, diet, and pollutants. It also includes genetic attributes that affect ability to metabolize specific compounds; stable attributes such as height or hair color; physiologic characteristics such as blood pressure; behaviors such as physical exercise; mental states such as stress or depression; the social environment, including poverty and discrimination; and participation in health care, such as disease screening and receipt of immunizations. As a consequence of this remarkable range of interests that fall within the scope of epidemiology, there is a corresponding diversity of methods for measuring exposure (Armstrong et al., 1992). Tools include biological assessment based on specimens of blood or urine, physical observation, assessment of the social and physical environment, review of paper or computerized records and a broad array of tools based on self-report and recall, including instruments to evaluate stress, diet, and tobacco use. The distinctive features of the exposure of interest pose specific challenges to accurate measurement, and thus there are many different strategies for evaluating exposure accuracy and misclassification. Nevertheless, some generic principles or questions can be described.

IDEAL VERSUS OPERATIONAL MEASURES OF EXPOSURE

The accuracy of an operational approach to exposure ascertainment is best defined in relation to the ideal measure, which would often if not always be impractical or unethical to obtain. If we are interested in alcohol intake, for example, we might wish to have an exact measure of the ounces of ethanol ingested over the individual's entire life. We may have a particular interest in when the exposure occurred, e.g., total ethanol ingested in the 10-year period prior to disease occurrence or total ethanol ingested from ages 30 to 39. Additional details of exposure might be important, for example, number of occasions at which five or more ounces of ethanol was ingested in a two-hour period. Establishing the benchmark of validity, preferably in specific, quantitative terms, is useful in evaluating how closely we are able to approximate that ideal, and conversely, in identifying sources and magnitude of distortion relative to that ideal measure. Epidemiologists often set modest, practical benchmarks for what is desired, confusing feasible goals with ideal goals, rather than seeking ways to overcome logistical constraints to better approximate the measure that is of real interest. Even in validation studies, in which a more intensive method of assessment can be applied to a subset of study participants, the comparison is usually between an inferior and superior method, not with the ideal measure.

Biologically Effective Exposure

Assuming the goal of the research is to understand the etiologic relationship between exposure and disease, the biological process by which exposure might cause disease is central to defining the ideal exposure indicator. All of the other

issues considered below are really just amplifications of this basic goal—
measure the exposure that is most pertinent to the etiology of the disease of interest. Though such a strategy may be obvious for exposures to chemicals or
viruses, it is equally applicable to psychological or social conditions that may influence the occurrence of disease. The overriding goal is to approximate the exposure measure that contributes to the specific etiologic process under investigation. Of course, in many if not all situations, the mechanisms of disease
causation will not be understood sufficiently to define the exact way in which
exposure may influence disease, but intelligent guesses should be within reach,
resulting in a range of hypothesized etiologic pathways that can be articulated to
define clearly the goals of exposure assessment.

In evaluating an exogenous agent such as exposure to DDT/DDE in the causation of breast cancer, we might begin by delineating the cascade leading from
exposure to disease: The use of DDT for pesticide control leads to persistent environmental contamination, which leads to absorption and persistence in the body,
which leads to a biological response that may affect the risk of developing breast
cancer. Residues of DDT and its degradation product, DDE, are ubiquitous in
the soil due to historical use and persistent contamination.

One option for an exposure measure would be average DDT/DDE levels in
the county of current residence. Obviously, this is an indirect measure of exposure: county averages may not apply directly to environmental levels where the
individual lives and works; the individuals of interest may not have always lived
in the county in which they resided at the time of their participation in the study;
and the present levels of contamination in the environment are likely to have differed in the past. For these reasons, this measure of environmental contamination is not likely to approximate individual exposure levels very accurately. Refinements in spatial resolution to finer geographic levels and incorporation of
individual residential history and historical levels of contamination in the area
would move us closer to the desired measure of exposure. Note that if our goal
was defined solely as the accurate characterization of the county's average exposure in the year 1995, we could carefully sample the environment, ensure that
the laboratory equipment for measuring DDT and DDE in soil samples was as
accurate as possible, and employ statistical methods that are optimal for characterizing the geographic area appropriately. Nevertheless, without consideration
of historical changes, residential changes, and individual behaviors that influence
exposure and excretion, even the perfect geographic descriptor will not necessarily provide a valuable indicator of the individual biologically effective exposure. Accuracy must be defined in relation to a specific benchmark.

Measurement of present-day blood levels of DDT/DDE in women with breast
cancer and suitably selected controls would reflect absorption and excretion over
a lifetime, integrating over the many subtle behavioral determinants of contact
with contaminated soil, food, water, and air, and better reflecting the dose that

has the potential to affect development of cancer. The temporal aspects of exposure relevant to disease etiology must still be considered, encouraging us to evaluate what the ideal measure would be. Perhaps the ideal measure would be a profile, over time, of DDT/DDE levels in breast tissue from puberty to the time of diagnosis, or over some more circumscribed period in that window, e.g., the interval 5–15 years past or the interval prior to first birth. By hypothesizing what the biologically effective exposure measure would be, we could evaluate conceptually, and to some extent empirically, the quality of our chosen measure of current serum level. Research can examine how closely serum measures generally correspond to levels in breast tissue. Archived serum specimens from the distant past can be examined to determine how past levels correspond to current levels and what factors influence the degree of concordance over time. If our only goal were to accurately measure the existing serum DDT/DDE levels, a necessary but not sufficient criterion for the desired measure, then we need only ensure that the laboratory techniques are suitable. As important as the technical accuracy of the chosen measure may be, the loss of information is often substantial in going from the correctly ascertained exposure to the conceptually optimal measure.

Defining the ideal exposure marker requires a focus on the exposure characteristics that have the greatest potential for having a biologic influence on the etiology of the disease. Often, exposure has many features of potential relevance, such as timing, intensity, duration, and the specific agents from within a group that require decisions and hypotheses regarding the biologically relevant form. As one moves outward from that unknown, biologically relevant form of exposure, and incorporates sources of variability in exposure that are not relevant to disease etiology, there is a loss of information that will tend to reduce the strength of association with disease. Assuming DDT in breast tissue in the interval 5–15 years past was capable of causing cancer, the association with DDT in present-day serum would be somewhat weaker because present-day levels would correlate imperfectly with integrated exposure over the desired time period. The association with DDT in the environment would be weaker still for the reasons noted previously. The quality of these surrogate measures, which epidemiologic studies *always* rely on to one degree or another, affects the ability to identify causes of disease. We are still able to make progress in identifying causes of disease even when we measure some aspect of exposure other than the ideal, but only if the measure we choose is strongly correlated with the right measure and the underlying association is sufficiently strong to be identifiable despite this shortcoming. We will observe some diluted measure of association, with the magnitude of dilution dependent on the degree of correlation between the ideal and actual values (Lagakos, 1988). If the ideal exposure measure is strongly related to disease, we may take comfort in still being able to observe some modest effect of a surrogate indicator of exposure on disease, but if the true relationship is weak, the effect may fall below a level at which it can be detected at all.

As biological markers become increasingly diverse and accessible, there can be confusion regarding where a refined exposure marker ends and an early disease marker begins. Indicators of a biological interaction between the exposure and target tissue, e.g., formation of DNA adducts, illustrate exposure biomarkers that come very close to a biologic response relevant to, if not part of, the process of disease causation. Biological changes indicative of early breast cancer would, empirically, be even more closely related to risk of clinical breast cancer than the most refined measure of exposure to DDT, but such events are increasingly removed from the environmental source and not directly amenable to intervention or prevention. Each step in the cascade from environmental agent to clinical disease is of scientific interest and therefore worthy of elucidation, but the conceptual distinction between exposure and disease needs to be retained for considering measures to alter exposure to reduce risk of disease.

Temporally Relevant Exposure

The timing of exposure relative to disease occurrence is among the most underappreciated aspects of exposure assessment and thus merits special emphasis. Some exposures are constant over time, such as genetic constitution or attributes defined at birth. However, exogenous exposures such as diet, medication use, social circumstances, and chemical pollutants vary over time, often substantially. Any choice of exposure measure implicitly or explicitly includes an assumption about the exposure interval that is relevant to disease etiology. The critical time window may be based on calendar time, age at exposure, or exposure relative to the occurrence of other exposures or events (Rothman, 1981). A corollary to the need to isolate the biologically relevant exposure is to pinpoint the etiologically relevant time window of exposure so that we can ignore etiologically irrelevant exposure that occurs outside that window. Inclusion of irrelevant exposure constitutes exposure misclassification relative to the ideal measure.

In examining the role of cigarette smoking in the causation of lung cancer, for example, we recognize that there is some interval between exposure and the occurrence of disease that is not relevant to its causation. The number of cigarettes smoked on the day of diagnosis is clearly not relevant, for example, nor are the cigarettes smoked during the period in which the tumor was present but undiagnosed. Under some hypothesized mechanisms, the exposure for months or years prior to the diagnosis may be irrelevant. In the face of such uncertainty, Rothman (1981) has argued for flexibility in evaluating temporal aspects of exposure. A series of reasoned hypotheses may be put forward based on alternative theories about disease causation.

In some instances, different timing of exposure corresponds to entirely different etiologic pathways. The role of physical exertion in relation to myocardial infarction appears to include an acute adverse effect, such that intense exertion is followed by some relatively brief period of increased risk (Siscovick et al., 1984; Albert et al., 2000), as well as a chronic beneficial effect, such that regular exercise over periods of months or years reduces risk of a myocardial infarction (Rockhill et al., 2001). The timing of the intense activity levels relative to the long-term history of activity may also be relevant, with a change from long-term inactivity to a higher level of activity a possible threat to health. Any attempt to measure physical activity in order to evaluate its association with risk of myocardial infarction would require carefully formulated etiologic hypotheses that address the temporal aspects of exposure and effect.

In other etiologic pathways, the critical exposure window may be defined not in relation to the timing of disease but based on stage of development. Regardless of when congenital malformations come to attention, precisely timed developmental events indicate the days and weeks of gestation in which certain defects can be produced by external insults (Kline et al., 1989). Similarly, it has been hypothesized that physical activity among adolescent girls is influential on their long-term risk of osteoporosis (US DHHS, 1996). For illustrative purposes, assume that this window of adolescence is the only period in which physical activity is pertinent to osteoporosis. A study that measured lifetime physical activity or physical activity from ages 40 to 49 would suffer from misclassification and observe the expected inverse association only to the extent that physical activity at those measured ages corresponded to physical activity in adolescence.

Optimal Level of Exposure Aggregation

Analogous to disease lumping and splitting, exposures can be conceptualized in a number of ways with regard to aggregation and disaggregation, depending on the etiologic hypothesis. The goal is to group together the contributors that share a specific etiologic pathway, leaving none out, but to exclude exposures that are irrelevant to that etiologic pathway. Focusing on only a subset of contributors to a given exposure index would constitute a lack of sensitivity in exposure assignment, and including some irrelevant elements in the construction of that index would represent a lack of specificity. In either case, relative to the optimal exposure category, it is misclassification.

For example, if we were interested in the possible effect of caffeine on risk of miscarriage, then the ideal measure of caffeine would be comprehensive and include all sources of dietary caffeine, such as coffee, tea, and chocolate, as well as caffeine-containing medications. Under the hypothesis that caffeine is the critical agent, study of caffeine from coffee alone would constitute underascertainment of exposure, and the exposure that was assigned would be lower to the extent that women were exposed to unmeasured sources of caffeine. A closely related but distinctive hypothesis however, concerns the possible effect of coffee on risk of miscarriage, in which constituents of the coffee other than caffeine are considered as potential etiologic agents. To address this hypothesis, aggregation of caffeinated and decaffeinated coffee would be justified. Under that hypothesis, coffee alone is the appropriate entity to study. Once the hypothesis is clearly formulated, then the ideal measure of exposure is defined, and the operational approaches to assessing exposure can be compared with the ideal.

Nutritional epidemiology provides an abundance of opportunities for creating exposure indices and demands clear hypotheses about the effective etiologic agent. Much research has been focused on specific micronutrients, such as beta-carotene or dietary fiber, and with such hypotheses, the goal is to comprehensively measure intake of that nutrient. An alternative approach is to acknowledge the multiplicity of constituents in foods, and develop hypotheses about fruit and vegetable intake, for example, or even more holistically, hypotheses about different patterns of diet. A hypothesis about beta-carotene and lung cancer is distinct from a hypothesis about fruit and vegetable intake and lung cancer, for example, with different demands on exposure assessment. Exposure indices must be defined with sufficient precision to indicate which potential components of exposure should be included and which should be excluded, and how the measure should be defined.

In practice, there are circumstances in which exposure is considered in groups that are not optimal for considering etiology but are optimal for practical reasons or for considering mitigation to reduce exposure. For example, there is increasingly clear evidence that small particles in the air (particulate air pollution) exacerbate chronic lung and heart disease and can cause premature mortality (Katsouyanni et al., 1997; Dominici et al., 2000). The size and chemical constituents of those particles differ markedly, and their impact on human disease may differ in relation to those characteristics as well. Technology now allows isolation of small particles, < 10 microns or < 2.5 microns, so that it is feasible to regulate and monitor compliance with regulation for the particle sizes thought to be most harmful to human health. It is not feasible however, to monitor the chemical constituents of those particles and thus regulations do not consider particle chemistry. We seek to reduce exposure to particulates, accepting that the effect of the mixture of particles with greater and lesser amounts of harmful constituents is accurately reflected in their average effect. Perhaps stronger associations would be found for subsets of particles defined by their chemical constitution, but the measured effect of particulates in the aggregate is still useful for identifying etiology and suggesting beneficial mitigation of exposure.

Operational Measures of Exposure

With a precise definition of the optimal exposure measure, or more plausibly, a set of exposure measures, each addressing a particular hypothesis, we can compare candidate operational measures of exposure to the ideal ones. The exact means by which the exposure indicator is constructed needs to be scrutinized, focusing on the operational details that go into the final assignment of individual exposure. The goal is to reveal the compromises that have been made, many without explicit consideration, and the resulting potential for disparity between the operational and ideal exposure measures.

For example, we may be interested in total ethanol intake over a lifetime in relation to cardiovascular disease endpoints, such as angina or myocardial infarction. Obviously, we will not have installed an alcohol meter at birth or directly observed alcohol intake over a lifetime. We may instead have self-report of typical weekly ingestion of beer, wine, and liquor averaged over adulthood, or intake of those beverages for specific periods of life, and use that information to construct a quantitative estimate of lifetime exposure. There is an abundance of opportunities for this operational measure to deviate from the ideal exposure measure, including inaccurate recall and intentional deception. Also there may be error even if the self-report is perfect in that there is likely to be variability in alcohol consumption over time and variable alcohol content of beverages. The etiologic process may require consideration of the amount of alcohol consumed on each occasion or drinking at different ages or different intervals relative to disease onset, introducing additional forms of misclassification when comparing the operational to the ideal measure.

Thus there are two ways in which the operational and ideal measures of exposure deviate from one another. One arises from conceptual problems in the approach to exposure assessment, such that a perfectly executed data collection effort would still result in an imperfect match with the etiologically relevant exposure. The error arises in the very choice of the operational definition of exposure. Second, superimposed on any conceptual misclassification is the more traditional misclassification based on errors in implementing the chosen approach. Environmental measurements contain sampling error and technical imprecision in characterizing chemical and physical agents, for example. Self-reported information on exposure inevitably introduces erroneous recall, which would exacerbate the inherent imperfections in the operational exposure definition. Recall may be distorted due to faulty memory, intentional deception, or bias related to the occurrence of disease in studies in which exposure is reported after disease occurrence. Laboratory data are often less subject to error in the conventional sense of imprecise measurement, but often more susceptible to conceptual error in not reflecting the exposure of ultimate interest.

A nearly ubiquitous challenge in collecting accurate data on exposure is the difficulty of gathering information over the potential etiologic period of interest. That is, the ideal definition often includes a time dimension over which exposure needs to be integrated or monitored. Even our most elegant tools, whether based on self-report, environmental measurements, or biological markers, rarely capture the exposure of interest over the period of interest. If we are interested in several years or decades of dietary intake of a specific nutrient, our options for data collection are limited. We can ask for people to use their memories to integrate over the interval, we can obtain more precise measurements at a point or several points over the interval, or some combination, such as a precise measure at one point and self-report regarding stability over a longer interval. In many instances, the most sophisticated, detailed, and accurate exposure indicators are only applicable to a brief period around the time of measurement. A rare exception to the generalization that lifetime exposure markers are unavailable is the collection of occupational ionizing radiation exposure through the use of film badges. These instruments, deployed at the time of hire and used throughout the period of employment, provide quarterly or annual measurements of all external ionizing radiation encountered. Subject to compliance and an interest restricted to occupational as opposed to other sources of ionizing radiation, the desired temporal information will be available from longitudinal data collection.

A variety of biochemical markers of tobacco use, for example, urinary or salivary cotinine, or carboxyhemoglobin, are precise indicators that are reflective of hours or at most a day of exposure. The alternative approach to assessing tobacco exposure is the ostensibly cruder measure of self-report, subject to the ability and willingness of respondents to recall their smoking behavior. If the ideal measure is lifetime (or long term) exposure, however, self-report is likely to be superior even to a series of biochemical measures only because the latter cannot integrate over time the way the participants' memories can. If the ideal exposure measure were lifetime inhalation of tar from tobacco combustion, the operational definition based on self-report of cigarettes smoked daily over specified periods of life is likely to be far more strongly correlated with that ideal measure than any present or recent biochemical markers of recent exposure. If our "gold standard" definition were inhalation of tar from tobacco combustion in the past 24 hours, the biochemical indicators would likely be far superior to self-report. The hypothesized temporal course of the relationship between exposure and disease should guide the selection of the optimal marker.

For those who generate research on challenging exposures (and nearly all exposures are challenging to measure), sufficient information should be provided on both the ideal and operational definition to compare them. While researchers are trained or even forced to reveal exactly what was done in the study, i.e., the operational exposure measure, they often neglect to be specific about the ideal exposure measure for addressing the hypothesis under study. In reviewing research reports, the often implicit definitions of the "gold standard" need to be extricated so that the actual methods of exposure assessment can be compared to the ideal. Readers should be watchful for the temptation on the part of researchers to state their goals in modest, attainable terms whereas the more etiologically appropriate index is less readily approximated. Problems can arise in the choice of the ideal exposure measure as well as in implementing that measure.

EVALUATION OF EXPOSURE MISCLASSIFICATION

All operational exposure measures are related only indirectly to the exposure of ultimate interest. Self-reported information clearly is removed from the etiologically effective exposures in that the verbal utterance in an interview does not constitute exposure nor does the checking of a box on a questionnaire constitute the exposure that results in disease. Even biological markers are to varying degrees proxies for the disease-causing factor, with compromises made with regard to the timing or site of assessment. Often, the measurement is taken at the feasible rather than ideal time (e.g., present versus past), and the assumption is made that the measure can be extrapolated to the critical time for addressing disease etiology. Similarly, collection of accessible specimens such as urine or blood is extrapolated to the exposure of interest in a less accessible site such as the kidneys or heart. As noted above, there is the everpresent potential for lumping too broadly, combining irrelevant with relevant exposures, or too narrowly, omitting key contributors to the exposure of interest.

Epidemiologists are well aware that use of imperfect exposure markers introduces error and should be viewed as opportunities for improvement in study methods. Sometimes we are deceived however, by advances in technology for biological or environmental evaluation, believing that laboratory sophistication automatically confers an advantage over the crudeness of self-report or paper records. We can lose sight of the fact that even measures that employ sophisticated technology also contain error relative to the desired information (Pearce et al., 1995). Even if the technology for measuring environmental or biological specimens is highly refined, the sources of error often arise at the point where the times and sites of collection of samples are decided. Accepting that epidemiology relies on indirect measures of the exposure of ultimate interest, the critical questions concern how effective the proxies are and the impact of the misclassification that they introduce relative to the unattainable "gold standard." The preferred option, of course, would be to obtain the ideal information and avoid the need to evaluate error and assess its impact. Accepting that this can never be achieved, there are a number of useful strategies for assessing the presence of exposure misclassification and the consequences of such errors on measures of association.

Compare Routine Measure to Superior Measures

In selecting the approach to evaluating exposure, some of the contenders must be dismissed due to lack of knowledge, unavailable technology, or ethical prohibitions. Among otherwise feasible options, however, some compromises are based on constraints that can, theoretically, be overcome, such as limited money, staff time, or respondent cooperation. Whatever routine exposure measure has been selected for the study, there are nearly always opportunities to obtain more sophisticated, accurate measures of exposure, even though there are remaining challenges that prevent attainment of the idealized gold standard. In designing a study, the investigator should consider options for assessing exposure, recognizing the tradeoffs between expanded study size and reduction in the level of exposure measurement accuracy that is attainable as a result of that increase in size. In many instances, small studies with accurate measurements as derived from repeated assessment of individuals or use of more prolonged sampling periods, for example, are more informative than larger studies that use less valid approaches (Phillips & Smith, 1993). Nevertheless, whatever the level of quality that was chosen, there is nearly always a better one that would have been feasible for a smaller study or one with a larger budget or longer timeline or more persuasive recruiters, and that superior measure constitutes a useful benchmark of comparison for the one that was routinely applied.

This strategy requires that the routine exposure assessment applied to all participants in the study be expanded by collecting more valid exposure data for a subset of study participants. In some cases, the more detailed information automatically has embedded within it the less sophisticated, routine measure. Diet inventories, for example, contain variable numbers of items depending on the amount of time one is willing to devote to the assessment, and the more items included, the better the measure is thought to be. The difference between a longer diet inventory and a shorter one can be assessed by collecting the full list and comparing the measure to what would have been found had only the shorter list been available. Similarly, if one is interested in exposure to environmental tobacco smoke and uses personal monitors, the duration of data collection might be 48 hours for all subjects except for a subset that is monitored using the exact same approach but for a full week.

More often, the routine and superior measures require distinct data collection efforts. Routine use of a questionnaire to be compared to a superior biological marker of exposure requires collection of both measures on a subset of participants. The questionnaire is not embedded within the biological marker in the same way a less complete food inventory is embedded within the more complete inventory. In either circumstance, with both the routine and superior measure available for the subset, the values can be compared to assess how closely the routine measure approximates the superior measure. With this information, estimates and judgments can be made as to what the results would have been if the superior measure had been applied routinely.

The more closely the routine exposure measure approximates the superior exposure measure, the less exposure misclassification is likely to be present. If they were perfectly correlated, then the "inferior" measure would simply represent a more efficient approach to gathering exactly the same information. More typically, there will be some inaccuracy in the routine measure relative to the more refined one, and the amount and pattern of inaccuracy can be assessed in a subset of study subjects. What this effort will not reveal is how close or distant both the routine and superior measures are from the ideal measure. They could be close to one another, giving the impression that the routine measure is quite good, yet both have substantial error relative to the unattainable ideal measure. Alternatively, there could be a major difference between the two, yet even the superior measure is far from optimal. What would be desirable but is rarely known is not just the ordinal ranking of the quality of the alternative measures but the absolute quality of each relative to the gold standard.

An important challenge to the interpretation of two measures that are presumed to be ordinal in quality is that the allegedly superior measure may just be different without really being better. When the basic strategies are similar, e.g., diet inventory or environmental measurements, and the superior measure has more detail or covers a more extended time period, the probability that it is better in absolute quality is quite high. When the approaches are qualitatively different, however, e.g., self-report versus biological marker, there is less certainty that the approaches can be rank-ordered as better and worse. Similarity between the superior and routine measure may give a false assurance regarding the quality of the routine measure if the allegedly superior measure really is not better. Worse yet, the ostensibly superior measure could be worse, so that a disparity is misinterpreted entirely. The common temptation is to accept any biological marker as superior to any form of self-report, and to downgrade confidence regarding the quality of self-report when they are not in close agreement. Biological markers of exposure often reflect a precise measure for a very brief period around the time of specimen collection, however, whereas self-report can represent an integration over long periods of time. Remembering that the ideal measure includes consideration of the etiologically relevant time period, it is not certain that a precise measure for the wrong time period from a biological marker is superior to an imprecise measure for the relevant time period based on self-report. Both strategies need to be compared to the ideal measure to the extent possible.

Assuming that there is a clear gradient in quality, what such comparisons between the inferior and superior measures provide is the basis for a quantitative assessment of the loss of information and expected reduction in measures of association based on the inferior measure relative to the superior one (Lagakos, 1988; Armstrong, 1990). Using the readily calculated correlation coefficient between the two measures, an estimate can be generated regarding how much of the information in the superior measure is lost by using the inferior one, using the expression $1 - r^2$, where r is the correlation coefficient. For example, if the correlation is 0.5, this expression equals 0.75, so that 75% of the information contained in the superior measure is lost by relying on the inferior one. Correlations of 1 and 0 correspond to values of 0% being lost and 100% being lost. Though a number of assumptions are made to justify this interpretation, it is a useful general rule of thumb.

An illustration of the loss of information in using an inferior compared to a superior exposure measure was provided by Baris et al. (1999) in a methodologic examination of exposure assignment methods for a study of residential magnetic fields and childhood leukemia. When children lived in two homes over the course of their lives, both were measured and integrated as a time-weighted average exposure, considered the "gold standard" relative to measurements in a single home. Various approaches to choosing the single home to measure were considered, including the duration of occupancy and whether or not it was currently occupied. Correlation coefficients between the gold standard and various surrogates (Table 8.1) indicate a range of values across the more limited measurement approaches,

TABLE 8.1. Pearson Correlation Coefficients Between Subjects' Estimated Time-Weighted Average Magnetic Field from Two Homes Measured, and Time-Weighted Averages Based on One Home Only or One Home Conjunction with Imputed Values for the Second Homes, National Cancer Institute Childhood Leukemia Study

SUBJECT'S TWA CALCULATED FROM DIFFERENT STRATEGIES	CORRELATION COEFFICIENT
TWA, two homes measured	1.00
Longer lived in homes only	0.95
Shorter lived in homes only	0.55
Former lived in homes only	0.90
Current lived in homes only	0.62
Longer lived in home plus shorter lived in homes imputed:	
With control mean*	0.95
With status specific mean†	0.95
Current lived in homes plus former lived in homes imputed:	
With control mean‡	0.62
With status specific mean§	0.62

*Shorter lived in homes were imputed from observed mean of longer lived in control homes.

†Shorter lived in homes were imputed from case mean of longer lived in homes (if case) or from control mean of longer lived in homes (if control).

‡Former lived in homes were imputed from observed mean of current lived in control homes.

§Former lived in homes were imputed from case mean of current lived in homes (if case) or from control mean of current lived in homes (if control).

Baris et al., 1999.

from 0.55 to 0.95. Among the simpler indices, the home that was lived in for the longer period provides the better proxy for the time-integrated measure, as expected. Counter to expectation, however, when the measures of association were computed using the various indices (Table 8.2), results for both former homes and currently occupied homes yielded results closer to the operational "gold standard" measure than the longest lived-in home. The relative risk in the highest exposure group was attenuated for all of the surrogate indices of exposure relative to the time-weighted average, suggesting that the extra expense of collecting data on multiple homes was a worthwhile investment of resources.

Examine Multiple Indicators of Exposure

It is preferable to have a single, perfect "gold standard" to serve as the referent for the routine exposure measure, or at least a measure that better approximates the "gold standard." It may still be informative however, to have another exposure proxy of similar quality to the routinely applied measure but differing in character, and thus in the nature of the error it contains. Neither the routine exposure measure nor the alternative measure in isolation is necessarily a better approximation of the exposure of interest, but we would expect them to be associated with one another to at least some extent because both are associated with the true exposure.

For example, in measuring exposure to environmental tobacco smoke over long periods of time, there are two basic strategies available: biochemical markers of short-term exposure and self-reported information on proximity to active smokers. The biochemical markers are precise indicators over short periods of time. Assuming that the measurement period represents a sample from the long-term period of etiologic interest, the accurate short-term measure has some value as a marker of long-term exposure. The self-report of proximity to smokers is capable of integration over the extended time period of etiologic interest, given that questions can be focused on specific periods of interest and the respondent can presumably reflect on and recall the period of interest. Self-report is vulnerable to the uncertainties of perception and recall, however, including potential biases in perceiving the presence of tobacco smoke and faulty memory in recalling those experiences. What type of association might we expect to observe between these markers, both of which are imperfect relative to the "gold standard," but for very different reasons? How do we interpret measures of their relationship to one another and the relationship of each marker to disease status?

First, it is important to remember that the accurate indicator of short-term exposure does not serve as the "gold standard" for the imprecise indicator of long-term exposure. Both are approaches to estimating the long-term exposure of etiologic interest, and both are inferior to concurrent measurement of exposure throughout the etiologic period as might be accomplished in a true prospective

TABLE 8.2. Odds Ratios and 95% Confidence Intervals for Magnetic Field Exposure and Acute Lymphocytic Leukemia from Different Residences, Categorised According to Initial Cutoff Points of Magnetic Field Exposure, National Cancer Institute Childhood Leukemia Study

Relative Risk for Acute Lymphoblastic Leukaemia Calculated With:

EXPOSURE CATEGORIES (μT)	TWA from Two Homes Measured				Measurement from Longer Lived in Home Only				Measurement from Former Lived in Home Only				Measurement from Currently Lived in Home Only			
	MEAN (μT)	CASES	OR	95% CI	MEAN (μT)	CASES	OR	95% CI	MEAN (μT)	CASES	OR	95% CI	MEAN (μT)	CASES	OR	95% CI
< 0.065	0.047	53	1.00	—	0.042	64	1.00	—	0.042	59	1.00	—	0.042	66	1.00	—
≥ 0.065–< 0.099	0.082	33	0.97	0.52 to 1.81	0.080	27	1.23	0.62 to 2.39	0.083	22	0.85	0.43 to 1.68	0.079	31	1.28	0.68 to 2.44
> 0.100–< 0.199	0.137	40	1.14	0.63 to 2.08	0.137	35	1.28	0.69 to 2.38	0.140	39	1.35	0.73 to 2.47	0.133	32	1.09	0.59 to 2.02
≥ 0.200	0.350	23	1.81	0.81 to 4.02	0.374	23	1.15	0.57 to 2.33	0.370	29	1.65	0.82 to 3.32	0.322	20	1.47	0.67 to 3.20
			P_{trend} = 0.2				P_{trend} = 0.3				P_{trend} = 0.1				P_{trend} = 0.4	

OR, odds ratio; CI, confidence interval; TWA, time-weighted average

Baris et al., 1999.

study. Because both are believed to be related to long-term exposure, however, one expects some association between the two measures and it would be troubling if they were completely unrelated. The magnitude of the association between two measures, even if both are associated with a third (e.g., the true value), however, can be quite small. Two variables can show a correlation coefficient as high as 0.7 with a third variable, for example, yet have a correlation of 0 with one another (Berkson, 1946). Thus, it would be possible for each of two proxies to be rather strongly related to the "gold standard," yet not related strongly to each other. In the absence of a "gold standard" measure, interpretation of the association between two imperfect indicators is thus of limited value in assessing the quality of either one.

Ideally, substantive understanding of each of the exposure measures could be used to create an integrated measure of exposure that takes advantage of the information provided by each. That is, with recognized strengths and deficiencies in each of two or more markers of exposure, those information sources might be combined into a single measure that is expected to be better than any of them would be in isolation. There is no generic approach to integrating these sources of exposure data because it depends on the way in which the information they provide is complementary. It might be known that when certain combinations of results occur, one measure should override the other. For exposures in which measurement is known to be highly insensitive, e.g., illicit drug use, we might accept that *any* of self-report, metabolites in urine, or metabolites in hair constitutes exposure. We might know that one measure is more accurate in a certain range of exposure or for certain respondents and another measure is better under other circumstances. For example, in comparing a biological measure with self-report, there may be known sources of interference from certain medications, unusual dietary habits, or illness. If self-report were negative, and the biological measure were positive but with an indication of a metabolic disease that can create false positive readings, one might simply override the biological marker for that individual and classify the person as negative. Similarly, there may be persons in whom the quality of self-report is thought to be fallible due to poor cooperation according to the interviewer, and we would then rely instead on the biological marker.

In the absence of substantive understanding of how errors in one measure or the other arises, one simplistic approach is to combine their information empirically into a composite variable, i.e., define exposed as positive on both markers or as positive on either of two markers. If the major problem is known to be one of sensitivity, then an algorithm might be applied in which being positive on either marker is used to infer that exposure is present. This will enhance the sensitivity relative to using either measure in isolation, and decrease the specificity. Alternatively, if specificity is the problem one wishes to minimize, classification as exposed may require being positive on both indicators, with only one being positive resulting in assignment as unexposed. Preferable to either extreme would be an examination of the pattern of results across all combinations of the two exposure measures, i.e., both positive, one measure positive and one measure negative, and both negative. Unless one or both of the measures is behaving very strangely, it would be expected that these levels would correspond to a monotonic gradient of true exposure, less subject to misclassification than use of either measure in isolation.

When one of the data sources on exposure can be viewed as a "gold standard," it provides an opportunity to better understand and ultimately refine the routine measure. For example, with a combination of self-reported exposure to environmental tobacco smoke over long periods in the past, and short-term biochemical markers, there is an opportunity to integrate the information to validate the self-report. Self-reported exposure can be generated over the time frame of ultimate interest, as well as for the brief time period reflected by the biochemical measure of exposure, i.e., the recent past. With that information and accepting the biochemical marker as a gold standard for the recent past, predictive models can be developed in which the self-reported information is optimized to estimate actual exposure. In the example of environmental tobacco smoke, self-report of exposure in the preceding 24 or 48 hours might be queried, for which the biochemical indicator would be a legitimate gold standard. With that quantitative prediction model now in hand, the questionnaire components for the period of etiologic relevance, typically a prolonged period in the past, can be weighted to generate a more valid estimate of historical exposure. The data would be used to determine which self-reported items are predictive of measured exposure to environmental tobacco smoke and the magnitude of the prediction, through the use of regression equations. Although there is no direct way to demonstrate that this extrapolation from prediction over short periods to prediction over long periods is valid, the availability of a "gold standard" for brief periods offers some assurance. The development of the predictive model linking self-reported exposure data to biological markers need not include all the study subjects and could be done on similar but not identical populations. The relationship between perceived experiences and actual exposure may well differ among different populations, however, suggesting that the validation be done on the study population or a group that is quite similar to the actual study subjects.

Multiple exposure indicators also may be used when it is unclear which is the most influential on the health outcome of interest. A sizable body of research has addressed particulate air pollution and health, particularly morbidity and mortality from cardiovascular and respiratory disease. As the research has evolved, there has been an increasing focus on the small particles, those < 10 $\mu g/m^3$ or < 2.5 $\mu g/m^3$ in diameter. In a large cohort study of participants in the American Cancer Society's Cancer Prevention II Study, air pollution measures in metropolitan areas were examined in relation to mortality through 1998 (Pope et al., 2002). To examine the nature of the relationship between particulate air pollution and mortality, a range of indices were considered, defined by calendar time of measurement, particle size, and sulfate content (Fig. 8.1). These results suggest once

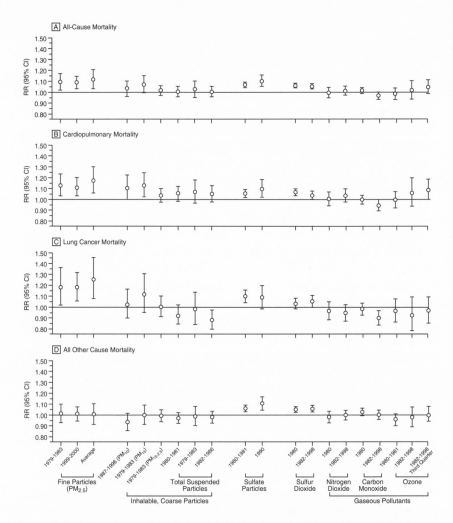

FIGURE 8.1. Adjusted mortality relative risk (RR) ratio evaluated at subject weighted mean concentration of particulate and gaseous air pollution in metropolitan areas, American Cancer Society Cancer Prevention II Study (Pope et al., 2002). PM$_{2.5}$ indicates particles measuring less than 2.5 μm in diameter; PM$_{10}$, particles measuring less than 10 μm in diameter; PM$_{15}$, particles measuring less than 15 μm in diameter; PM$_{15-2.5}$, particles measuring between 2.5 and 15 μm in diameter; and CI, confidence interval.

again that the fine particles (< 2.5 μm) are more clearly associated with mortality from cardiopulmonary disease, lung cancer, and total mortality, as compared to inhalable coarse particles or total suspended particulates. The associations for measurements in different calendar times are similar to one another, and sulfate particles are similar to fine particles in their effects. Examination of multiple indices suggests that the associations are rather consistent across measurement period but specific to fine particles.

Examine Gradient of Exposure Data Quality

It is often possible to construct an ordinal gradient of exposure classification accuracy. Where a variety of alternative exposure measures are available or can be constructed, there is the opportunity to examine the measure of exposure–disease association across a series of alternative exposure assessment methods. The more valid exposure indicator should yield the more valid measure of association, and data for a series of markers that can be rank-ordered from better to worse provide the opportunity to extrapolate even when all available measures are imperfect to one degree or another. That is, the spectrum of quality in exposure data will often be incomplete, lacking the true "gold standard" exposure measure of ultimate interest, but observing the pattern of association across a gradient of measures of varying quality may help to speculate more accurately about what would have been observed had the "gold standard" been available. This is a form of dose-response analysis, where the dose measure is not the amount of exposure received but rather the probability that exposure is accurately classified.

If measures of increasing quality show a gradient of increasing magnitude of association with disease, this suggests that an association of presumably greater magnitude would have been observed if a superior exposure measure outside the range of what was feasible had been obtained. In contrast, if the spectrum of available exposure measures shows no clear pattern of differences in the magnitude of association with disease, or indicates that the better measures of exposure show weaker associations, it may be inferred that a causal association is less likely to be present. In order to assess the influence of exposure measures of varying quality, there must, of course, be such a spectrum available. In addition, the interpretation of the results must consider the possibility that what is thought to constitute a gradient in quality of exposure data may not actually be a gradient. That is, the assessment of which measures are better and worse is subject to error.

Consider a study to evaluate the role of socioeconomic status in relation to prevalence of hypertension, where multiple measures of socioeconomic status of varying quality are available. If median income for the census tract in which the individual resides shows a relative risk of 1.5, contrasting lowest and highest socioeconomic levels, individual level of education has a relative risk of 2.0 comparing least to most educated, and income relative to poverty level indicates a relative risk of 2.5 from lowest to highest, one might infer that a measure that truly captures the underlying construct of socioeconomic deprivation would show a more marked gradient in risk. That is, the etiologically critical aspects of socioeconomic status are elusive to define and measure, but we might accept that the average income in the area, educational level, and personal income form a gradient in quality with an expected (but unproven) stronger association if we could derive the ideal measure. Observing such a pattern is consistent with the hypothesis that there is a causal association between socioeconomic status and hypertension and that all of the available measures reflect the magnitude of that association imperfectly.

Examine Subsets of the Population with Differing Exposure Data Quality

Accuracy of exposure assignment may vary in predictable ways in relation to attributes such as gender, education, or age. Based on previously reported research or based on validation studies contained within the study of interest, groups may be defined for whom the routine exposure measure is more likely to be valid than it is for other groups in the study. Younger persons may show a greater or lesser concordance of the routine and superior exposure measures than older persons, or women may report more or less accurately than men. Often, groups expected to have superior cognitive function, e.g., younger participants versus the elderly, or those without a history of alcohol and drug abuse compared to those with such a history, are likely to provide better quality information through recall and self-report. In fact, when the disease itself is associated with cognitive decline, e.g., studies of chronic neurodegenerative disease, case–control studies are susceptible to bias because cases provide data of inferior accuracy relative to controls. Some individuals in the study may have experienced the etiologically relevant period in the more distant past than others. All other considerations equal, those who are reporting for a more recent calendar period may well provide better data than those reporting for a more remote time.

Physiologic differences among individuals may also make the exposure measure more accurate for some than others. Differences arising from genetic variation or induced metabolic changes can create variation in the biologically effective dose for a given level of exogenous exposure. Depending on the particular exposure of interest, a variety of hypotheses might be put forward regarding subgroups of participants in whom the accuracy of data would be higher or lower. For example, in addressing the question of whether historical exposure to organochlorines such as DDT and PCBs may be related to the development of breast cancer, a major challenge is in accurately reconstructing historical exposure. In case–control studies, in particular, measurements of present-day serum residues of the chemicals of interest serve as an exposure indicator for lifetime exposure history. While there are a number of factors that influence the changes in body stores and serum levels over time, lactation is a primary means by which such organochlorines are excreted. All other considerations equal, serum organochlorines in women who have lactated are less indicative of long-term historical exposure levels than for women who have not.

This understanding of lactation as a modifier of exposure was exploited in recent studies of organochlorines and breast cancer to define strata in which the present-day serum markers are more valid markers of long-term exposure (Millikan et al., 2000). The association between serum levels of DDE and PCBs were examined in relation to breast cancer in strata of women who were nulliparous, parous but never breastfed, and those who were parous and had breastfed (Table 8.3). These data suggest a weak positive association, though without a dose-response gradient, limited to women who had never breastfed, i.e., the first two strata. Among those who had breastfed, the odds ratios were close to or some-

TABLE 8.3. Odds Ratios for Lipid-Adjusted DDE and PCBs and Breast Cancer, Stratified by Parity and History of Breastfeeding, North Carolina, 1993–1996

			Referent	
	CASES	CONTROLS	OR* (95% CI)	OR† (95% CI)
Nulliparous				
DDE‡				
< 0.394	41	25		
0.394 to < 1.044	36	23	1.28 (0.59–2.78)	1.24 (0.54–2.82)
≥ 1.044	35	17	1.87 (0.67–5.20)	1.48 (0.49–4.46)
Total PCBs§				
< 0.283	37	25		
0.283 to < 0.469	39	21	1.51 (0.69–3.33)	2.06 (0.88–4.85)
≥ 0.469	36	19	1.74 (0.67–4.54)	1.62 (0.57–4.58)
Parous, Never Breastfed				
DDE				
< 0.394	131	102		
0.394 to < 1.044	122	123	0.86 (0.59–1.26)	0.96 (0.65–1.42)
≥ 1.044	134	111	1.07 (0.91–2.15)	1.23 (0.80–1.89)
Total PCBs				
< 0.283	115	112		
0.283 to < 0.469	159	125	1.51 (1.04–2.20)	1.50 (1.01–2.23)
≥ 0.469	113	99	1.40 (0.91–2.15)	1.30 (0.82–2.06)
Parous, Ever Breastfed				
DDE				
< 0.394	102	93		
0.394 to < 1.044	73	73	0.94 (0.60–1.48)	1.16 (0.70–1.90)
≥ 1.044	74	92	0.71 (0.41–1.21)	0.80 (0.45–1.44)
Total PCBs				
< 0.283	87	82		
0.283 to < 0.469	68	74	0.92 (0.58–1.47)	0.90 (0.55–1.48)
≥ 0.469	94	102	0.95 (0.57–1.57)	0.84 (0.49–1.44)

*Adjusted for age, age-squared, and race.

†Adjusted for age, age-squared, race, menopausal status, BMI, body mass index, HRT, hormone replacement therapy use, and income.

‡p,p'-DDE in μg/g lipid.

§Total PCBs in μg/g lipid.

Millikan et al., 2000.

what below the null. Such results, though suggestive at most, may be reflective of the superiority of the serum measures as an exposure indicator for women who had never breastfed and accurately reflect a small increase in risk associated with the exposure.

As illustrated by the above example, information on predictors of accuracy in exposure classification can be used to create homogeneous strata across which the validity of exposure data should vary in predictable ways. All other influences being equal, those strata in which the exposure data are better would be expected to yield more accurate measures of association with disease than those strata in which the exposure data are more prone to error. Identifying gradients in the estimated validity of the exposure measure and examining patterns of association across those gradients serves two purposes—it can provide useful information to evaluate the impact of exposure misclassification and also generate estimates for subsets of persons in whom the error is least severe. Note that it is not helpful to adjust for indicators of data quality as though they were confounding factors, but rather to stratify and determine whether measures of association differ across levels of hypothesized exposure data quality.

The quality of women's self-reported information on reproductive history and childhood social class was evaluated in a case–control study of Hodgkin's disease in northern California using the traditional approach of reinterviewing some time after the initial interview (Lin et al., 2002). Twenty-two cases and 24 controls were reinterviewed approximately eight months after their initial interview, and agreement was characterized by kappa coefficients for categorical variables and intraclass correlation coefficients for continuous measures. Whereas cases and controls showed similar agreement, education was rather strongly associated with the magnitude of agreement (Table 8.4). Across virtually all the measures, women who had more than a high school education showed better agreement than women of lower educational level, suggesting that the more informative results from the main study would be found within the upper educational stratum.

Non-specific markers of exposure data quality such as age or education may also yield strata that differ in the magnitude of association for reasons other than the one of interest. There may be true effect measure modification by those attributes, in which exposure really has a different impact on the young compared to the old, or there may be other biases related to non-response or disease misclassification that cause the association to differ. When the identification of persons who differ in the quality of their exposure assignment is based on specific factors related to exposure, such as having been chosen for a more thorough protocol or having attended a clinic or worked in a factory in which more extensive exposure data were available, then the observed pattern of association is more likely to be reflective of the accuracy of the exposure marker as opposed to other correlates of the stratification factor.

TABLE 8.4. Kappa or Intraclass Correlation Coefficients Among Subjects (n = 46) Reinterviewed between 1992 and 1995 in a Case-Control Study of Hodgkin's Disease, Stratified by Education, Northern California

	Kappa or Intraclass Correlation Coefficient*	
VARIABLE	HIGH SCHOOL OR LESS (N = 9)	MORE THAN HIGH SCHOOL (N = 37)
Age at first period	0.827 (*n* = 9)	0.920 (*n* = 33)
Age at first period†	0.541 (*n* = 5)	0.848 (*n* = 27)
Number of pregnancies	0.584 (*n* = 8)	0.823 (*n* = 37)
Number of live births	0.632 (*n* = 8)	0.887 (*n* = 37)
Use of birth control pills or shots	0.769 (*n* = 9)	0.877 (*n* = 37)
Number of playmates at age 8	0.158 (*n* = 8)	0.779 (*n* = 36)
Birth weight in pounds	0.943 (*n* = 5)	0.966 (*n* = 29)
History of mononucleosis	0.000 (*n* = 9)	0.907 (*n* = 37)
Mean reliability‡	0.558	0.876
(95% CI)	(0.345, 0.735)	(0.837, 0.912)

*Calculation of kappa and intraclass correlation coefficients does not include missing or unknown responses.

†Calculated by subtracting year of birth from reported year at first period.

‡Bootstrapped difference between means (more than high school-high school or less) and 95% CI: 0.319 (0.147, 0.521).

CI, confidence interval.

Lin et al., 2002.

Evaluate Known Predictors of Exposure

Although the nature of the association between exposure and the disease of interest is uncertain to at least some extent, or there would be no motivation to conduct the study, there may be well-established predictors of exposure that *are* known with certainty. If accurately assessed exposure can safely be assumed to have certain such predictors, assessing whether the expected associations with exposure are present would help to indicate whether the exposure data are valid.

Exposure predictors are generally not of direct interest in relation to disease, so that this information will not always be collected unless the application of such information to the validation of exposure measurement is anticipated. The basis for the linkage between the antecedent and the exposure need not be causal, in that a well-established non-causal statistical predictor would serve the same purpose of helping to indicate that exposure has (or has not) been measured successfully. When such a predictor of exposure is available, and the expected relation to exposure is very strong, the predictor may even be a useful proxy measure of exposure.

For example, assessment of the use of illicit drugs is a great challenge. It is well known however, that a strong predictor, and perhaps a causal determinant, is the pattern of drug use among friends. Therefore, it would be expected that those who are using illicit drugs would also report having friends who do so. Thus, to avoid at least part of the sensitivity and stigma associated with such behavior, questionnaires might include items pertaining to drug use among friends, something that respondents may be more willing to admit to than their own drug use. Such information can be used to determine whether the expected positive association is found with self-reported drug use, and also to create a category of uncertain drug use when the individual reports not using drugs but having friends who do so.

Another illustration of ascertaining and using information on the predictors of exposure is often applied in the assessment of use of therapeutic medications. There are certain illnesses or symptoms that serve as the reasons for using those medications, and the credibility of reports of drug use (or even non-use) can be evaluated to some extent by acquiring information on the diseases that the drug is used to treat. When a respondent reports having an illness that is known to be an indicator for using a specific medication, along with recall of using that medication, confidence is enhanced that they are accurately reporting the medication use. Those who had an illness that should have resulted in use of the drug but did not report doing so, and those who reported using the medication but without having reported an illness for which that medication is normally used, would be assigned a less certain exposure status.

In a study of the potential association between serum selenium and the risk of lung and prostate cancer among cigarette smokers, Goodman et al. (2001) provided a rather detailed analysis of predictors of serum selenium concentrations (Table 8.5). In addition to addressing concerns with the comparability of collection and storage methods across study sites, they were able to corroborate the expected reduction in serum selenium levels associated with intensity and recency of cigarette smoking. Even though the background knowledge is limited to help anticipate what patterns to expect, confirming the inverse association with smoking adds confidence that the measurements were done properly and are more likely to be capturing the desired exposure.

Even when the linkage of antecedent to exposure is less direct, as in the case of social and demographic predictors, there may still be value in assessing exposure predictors as a means of evaluating the accuracy of exposure information. Weaker associations with exposure or those that are less certain will be less contributory but can help to provide at least some minimal assurance that the exposure information is reasonable. If assessing the consequences of otitis media in children on subsequent development, the known positive association of the exposure with attendance in day care and sibship size and patterns of occurrence by age (Hardy & Fowler, 1993; Zeisel et al., 1999) may be helpful in verifying that otitis media has been accurately documented. As always, when the data conflict with prior expectations, the possibility that prior expectations were wrong

TABLE 8.5. Adjusted Mean Serum Selenium (μg/dl) Concentration in Control
Participants, Carotene and Retinol Efficacy Trial, 1985–1999

	ADJUSTED MEAN (SE)*	P†
Gender		0.30
Male	11.55 (0.07)	
Female	11.75 (0.17)	
Race		0.99
White	11.58 (0.07)	
African American	11.57 (0.32)	
Other/Unknown	11.64 (0.37)	
Exposure Population		0.06
Asbestos	11.31 (0.16)	
Heavy smokers	11.72 (0.09)	
Study Center		0.0001
Baltimore	9.89 (0.27)	
Irvine	10.76 (0.22)	
New Haven	11.20 (0.28)	
Portland	11.96 (0.13)	
San Francisco	10.99 (0.30)	
Seattle	12.01 (0.10)	
Blood Draw Smoking Status		0.0001
Current	11.34 (0.09)	
Former	11.86 (0.09)	

*Adjusted means from model including all variables with $p < 0.1$ except years quit smoking for the
heavy-smoker population. Adjusted means for blood draw year ($p = 0.28$) not given because this
was a linear variable in the model.
†p for test of heterogeneity.
SE, standard error.
Goodman et al., 2001.

needs to be considered as an alternative to the inference that the data are in
error.

Evaluate Known Consequences of Exposure

In some instances, exposures are known to have specific health consequences,
and verification of the expected associations with those other outcomes offers a
means of assessing the accuracy of exposure assessment. Presumably the principal research question concerns potential health consequences of exposure that

are *not* fully understood or the study would be of little value. When data can be obtained to assess whether strongly expected associations with exposure are found, in the same sense as a positive control in experimental studies, confidence regarding the validity of exposure measurement is enhanced. If expected associations are not found, serious concern is raised about whether the exposure is reflective of the construct that was intended.

In a cohort study designed to examine the effect of heavy alcohol use on the risk of myocardial infarction, we might examine the association between our measure of heavy alcohol use and risk of cirrhosis, motor vehicle injuries, or depression, since these are established with certainty as being associated with heavy alcohol use. If feasible, we might evaluate subclinical effects of alcohol on liver function. If the study participants classified as heavy alcohol users did not show any increased risk for health problems known to be associated with heavy alcohol use, the validity of our assessment of alcohol use would be called into question. If the expected associations were found, then confidence in the accuracy of the measure would be enhanced.

An examination of the effect of exercise on depression made use of known consequences of physical activity to address the validity of the assessment, illustrating this strategy. In a prospective cohort study of older men and women in Southern California, the Rancho Bernardo Study (Kritz-Silverstein et al., 2001), exercise was addressed solely with the question "Do you regularly engage in strenuous exercise or hard physical labor?" Given the simplicity and brevity of this query, it is reasonable to ask whether it has successfully isolated groups with truly differing activity levels. Building on previous analyses from this cohort, they were able to refer back to an examination of predictors of cardiovascular health. Reaven et al. (1990) examined a number of correlates and potential consequences of self-reported engagement in physical activity (Table 8.6). There was clear evidence of a lower heart rate and higher measure of HDL cholesterol among men and women who responded affirmatively to the question about regular exercise. Though differences were not large, they do indicate some validity to the question in distinguishing groups who truly differ in level of physical activity. Note that the ability to make this inference depends on the knowledge that activity is causally related to these measures, which must come from evidence obtained outside the study.

Ideally, we would like to go beyond this qualitative use of the information to increase or decrease confidence in the accuracy of exposure measures and actually quantify the quality of exposure data. Few exposure–disease associations are understood with sufficient precision however, to enable us to go beyond verifying their presence and examine whether the actual magnitude of association is at the predicted level or whether exposure misclassification has resulted in attrition of the association. For the few exposure–disease associations for which the magnitude of association is known with some certainty, e.g., smoking and lung can-

TABLE 8.6. Relation Between Regular Exercise Status and Mean Plasma Lipid Levels Lipoprotein Levels and Other Variables Adjusted for Age in Men and Women Aged 50 to 89 Who Were Not Currently Using Cholesterol-Lowering Medications, Rancho Bernardo, California, 1984–1987

	Regular Exercise in Men ($n = 1019$)			Regular Exercise in Women ($n = 1273$)		
	NO	YES	P VALUE	NO	YES	P VALUE
Other Variables						
Age* (year)	72.0	67.4	< 0.001	70.8	67.6	< 0.001
BMI	26.1	25.8	0.12	24.6	24.1	0.10
WHR	0.918	0.909	0.03	0.798	0.788	0.04
Cigarettes (per day)	2.8	0.5	< 0.001	2.3	2.0	0.53
Alcohol (mL/week)	131.6	115.0	0.14	78.2	81.3	0.69
Heart rate (beats per minute)	61.9	58.9	< 0.001	64.5	62.0	< 0.001
PME use (% who use)	—	—	—	27.0	34.0	0.03
Lipid and Lipoprotein Levels (mg/dL)						
Cholesterol	210.1	209.3	0.76	228.0	231.7	0.19
HDL	52.7	55.9	< 0.01	67.5	72.0	0.001
LDL	132.2	132.8	0.79	137.6	137.3	0.93
Triglyceride	108.3	91.7	< 0.001	102.7	99.2	0.37
n	758	261		1022	251	

BMI, body mass index; WHR, waist-to-hip ratio; PME, postmenopausal estrogen use; HDL, high-density lipoproteins; LDL, low-density lipoproteins.
*Age is unadjusted.
Reaven et al., 1990.

cer, and the misclassification can be assumed to be nondifferential with respect to disease, estimates of the amount of exposure misclassification required to observe a diluted association of a given magnitude can be derived (Kleinbaum et al., 1982; Copeland et al., 1977). The need for a series of assumptions regarding the expected magnitude of association, freedom from other sources of error, and applicability to the specific study population of interest limit the quantitative evaluation. Nevertheless, the concept may be helpful in the interpretation of the patterns of association between exposure and its known consequences.

Examine Dose-Response Gradients

If we are able to specify the etiologically relevant measure of the amount of exposure, and the amount of that exposure varies over the range that affects disease risk, then, by definition, more of that exposure will result in a greater probability of developing the disease. We will observe a dose-response gradient, in which increasing exposure results in an increasing risk of disease. The restrictions and uncertainties inherent in this evaluation should be recognized (Weiss, 1981). The critical aspect of the exposure that will yield increasing risk of disease may not be obvious, with the default approach based solely on some index of cumulative dose subject to uncertainty and error. What may be more important than the total amount of exposure is the form of the exposure, its biological availability, peak exposures, when it occurs, etc. A rather detailed understanding of the biologic process linking exposure and disease is required to quantify the relevant dose accurately. Furthermore, the shape of the dose-response function, if one is present at all, will vary across levels of exposure, potentially having a subthreshold range in which there is no response with increasing dose as well as ranges in which the maximum response has been attained and dose no longer matters. If the variation in the exposure levels that are available to study are all below or above the range in which disease risk responds to varying exposure, then no dose-response gradient will be found. Nonetheless, the potential value in identifying gradients in disease risk in relation to varying levels of exposure is always worthy of careful evaluation. When such a gradient is observed, it is informative and can support a causal hypothesis, but when it is absent, a causal association is by no means negated.

The hypothesized etiologic relationship under study should include at least a general specification of the type of exposure that would be expected to increase the risk of disease. The hypothesis and available data need to be scrutinized carefully for clues to the aspects of exposure that would be expected to generate stronger relations with disease. Total amount of exposure, generally measured as intensity integrated over time, is commonly used. Even in the absence of any measures of intensity, the duration of exposure may be relevant. More complex measures such as maximum intensity or average intensity over a given time period may also be considered.

For example, assume we are evaluating the relationship between oral contraceptive use and the development of breast cancer. If the hypothesis suggests that *dose* be defined by cumulative amount of unopposed estrogen, we would examine specific formulations of oral contraception and the duration of time over which those formulations were used. If the hypothesis concerns the suppression of ovulation, then the total number of months of use might be relevant. If the hypothesis concerned a permanent change in breast tissue brought about by oral contraceptive use prior to first childbirth, we would construct a different dose measure, one that is specific to the interval between becoming sexually active and first pregnancy.

In a study of oral contraceptives and breast cancer in young women (< 45 years of age), Brinton et al. (1995) examined several such dose measures. A multisite case–control study enrolled 1648 breast cancer cases and 1505 controls through random-digit dialing with complete data for analysis of oral contraceptive use. To examine varying combinations of duration of use and timing of use (by calendar time and by age), relative risks were calculated for a number of different dose measures (Table 8.7). Except for some indication of increased risk with more recent use, no striking patterns relative to duration and timing of oral contraceptive use were identified.

There is no universally applicable optimal measure because the specific features of the etiologic hypothesis lead to different ideal exposure measures. Multiple hypotheses of interest can be evaluated in the same study, each hypothesis leading to a specific exposure measure. In many cases, the various indices of exposure will be highly correlated with one another. On the positive side, even if we specify the wrong index of exposure (relative to the etiologically effective

TABLE 8.7. Relative Risks and 95% Confidence Intervals of Breast Cancer by Combined Measures of Oral Contraceptive Use Patterns: Women Younger Than 45 Years of Age, Multicenter Case-Control Study, 1990–1992

	Used 6 months to < 5 years		Used 5–9 years		Used ≥ 10 years	
	NO.	RR (95% CI)	NO.	RR (95% CI)	NO.	RR (95% CI)
No. of Years Since First Use						
< 15	136	1.44 (1.1–1.9)	66	1.55 (1.0–2.3)	22	1.27 (0.7–2.4)
15–19	221	1.14 (0.9–1.4)	120	1.45 (1.1–2.0)	93	1.58 (1.1–2.2)
≥ 20	292	1.29 (1.0–1.6)	190	1.10 (0.8–1.4)	119	1.11 (0.8–1.5)
No. of Years Since Last Use						
< 5	80	1.66 (1.1–2.4)	87	1.49 (1.0–2.1)	131	1.37 (1.0–1.8)
5–9	66	1.28 (0.9–1.9)	71	1.49 (1.0–2.2)	66	1.13 (0.8–1.7)
≥ 10	503	1.21 (0.9–1.5)	218	1.14 (0.9–1.5)	37	1.34 (0.8–2.3)
Age at First Use, Years						
< 18	79	1.04 (0.7–1.5)	80	1.55 (1.1–2.2)	75	1.47 (1.0–2.2)
18–21	342	1.32 (1.1–1.6)	224	1.21 (0.9–1.5)	122	1.12 (0.8–1.5)
≥ 22	228	1.29 (1.0–1.6)	72	1.21 (0.8–1.8)	37	1.68 (0.9–3.0)

*Adjusted for study site, age, race, number of births, and age at first birth. All risks relative to women with no use of oral contraceptives or use for less than 6 months (389 patients and 431 control subjects).

RR, relative risk; CI, confidence interval.

Brinton et al., 1995.

measure), it will be sufficiently correlated with the correct one to observe a dose-response gradient. On the other hand, correlations among candidate indices of exposure make it difficult or sometimes impossible to isolate the critical aspect of exposure.

ASSESSMENT OF WHETHER EXPOSURE MISCLASSIFICATION IS DIFFERENTIAL OR NONDIFFERENTIAL

Definitions

Consideration of the *pattern* of error is critical to evaluating its likely impact on measures of association. The most important question is whether the pattern of error in exposure ascertainment varies in relation to disease status. If the nature of the error is identical for persons with and without the disease of interest, the misclassification is referred to as nondifferential. If the pattern of exposure misclassification varies in relation to disease status, it is called differential misclassification. In the absence of other forms of error, nondifferential misclassification of a dichotomous exposure indicator leads to a predictable bias towards the null value for the measure of the exposure–disease association (Copeland et al., 1977). A number of exceptions to this principle have been identified, for example, multiple exposure levels in which misclassification may occur across non-adjacent categories (Dosemeci et al., 1990) and categorization of a continuous measure (Greenland, 1995). Nonetheless, the determination of whether disease status is affecting the pattern of error in exposure assignment remains a critical step in assessing the potential consequences of misclassification. When the quality of exposure assignment differs in relation to disease status, there are no readily predictable consequences and the direction of bias needs to be assessed on a case-by-case basis. In many, even most, cases of non-differential misclassification, the bias tends to be toward the null value.

The source of exposure misclassification that arises from the disparity between the ideal, etiologically relevant exposure indicator and the feasible, operational definition of exposure would for the most part apply equally to persons with and without disease. That is, inaccuracy in exposure assessment that results from inherent limitations in the ability to capture the construct of interest would usually be independent of disease status. In contrast, the errors that arise going from the operational definition to the acquisition of the relevant data through monitoring, interviews, and specimen collection are often susceptible to distortion related to the past or even future occurrence of disease. There are almost always disparities between the operational definition of exposure and the information on which that assignment is based, and the processes by which such errors arise (recall, perception, behaviors, physiology) often differ in relation to disease status.

Mechanisms of Differential Exposure Misclassification

Disease May Distort Reporting or Perception of Exposure. Assuming a given amount or level of exposure has occurred, there must be some mechanism by which information on that exposure is ascertained. Questionnaires or interviews are usually at least a component of the exposure assessment process, whether done in a clinical setting and recorded in a medical record, elicited by an interviewer exclusively for the study, or through a mailed questionnaire. The respondent is asked to tell about his or her exposure, either directly or indirectly. Therefore, the opportunity for their representation of that exposure to be influenced by current or past health experience needs to be scrutinized.

One classic mechanism by which disease distorts reporting of exposure is through conscious concerns with the potential exposure–disease association under study. If an individual has heard or believes that exposure causes a disease, and he or she is suffering from that disease, he or she may be more inclined to believe and report that he or she was exposed. What is only a vague memory may be reported as fact, or rumination about whether he or she did or did not have the putative causal exposure may result in erroneously reporting that he or she did. While this phenomenon is appropriately invoked as a concern in studies that require reporting of exposure after disease onset, usually case–control studies, the circumstances under which it would occur are limited. Although there is much speculation about disease-inspired reporting of exposure because it seems reasonable to anticipate it, there are few instances in which this biased reporting has been documented.

One of the issues of concern has been the reporting of exposure to medications during pregnancy in relation to the risk of having a child with a congenital defect (Klemetti & Saxén, 1967). Mothers who have suffered the emotional trauma of having an affected child are postulated to overreport use of medications that they did not truly take. A number of studies indicate that recall of medications and many other exposures during pregnancy is often incomplete, but overreporting is quite rare (Werler et al., 1989). In addition, the patterns of erroneous underreporting tend to be similar among those with and without the disease. The susceptibility to differentially incomplete reporting depends in large part on how susceptible the exposure is to incomplete reporting more generally. Recall of relatively inconsequential events, such as taking cold medications during pregnancy, is highly vulnerable to faulty, often incomplete, recall. In contrast, recall of whether medications to control epilepsy were taken during pregnancy is likely to be much more comprehensively recalled and thus is less likely to differ for those with and without an adverse health outcome.

In order for the completeness of recall to be affected by the health outcome, the respondent must consciously or unconsciously establish a link between the exposure and outcome. Therefore, the potential for biased reporting of exposure depends in part on perception among respondents of a link between exposure and disease, and those relations that have a high level of media attention and public interest are therefore more vulnerable. Many putative associations gather widespread public interest and awareness, making it difficult to elicit information without some contamination based on the participants' expectations. Investigators sometimes will ask directly if the participant has heard about or believes that the exposure of interest can cause the disease under study, allowing for stratification by those who do and do not believe it does. Although it can be argued that those lacking suspicion would generate the more accurate responses, it could also be hypothesized that those who are most attentive to media reports are also the most attentive to their own exposures and provide the more accurate data.

An additional determinant of susceptibility to biased recall is the degree of subjectivity in defining the exposure. Events such as prior surgery or level of education, for example, are unambiguous and not subject to varying interpretation. In contrast, history of diseases based on self-diagnosis, such as frequent headaches or conditions that are inherently subjective such as perceived stress are much more vulnerable to differential misclassification in that the reporting contains an element of judgment.

There are several approaches to evaluating how likely it is that such biased recall has occurred and if it has occurred, how much it has affected the study results. As always, the opportunity to validate reported exposure is optimal, in this case requiring validation of reports from a sufficient number of persons with and without the disease to contrast the two groups. Both the *absolute* level of accuracy, as an indicator of potential bias due to exposure misclassification generally, and *relative* level of accuracy among those with and without disease, as an indicator of potential bias due to differential exposure misclassification, are of interest. The closer the validation measure is to the gold standard, the better, but even a measure of similar quality that is less vulnerable to distortion due to disease may be helpful. That is, an equally fallible exposure indicator that could not possibly be affected by development of disease, such as record-based exposure ascertained long before disease development, can be compared to self-reported exposure among cases and non-cases to determine whether there is evidence of differential error, even if the absolute level of error is not known.

Another approach is to examine some exposures that are very unlikely to affect the occurrence of disease but otherwise meet all the criteria for biased reporting. Exposures that are widely perceived as being related to disease causation are most vulnerable to reporting error. If data on such an exposure or ideally, multiple exposures, are available, and show no evidence of differing in relation to disease status, this would provide reassurance that it is unlikely to be present for exposures that are less widely perceived as being related to disease or more objective in nature. If there is evidence of recall bias for those exposures most susceptible to biased reporting, then further examination of the potential for bias in the measurement of exposures of interest is warranted. Data on a spectrum of exposures can be helpful in looking for patterns of this sort.

Often, this can be readily incorporated into study of multiple specific agents, e.g., medications, dietary constituents. Even if the true interest is in a single medication or a narrow class of medications, for example, the investigators might obtain a somewhat longer list to use the other drugs as markers of susceptibility to differential misclassification. That is, if medications thought to be very unlikely to cause disease are nevertheless reported more commonly by those with disease than those without, differential exposure misclassification for those drugs as well as the ones of primary interest might be inferred as being more probable. Application of this strategy requires placebo exposures that are perceived by the public to be potential causes but unlikely to actually affect disease.

An example from the literature serves to illustrate several of these pathways for differential exposure misclassification. The possibility that head trauma may affect risk of developing brain tumors has been evaluated rather extensively (Ahlbom et al., 1986; Burch et al., 1987), and always in case–control studies. This is the sort of hypothesis that is more intuitively appealing to the public than to most investigators, who are skeptical about whether a plausible mechanism might link physical trauma to tumor development. In a series of case–control studies reporting a positive association, there is a persistent concern with over-reporting by cases. In order to address that possibility, more objective measures of head trauma have been sought by restricting the severity. Whereas recall of minor bumps on the head over one's life may be highly vulnerable to distortion, memory of head trauma resulting in loss of consciousness or medical treatment is less susceptible to individual interpretation and selective recall. The ratio of reports of major, verifiable head trauma to unverifiable minor head trauma might be examined for cases and controls. Other ostensibly significant exposures in the head area might be queried as markers of biased reporting, e.g., cuts, insect bites. The proportion of participants who believe that head trauma may play a role in the development of brain tumors would be of interest, giving some sense of the level of vulnerability to biased reporting.

Disease May Distort the Measure of Exposure. Analogous to the phenomenon in which the occurrence of disease may alter perception or self-report of exposure, disease may alter biological measures of exposure if those measures are taken after or even near the time of disease onset. Despite many attractive features of biological markers of exposure, the question of whether their accuracy has somehow been altered by the disease of interest deserves careful appraisal. For diseases that develop over extended periods of time before becoming clinically apparent, including many chronic diseases such as neurodegenerative disease, cancer, and atherosclerotic heart disease, measures taken months or even several years before the manifestation of disease could reflect, in part, the evolving disease itself. Early stages of disease or disease precursors could alter the measure of exposure and produce an association between measured exposure and disease that has no etiologic significance.

Research on chlorinated hydrocarbons and breast cancer illustrates the concerns that can arise about whether the disease or its treatment might affect measured serum levels of DDT, DDE, and other stored compounds (Ahlborg et al., 1995). If, in fact, early stages of breast cancer result in the release of some of the persistent organochlorines that are stored in fat tissue, then women who go on to develop clinically apparent breast cancer will have had some period prior to diagnosis during which blood levels of those compounds were elevated, solely as a result of the early disease process. A prospective study that uses measurements obtained in the period shortly before case diagnosis could be affected. In a case–control study in which blood levels of organochlorines are measured after diagnosis and treatment of disease, there is even greater susceptibility to having case–control differences arise as a result of metabolic changes among cases. The problem arises when the measure of exposure is also, in part, reflecting the consequence of the disease itself.

One way to evaluate the potential influence of disease on measures of exposure is through a thorough understanding of the biological determinants of the exposure marker, allowing assessment of whether the disease process would be expected to modify the measure. Obviously, this requires substantive knowledge about the often complex pathways affecting the measure and a thorough understanding of the biologic effects over the course of disease development. In the case of breast cancer and chlorinated hydrocarbons, the pathways are quite complex and make it difficult to predict the combined effect of the disease on metabolism, influence of disease-associated weight loss, etc.

A better approach is to empirically assess the influence of disease on the exposure marker, through obtaining measurements before the disease has occurred, ideally even before the time when disease precursors would have been present, as well as after disease onset. The interest is in exposure during the etiologic period before the disease has begun to develop, so the measure prior to the onset of the disease can be viewed as the "gold standard" and the accuracy of the measure taken after onset can be evaluated for its adequacy as a proxy. This requires having stored specimens for diseases that are relatively rare and develop over long periods of time, so that a sufficient number of prediagnosis measurements are available. One study was able to use specimens obtained long before the manifestation of disease (Krieger et al., 1994), but did not report any comparisons of prediagnosis with postdiagnosis measures from the same women. One study did evaluate the effect of treatment for breast cancer on such markers (Gammon et al., 1996), and verified that the values just prior to initiation of treatment were quite similar to those observed shortly after treatment began, addressing at least one of the hypothesized steps at which distortion might arise.

Even if the ideal data are not available, strategies exist for indirectly assessing the likely impact, if any, of disease on the measure of exposure. The disease may have varying degrees of severity, with influences on exposure measures more likely for severe than mild forms of the disease. For example, breast cancer ranges from carcinoma *in situ*, which should have little if any widespread biologic effects, to metastatic disease, with profound systemic consequences. If the association between chlorinated hydrocarbons and breast cancer were similar across the spectrum of disease severity, it would be unlikely to merely reflect metabolic changes associated with disease given that the severity of those metabolic changes would be quite variable *among* breast cancer cases. Examining the pattern of results across the spectrum of disease severity would reveal the extent to which the disease process had altered measurements, with results for the least severe disease (carcinoma *in situ*) most valid and the results for late-stage disease least valid.

The timing of exposure ascertainment relative to the onset of disease has been examined as well to indicate the likely magnitude of distortion. A series of studies in the 1970s and early 1980s had suggested that low levels of serum cholesterol were related to development of a number of types of cancer, with cholesterol assessed prior to the onset of disease (Kritchevsky & Kritchevsky, 1992). Nonetheless, there was great concern with the possibility that even cancer in its early, preclinical stage may have affected the serum cholesterol levels. Under this scenario, low levels of cholesterol followed within a limited period, say 6 to 12 months, by the diagnosis of cancer, may have been low due to the developing cancer itself. The approach taken to assess this problem has been to examine risk stratified by time since the measurement in longitudinal studies, in order to determine whether the pattern of association with disease differs across time. It would be more plausible that preclinical cancer that became manifest in the first 6 months following cholesterol measurement had affected the cholesterol measure than it would for cancers diagnosed 5 years or 10 years after cholesterol measurement.

Disease May Cause Exposure. For certain types of exposure, it is possible for early disease not just to distort the measure of exposure, as described above, but also to actually cause the exposure. This is especially problematic for exposures that are closely linked to the early symptoms of the disease of concern, which may include medications taken for those symptoms or variants of the symptoms themselves. Prior to being diagnosed, early disease may lead to events or behaviors that can be mistakenly thought to have etiologic significance. The causal sequence is one in which preclinical disease results in exposure, and then the disease evolves to become clinically recognized.

Among the candidate influences on the etiology of brain tumors are a number of diseases or medications, including the role of epilepsy and drugs used to control epilepsy (White et al., 1979; Shirts et al., 1986). It is clear that epilepsy precedes the diagnosis of brain tumors, and medications commonly used to treat epilepsy are more commonly taken prior to diagnosis by brain tumor cases than controls in case–control studies. What is not clear is whether the early symptoms of brain tumors, which are notoriously difficult to diagnose accurately in their early stages, include epilepsy, such that the disease of interest (brain tumor) is causing the exposure (epilepsy and its treatments). Similar issues arise in studying medications used to treat early symptoms of a disease, e.g., over-the-counter medications for gastrointestinal disturbance as a possible cause of colon cancer.

Similarly, undiagnosed chronic disease has the potential to distort certain exposures of interest as potential causes, illustrated in a recent study of depression as a potential influence on the risk of cancer. In a large cohort study in Denmark, Dalton et al. (2002) evaluated the association between depression and other affective disorders in relation to the incidence of cancer. By stratifying their results by years of follow-up (Table 8.8), they were able to consider the time course of depression and cancer incidence to better understand the etiologic significance of the results. Focusing on the results for the total cohort, note that brain cancer risk was substantially elevated for the first year of follow-up only, returning to near baseline thereafter. Although it could be hypothesized that depression is causally related to brain cancer with a short latency, it seems much more likely that undiagnosed brain cancer was a cause of the depressive symptoms given what is known about the time course of cancer development. That is, the disease of interest, brain cancer, undiagnosed at the time of entry into the cohort, may well have caused the exposure of interest, depression. The likelihood that undiagnosed brain cancer becomes manifest many years after entry, distorting measures of association years later, is much less plausible so that the overall pattern is suggestive of reverse causality.

Identification of Subgroups with Nondifferential Exposure Misclassification

Because the effects of errors in exposure that are the same for diseased and non-diseased individuals tend to produce more predictable errors, often leading to bias toward the null value, there is value in trying to create strata in which the error is likely to be nondifferential. It would be preferable, of course, to avoid error altogether, but stratification to achieve nondifferential misclassification is still of benefit.

When a determinant of exposure accuracy, for example, educational level, is also associated with disease, the results will be distorted due to differential misclassification of exposure if education is ignored. In other words, the imbalance in educational levels among those with and without disease, and the association between educational level and accuracy of reported exposure, results in differ-

TABLE 8.8. Standardized Incidence Ratios for All Types of Cancer Combined and for Tobacco-Related Cancers, by Diagnostic Group, in Patients Hospitalized with an Effective Disorder in Denmark, 1969–1993

											Portion of Follow-up Period			
	Total			First Year of Follow-up			1–9 Years of Follow-up			≥10 Years of Follow-up				
DIAGNOSIS	OBS	SIR*	95% CI	OBS	SIR	95% CI	OBS	SIR	95%CI	OBS	SIR	95% CI		
Total Cohort	9922	1.05	1.03, 1.07	654	1.19	1.11, 1.29	4655	1.02	0.99, 1.05	4613	1.07	1.03, 1.10		
Tobacco-related cancers†	2813	1.21	1.16, 1.25	182	1.37	1.18, 1.59	1224	1.09	1.03, 1.16	1407	1.30	1.23, 1.37		
Non-tobacco-related cancers	7109	1.00	0.98, 1.02	472	1.14	1.04, 1.25	3431	1.00	0.97, 1.03	3206	0.99	0.95, 1.02		
Brain cancer	277	1.18	1.00, 1.32	46	3.27	2.39, 4.36	142	1.24	1.04, 1.46	89	0.84	0.67, 1.03		
Other	6832	0.99	0.97, 1.02	426	1.06	0.97, 1.17	3289	0.99	0.96, 1.02	3117	0.99	0.96, 1.03		
Diagnostic Level‡														
Bipolar psychosis	1217	0.99	0.93, 1.03	62	1.16	0.89, 1.49	557	1.00	0.92, 1.09	598	0.94	0.87, 1.02		
Tobacco-related cancers†	292	0.92	0.82, 1.04	18	1.30	0.77, 2.06	133	0.94	0.78, 1.11	141	0.88	0.74, 1.04		
Non-tobacco-related cancers	925	1.00	0.93, 1.06	44	1.11	0.80, 1.48	424	1.02	0.93, 1.12	457	0.97	0.88, 1.06		
Brain cancer	26	0.82	0.53, 1.20	4	2.72	0.73, 6.97	12	0.81	0.42, 1.42	10	0.64	0.31, 1.17		
Other	899	1.00	0.94, 1.07	40	1.04	0.75, 1.42	412	1.03	0.93, 1.13	447	0.98	0.89, 1.07		
Unipolar Psychosis	4345	0.98	0.95, 1.01	290	1.00	0.89, 1.12	2176	0.94	0.90, 0.98	1879	1.03	0.99, 1.08		
Tobacco-related cancers†	1144	1.05	0.99, 1.11	76	1.07	0.84, 1.34	538	0.95	0.87, 1.03	530	1.18	1.08, 1.29		
Non-tobacco-related cancers	3201	0.96	0.93, 1.00	214	0.98	0.85, 1.12	1638	0.94	0.90, 0.99	1349	0.98	0.93, 1.04		
Brain cancer	119	1.19	0.99, 1.43	21	3.10	1.92, 4.75	58	1.11	0.84, 1.43	40	0.99	0.70, 1.34		
Other	3082	0.96	0.92, 0.99	193	0.91	0.79, 1.05	1580	0.94	0.89, 0.99	1309	0.98	0.93, 1.04		

(continued)

TABLE 8.8. Standardized Incidence Ratios for All Types of Cancer Combined and for Tobacco-Related Cancers, by Diagnostic Group, in Patients Hospitalized with an Effective Disorder in Denmark, 1969–1993 (continued)

| | Portion of Follow-up Period | | | | | | | | | | |
| | Total | | | First Year of Follow-up | | | 1–9 Years of Follow-up | | | ≥10 Years of Follow-up | | |
DIAGNOSIS	OBS	SIR*	95% CI	OBS	SIR	95% CI	OBS	SIR	95%CI	OBS	SIR	95% CI
Reactive Depression	2075	1.13	1.08, 1.18	184	1.62	1.39, 1.87	997	1.12	1.05, 1.19	894	1.07	1.00, 1.14
Tobacco-related cancers†	663	1.41	1.30, 1.52	58	2.03	1.54, 2.62	297	1.32	1.17, 1.48	308	1.43	1.27, 1.59
Non-tobacco-related cancers	1412	1.03	0.98, 1.09	126	1.48	1.23, 1.76	700	1.06	0.98, 1.14	586	0.95	0.87, 1.02
Brain cancer	59	1.20	0.92, 1.55	14	4.55	2.48, 7.63	29	1.21	0.81, 1.74	16	0.73	0.42, 1.18
Other	1353	1.03	0.97, 1.08	112	1.36	1.12, 1.64	671	1.05	0.97, 1.13	570	0.95	0.88, 1.03
Dysthymia	2285	1.18	1.13, 1.23	118	1.32	1.09, 1.58	925	1.15	1.08, 1.23	1242	1.19	1.13, 1.26
Tobacco-related cancers†	714	1.56	1.45, 1.68	30	1.58	1.07, 2.26	256	1.40	1.24, 1.59	428	1.68	1.52, 1.84
Non-tobacco-related cancers	1571	1.06	1.01, 1.12	88	1.25	1.00, 1.54	669	1.07	0.99, 1.16	814	1.04	0.97, 1.11
Brain cancer	73	1.34	1.05, 1.68	7	2.54	1.02, 5.24	43	1.80	1.30, 2.43	23	0.82	0.52, 1.23
Other	1498	1.05	1.00, 1.11	81	1.19	0.95, 1.48	626	1.04	0.97, 1.13	791	1.04	0.97, 1.12

*Observed number of cases/expected number of cases. The expected number of cases was the number of cancer cases expected on the basis of age-, sex-, and calendar-year-specific incidence rates of first primary cancers in Denmark.

†Cancers of the buccal cavity, larynx, lung, esophagus, pancreas, kidney, and urinary bladder.

‡Bipolar psychosis: ICD-8 codes 296.39, 296.19, and 298.19; unipolar psychosis: ICD-8 codes 296.09, 296.29, 296.89, and 296.99; reactive depression: ICD-8 code 298.09; dysthymia: ICD-8 codes 300.49 and 301.19.

Obs, observed; SIR, standardized incidence ratio; CI, confidence interval; ICD-8, *International Classification of Diseases*, Eighth Revision.

Dalton et al., 2002.

ential misclassification of exposure. The solution in this example is simple: stratify on educational level and examine the exposure–disease association within education strata. Within the strata, the accuracy of reporting exposure is more homogeneous in that one source of variability has been controlled, so that remaining errors are more nondifferential in character. There may be other contributors to differential exposure accuracy that remain or educational level may have been the sole basis for the differential. Regardless, stratification by education will be beneficial.

Note that education, in this example, is a marker of accuracy, not a confounder, and should therefore not be adjusted. In fact, under the assumption that more highly educated respondents provide more accurate data, the expectation would be that the most accurate results would be obtained in the high education stratum (less nondifferential misclassification). In order to implement this strategy, the markers of classification accuracy must be known, measured, and not too strongly related to disease status. At the extreme, if the marker of accuracy is perfectly correlated with disease status, it cannot be separated from disease in the analysis.

INTEGRATED ASSESSMENT OF POTENTIAL FOR BIAS DUE TO EXPOSURE MISCLASSIFICATION

Exposure misclassification has been recognized as ubiquitous in epidemiologic studies (Rothman & Greenland, 1998; Armstrong et al., 1992), and thus the focus is on the magnitude and severity of exposure misclassification in the interpretation of epidemiologic study results. Clearly, accuracy of exposure measurement deserves great attention in the study design phase. Inaccuracy arises through diverse pathways, and all the conceptual and practical limitations that produce a disparity between the operational measure and the ideal measure of exposure need to be considered. Investigators may be reluctant to articulate precisely what they would truly like to know, in that such honesty reveals how much they have to compromise to arrive at a feasible study plan. In particular, the insurmountable limitations in exposure assessment are often ignored or downplayed simply because there is little that can be done to address them. The hypothesis under study often directs attention to a specific pathway, with the ideal exposure measure the one that is biologically and temporally matched to the disease process. Decisions about lumping and splitting exposure are analogous to those for disease: select the level of aggregation that is pertinent to the hypothesized etiologic pathway.

Given a completed study, the presence of exposure misclassification and its influence on the measure of association should be evaluated. Where possible, measures that are superior to those routinely obtained should be sought, allowing a comparison between them to better assess the quality of the routine measure. Assessing such accuracy for those with and without disease can reveal differential exposure misclassification. In addition, by examining results across a spectrum of exposure measures of differing quality, inferences can be made about how results might look with a more perfect indicator. Even when there are not demonstrably superior measures of exposure available, useful information can be obtained through multiple, imperfect exposure measures that can then be combined in a variety of ways or compared. Consideration of known exposure determinants or consequences can help to assess the extent to which the measure is functioning as desired.

The potential for differential exposure misclassification deserves special attention, given that its influences on measures of effect are not readily predictable. The presence of disease may influence the way people report or interpret exposure, a problem that occurs when disease onset precedes exposure ascertainment. Distinct from the awareness of the disease affecting exposure, the biologic process of the disease, even at early, preclinical stages may alter biologic exposure measures. Sometimes, symptoms associated with the early stages of undiagnosed disease actually cause the exposure to occur, such as the use of medications to treat preclinical symptoms. Opportunities to convert differential to non-differential exposure misclassification should be pursued where possible by stratifying on disease predictors that also affect exposure data quality.

Measurement technologies have different strengths and pitfalls, and these considerations have been discussed in great detail (Armstrong et al., 1992). Self-reported exposure has obvious potential for error, due to the fallibility of human memory and cognition, and the possible influence of the disease process on such error needs to be carefully examined. Biological measures, ostensibly more precise in one sense, also have pitfalls, most notably a limited ability to reflect the etiologic period of interest and susceptibility to distortion by the disease itself. As new, increasingly elaborate technologies become available to assess exposure, whether based on molecular biology or more cognitively sophisticated interviewing strategies, the guiding question remains the same: How well does the operational measure of exposure approximate the ideal?

REFERENCES

Ahlbom A, Navier IL, Norell S, Olin R Spannare B. Nonoccupational risk indicators for astrocytomas in adults. Am J Epidemiol 1986;124:334–337.

Ahlborg UF, Lipworth L, Titus-Ernstoff L, Hsieh C-C, Hanberg A, Baron J, Trichopoulos D, Adami H-O. Organochlorine compound in relation to breast cancer, endometrial cancer, and endometriosis: An assessment of the biological and epidemiological evidence. Crit Rev Toxicol 1995;25:463–531.

Albert C, Mittleman M, Chae C, Lee I, Hennekens C, Manson J. Triggering of sudden death from cardiac causes by vigorous exercise. N Engl J Med 2000;343:1355–1361.

Armstrong BG. The effects of measurement errors on relative risk regressions. Am J Epidemiol 1990;132:1176–1184.

Armstrong BK, White E, Saracci R. Principles of exposure measurement in epidemiology. New York: Oxford University Press, 1992.

Baris D, Linet MS, Tarone RE, Kleinerman RA, Hatch EE, Kaune WT, Robison LL, Lubin J, Wacholder S. Residential exposure to magnetic fields: an empirical assessment of alternative measurement strategies. Occup Environ Med 1999;56:562–566.

Berkson J. Limitations of the application of the fourfold table to hospital data. Biomet Bull 1946;2:47–53.

Brinton LA, Daling JR, Liff JM, Schoenberg JB, Malone KE, Stanford JL, Coates RJ, Gammon MD, Hanson L, Hoover RN. Oral contraceptives and breast cancer risk among younger women. J Natl Cancer Inst 1995;87:827–835.

Burch JD, Craib KJP, Choi BCK, Miller AB, Risch HA, Howe GR. An exploratory case-control study of brain tumors in adults. J Natl Cancer Inst 1987;78:601–609.

Copeland KT, Checkoway H, Holbrook RH, McMichael AJ. Bias due to misclassification in the estimate of relative risk. Am J Epidemiol 1977;105:488–495.

Dalton SO, Mellemkjaer L, Olsen JH, Mortensen PB, Johansen C. Depression and cancer risk: a register-based study of patients hospitalized with affective disorders, Denmark, 1969–1993. Am J Epidemiol 2002;155:1088–1095.

Dominici F, Samet J, Zeger SL. Combining evidence on air pollution and daily mortality from the largest 20 U.S. cities: a hierarchical modeling strategy. J Roy Stat Soc Ser A 2000;163:263–302.

Dosemeci M, Wacholder S, Lubin J. Does nondifferential misclassification of exposure always bias a true effect toward the null value? Am J Epidemiol 1990;132:746–749.

Gammon M, Wolff M, Neugut A, Terry M, Britton J, Greenebaum E, Hibshoosh H, Levin B, Wang Q, Santella R. Treatment for breast cancer and blood levels of chlorinated hydrocarbons. Cancer Epidemiol Biomark Prev 1996;5:467–471.

Goodman GE, Schaffer S, Bankson DD, Hughes MP, Omenn GS, Carotene and Retinol Efficacy Trial Co-Investigators. Predictors of serum selenium in cigarette smokers and the lack of association with lung and prostate cancer. Cancer Epidemiol Biomark Prev 2001;10:1069–1076.

Greenland S. Avoiding power loss associated with categorization and ordinal scores in dose-response and trend analysis. Epidemiology 1995;6:450–454.

Hardy AM, Fowler MG. Child care arrangements and repeated ear infections in young children. Am J Public Health 1993;83:1321–1325.

Katsouyanni K, Touloumi G, Spix C, et al. Short-term effects of ambient sulfur dioxide and particulate matter on mortality in 12 European cities: results from time series data from the APHEA project. BMJ 1997;314:1658–1663.

Kleinbaum DG, Kupper LL, Morgenstern H. Epidemiologic research: principles and quantitative methods. Belmont, California: Lifetime Learning Publications, 1982.

Klemetti A, Saxén L. Prospective versus retrospective approach in the search for environmental causes of malformations. Am J Pub Health 1967;57:2071–2075.

Kline J, Stein Z, Susser M. Conception to birth: Epidemiology of prenatal development. New York: Oxford University Press, 1989:28–30.

Krieger N, Wolff M, Hiatt R, Rivera M, Vogelman J, Orentreich N. Breast cancer and serum organochlorines: a prospective study among white, black and Asian women. J Natl Cancer Inst 1994;86:589–599.

Kritchevsky SB, Kritchevsky D. Serum cholesterol and cancer risk: an epidemiologic perspective. Annu Rev Nutr 1992;12:391–416.

Kritz-Silverstein D, Barrett-Connor E, Corbeau C. Cross-sectional and prospective study of exercise and depressed mood in the elderly. The Rancho Bernardo Study. Am J Epidemiol 2001;153:596–603.

Lagakos SW. Effects of mismodelling and mismeasuring explanatory variables in tests of their association with a response variable. Stat Med 1988;7:257–274.

Lin SS, Glaser SL, Stewart SL. Reliability of self-reported reproductive factors and childhood social class indicators in a case-control study of women. Ann Epidemiol 2002;12:242–247.

Millikan R, DeVoto E, Duell EJ, Tse C-K, Savitz DA, Beach J, Edmiston S, Jackson S, Newman B. Dichlorodiphenyldichloroethene, polychlorinated biphenyls, and breast cancer among African-American and white women in North Carolina. Cancer Epidemiol Biomark Prev 2000;9:1233–1240.

Pearce N, Sanjose S, Boffetta P, Kogevinas M, Saracci R, Savitz D. Limitations of biomarkers of exposure in cancer epidemiology. Epidemiology 1995,6:190–194.

Phillips AN, Smith GD. The design of prospective epidemiological studies: more subjects or better measurements? J Clin Epidemiol 1993;10:1203–1211.

Pope CA III, Burnett RT, Thun MT, Calle EE, Krewski D, Ito K, Thurston GD. Lung cancer, cardiopulmonary mortality, and long-term exposure to fine particulate air pollution. JAMA 2002;287:1132–1141.

Reaven PD, McPhillips JB, Barrett-Connor EL, Criqui MH. Leisure time exercise and lipid and lipoprotein levels in an older population. J Am Geriatr Soc 1990;38:847–854.

Rockhill B, Willett WC, Manson JE, et al. Physical activity and mortality: a prospective study among women. Am J Public Health 2001;91:578–583.

Rothman KJ. Induction and latent periods. Am J Epidemiol 1981;114:253–259.

Rothman KJ, Greenland S. Modern epidemiology, Second edition. Philadelphia: Lippincott-Raven Publishers, 1998.

Shirts SB, Annegers JF, Houser WA, Kurland LT. Cancer incidence in a cohort of patients with severe seizure disorders. J Natl Cancer Inst 1986;77:83–87.

Siscovick D, Weiss N, Fletcher R, Lasky T. The incidence of primary cardiac arrest during vigorous exercise. N Engl J Med 1984;311:874–877.

US DHHS. Physical activity and health: A report of the Surgeon General. Atlanta, GA: US Department of Health and Human Services, Centers for Disease Control and Prevention, National Center for Chronic Disease Prevention and Health Promotion, 1996.

Weiss NS. Inferring causal relationships. Elaboration of the criterion of dose-response. Am J Epidemiol 1981;113:487–490

Werler MM, Pober BR, Nelson K, Holmes LB. Reporting accuracy among mothers of malformed and nonmalformed infants. Am J Epidemiol 1989;129:415–421.

White SJ, McClean AEM, Howland C. Anticonvulsant drugs and cancer: a cohort study in patients with severe epilepsy. Lancet 1979;2:458–460.

Zeisel SA, Roberts JE, Neebe EC, Riggins R Jr, Henderson F. A longitudinal study of otitis media with effusion among 2- to 5-year-old African-American children in child care. Pediatrics 1999;103:15–19.

9

MEASUREMENT AND CLASSIFICATION
OF DISEASE

In this chapter, the challenges that arise in accurately identifying the occurrence
of disease, or more broadly, health outcomes, are considered. Also, consideration is given to the methods for detecting such errors and quantifying their impact on measures of association. Some amount of error in assessment is inevitable,
with the extent of such error dependent on the nature of the health outcome of
interest, the ability to apply definitive (sometimes invasive) tests to all participants, and human and instrument error associated with gathering and interpreting the information needed to assess the outcome.

FRAMEWORK FOR EVALUATING DISEASE MISCLASSIFICATION

Misclassification or measurement error refers to a phenomenon in which the values assigned to study variables (exposure, disease, or confounders) are incorrect
relative to their true values. For a dichotomous measure of disease, some persons who in fact have the disease are misidentified as disease-free or those who
are free of the disease are falsely labeled as having the disease. For measures
with multiple categories, individuals are assigned the wrong level of the variable, or for measures that are continuous, e.g., blood pressure, serum glucose,
the quantitative score they are given is in error relative to their actual score.

The consequence of misclassification on the measure of association is some-times referred to as information bias. The concept applies as much to continu-ous as to categorical variables, though the terminology differs slightly—with con-tinuous measures, we usually describe the phenomenon as measurement error, in which the true and measured values differ from one another. The closer the true and measured values are to one another, on average, the less measurement error exists. In the case of categorical variables, we consider the probabilities of clas-sifying an individual into the correct category and failure to do so as misclassi-fication. The methodological literature often focuses on dichotomous variables and uses terminology derived from the concepts of screening for disease: sensi-tivity refers to the proportion of subjects with the attribute who are correctly iden-tified as having the attribute and specificity refers to the proportion of subjects without the attribute who are correctly identified as lacking it. In the screening literature, these terms are used to evaluate the accuracy of an imperfect indica-tor of disease relative to the gold standard diagnosis, whereas in the application to misclassification, the routinely applied measure is the counterpart of a screen-ing test that is evaluated against a superior, ideally perfect, indicator of the pres-ence or absence of disease.

Typically, disease is categorized into a dichotomy, present or absent, even though the underlying biological phenomenon often falls along a continuum, as discussed below. Most of the discussion in this chapter is focused on dichoto-mous measures of disease, in part for simplicity but also because many health events truly are present or absent. Death is perhaps the most distinctly dichoto-mous, and even where there is a biological phenomenon on a continuous scale (blood pressure, glucose tolerance), clinical medicine often considers disease to be present when some threshold is exceeded and the value falls outside the nor-mal range. All the concepts that are developed for disease dichotomies would apply to health outcomes measured in multiple categories and continuously as well.

SOURCES OF DISEASE MISCLASSIFICATION

The most obvious source of disease misclassification is outright error, for ex-ample, a clerical error in which a healthy person is assigned the wrong labora-tory result and is incorrectly labeled as diseased. Conversely, an individual who truly has a disease may be examined, but through clinician oversight, critical symptoms are not queried or the appropriate diagnostic tests are not conducted. This oversight results in a false negative diagnosis and the patient is erroneously labeled as being free of disease. In the conventional table of a dichotomous dis-ease cross-classified with exposure, the person who belongs in the diseased cell is placed in the non-diseased cell or vice versa.

There are many variations and complexities in disease ascertainment that result in some form of misclassification. One level beyond simple errors at the individual level is error in the very definition of disease that is chosen and applied in the study. Sometimes the rules for disease ascertainment, even if followed precisely, predictably generate false positive and false negative diagnoses. For many diseases, such as rheumatoid arthritis or Alzheimer's disease, the diagnosis requires meeting a specified number of predesignated signs and symptoms, which has the virtue of providing a systematic, objective method of classification. Systematic and objective does not necessarily mean valid, however, only reliable. At best, such criteria are probabilistic in nature, with cases that are identified by meeting the diagnostic criteria likely or even very likely to be diseased, and those assigned as noncases very likely to be free of the disease. Even when the rules are followed precisely however, some proportion of false positives and false negatives are inevitable. Often, the diagnosis based on a constellation of symptoms is truly the best that can be done on living patients, but sometimes there is an opportunity to evaluate the validity of the diagnosis at some future date when diagnostic information is refined. Where a definitive diagnosis can be made after death, as in Alzheimer's disease, the diagnostic accuracy based on applying clinical criteria can be quantified. In other instances, such as many psychiatric diagnoses, there is no such anchor of certainty so that the patient's true status is unknown and the effectiveness of the diagnostic criteria is not readily measured.

As a reminder that disease assignment can be a fallible process, expert committees periodically evaluate diagnostic criteria and modify them as concepts and empirical evidence evolve. Clearly, either the initial criteria, the revised criteria, or both had to contain systematic error relative to the unknown gold standard. If, in fact, some of those signs and symptoms should not have been included as criteria or if some components of the diagnosis that should have been included were omitted, errors of diagnosis must have resulted from proper application of the rules. Even an optimally designed checklist has probabilistic elements in that a given constellation of symptoms cannot definitively lead to a specific diagnosis and exclude all others. Regardless of the origins of the problem, under this scenario all relevant signs and symptoms will be elicited properly, recorded accurately, and integrated according to the best rules available, yet a certain fraction of persons labeled as diseased will not have the disease and some of those labeled as non-diseased will actually have it.

Beyond the likelihood of error in properly applied operational definitions of disease, the actual process by which individuals come to be identified as cases in a study provides many additional opportunities for errors to arise. Typically, a sequence of events and decisions are made to become a diagnosed case such that overcoming one hurdle is required to proceed with the next on the pathway leading to disease identification and inclusion as a case in the study. These include both technical considerations based on disease signs and symptoms, but also hurdles defined by recognition of symptoms and clinician insights.

False positives tend to be more readily identified and corrected than false negatives. False positives are often less likely because those who meet a given milestone on the path to diagnosis are evaluated more intensively at the next stage and can thus be weeded out at any point along the way. On the other hand, failure to identify a person as needing further scrutiny in any step along the pathway to diagnosis can result in elimination from further consideration and a false negative diagnosis. Once a potential case of disease comes to the attention of the health care system, substantial effort can be devoted to verifying the presence of disease as a prelude to choosing among treatment options.

Optimally, a series of sequential screening efforts of increasing cost and sophistication is designed to end up with true cases, starting with a rather wide net that is highly sensitive and not terribly specific, and proceeding to increasingly specific measures. If the early stages of screening are not highly sensitive, then false negative errors will occur and not have the opportunity to be identified given that potential cases will leave the diagnostic pathway. Once such an error is made in the early phase of identifying disease, it is inefficient for the massive numbers of presumptively negative individuals to be re-evaluated to confirm the absence of disease. People do not always recognize symptoms, they may fail to seek treatment for the symptoms they do recognize, and even after seeking treatment, they may not be diagnosed accurately. Each of these steps in reaching a diagnosis constitutes the basis for terminating the search, affording numerous opportunities for underascertainment.

Many diseases, defined as a specific biologic condition, are simply not amenable to comprehensive ascertainment for logistical reasons. For example, a sizable proportion (perhaps 10%–15%) of couples are incapable of reproducing, and some fraction of that infertility is attributable to blockage in the fallopian tubes, preventing the transport of the ovum from the ovary to the uterus. This specific biologic problem, obstruction of the fallopian tubes, is considered as the disease of interest in this illustration. Under the right set of circumstances, such couples will be accurately diagnosed as having infertility and further diagnostic assessment will result in identification of occlusion of the fallopian tubes as the underlying basis for the infertility. In order for this diagnosis to be made, however, the otherwise asymptomatic individual has to meet a number of criteria that are dependent in part on choices and desires. The intent to have a child has to be present. Persons who are not sexually active, those sexually active but using contraception, and even those who engage in unprotected intercourse without the intent of becoming pregnant would not define themselves as infertile and would thus not undergo medical evaluation and diagnosis. Many women who in fact have occlusion of the fallopian tubes are not diagnosed because they do not seek the medical attention required to be diagnosed (Marchbanks et al., 1989).

In principle, the problem could be circumvented by conducting the definitive evaluation on all women in a given population, regardless of their reproductive intentions, but the application of such procedures would be questionable on ethical and logistical grounds. The problem of undiscovered cases due to the lack of interest in conceiving cannot readily be overcome. Under the right conditions, the underlying medical problem would be revealed, but the biological problem is not a clinical or health problem until that occurs. It could be argued that a defining element of tubal infertility is the self-identification of infertility, not just the underlying biological condition.

Another mechanism resulting in systematic and often substantial underdiagnosis is when the biological condition often remains asymptomatic, as in most cases of prostate cancer in older men or atherosclerosis that falls below the threshold of producing symptoms. Advanced technologies capable of non-invasive assessment are being developed to comprehensively screen and identify such conditions, but under routine clinical care, false negatives (assuming that the underlying pathophysiologic process is defined as the disease of interest) are quite common.

Misclassification is only avoided by defining the disease, somewhat arbitrarily, as the combination of an underlying biologic condition *and* the symptoms that lead to its diagnosis. When the prevalence of subclinical disease is high, the distinction between those who are identified as diseased and those who are not is often based on decisions and behaviors unrelated to the disease process of interest. Some diagnoses may be incidental in the course of being evaluated for other health problems. To some extent, identification may reflect the idiosyncrasies that make some individuals perceive and report symptoms for a given condition whereas other individuals, with an ostensibly identical condition, do not. A particular challenge this can introduce is that any factors that are related to the tendency to be diagnosed can be mistaken as risk factors for the development of the disease. If wine consumption were positively associated with the desire to have children, for example, then wine consumption might well be associated with increased risk of *diagnosed* tubal infertility.

Poor choice of the quantitative scale on which disease is classified can introduce another form of misclassification, if the clinical classification methods conflict with the underlying biological phenomenon. Blood pressure follows a continuous distribution and it appears that the risk of adverse health consequences increases continuously with rising blood pressure (Rose, 1985). For the purpose of determining treatment, however, a dichotomous category of hypertension is established, and this may well be an entirely appropriate decision rule regarding the point at which the benefits of treatment outweigh the risks. Even here, however, a diagnosis of borderline hypertension suggests recognition that the dichotomy is arbitrary. Labeling those who fall below the threshold for diagnosing hypertension as disease free and those who fall over the threshold as diseased constitutes a form of misclassification, insofar as the disease of hypertension is defined in order to accurately reflect the relationship of blood pressure to heart disease and stroke. Choosing an operational definition of the disease variable that is not optimal for evaluating the consequences of the condition represents a form of misclassification, whether it involves inappropriately dichotomizing, setting the wrong cutpoint for a dichotomy, or evaluating a continuum when in reality a dichotomy is more useful.

Another continuum, gestational age at the time of delivery, is often dichotomized at 37 weeks' completed gestation as preterm delivery (diseased) versus term delivery (non-diseased). If one uses the prediction of infant health and survival as the gold standard for classification of gestational age at delivery into preterm versus term, the dichotomy has some merits in that risk increases markedly prior to completion of 37 weeks' gestation but there is little discernible benefit to advancing beyond 38 weeks. The grouping of very early (e.g., < 32 weeks' gestation) infants with marginally early births (e.g., 35–36 weeks' gestation) is problematic however, because the risk of infant death is many times higher for very early as compared to marginally early births. Examination of determinants of the entire spectrum of gestational age, tempting because of seemingly improved statistical power to evaluate a continuous measure, would not be a good strategy in this case. After 37 weeks, duration of gestation has little impact on survival (until the extreme high end of postterm births), and a continuous measure will be dominated by differences in the range of 37–41 weeks given that that is when most births occur but it is a period in which differences in duration of gestation are clinically inconsequential. In this case, the problem with a dichotomy of 37 weeks' gestation is the implication that births prior to that cutpoint are equally at risk, when they are not, and the problem with a continuous measure is that it implies duration of gestation across the entire spectrum, including the over 37 week period is important, when it is not. Some more complex definition of the outcome may be more appropriate, e.g., multiple categories below 37 weeks' gestation.

The exposure of interest, or more generally, the etiologic process under study, is also pertinent to defining and measuring disease. A phenomenon like mental retardation has some features of a continuum of intellectual and cognitive ability, with an arbitrary cutpoint, as well as some features of a true dichotomy, in which severe cases are not simply part of the normal distribution but rather a distinct entity. For studying possible influences on the etiology of mental retardation, we need to be explicit about which condition is of interest. Lead exposure, within the range typically encountered, is thought to result in a modest diminution in intellectual function across the entire spectrum (Schwartz, 1994), with an increased proportion of children expected to fall into the range defined as mentally retarded because the whole distribution is shifted downward. In this instance, the most informative outcome would be the continuous measure of intellectual function such as IQ score or the proportion below a threshold for mild retardation. On the other hand, in the case of certain viral infections during pregnancy, such as rubella, severe losses of intellectual ability would be anticipated, so that the proper disease endpoint for study is the dichotomy severe mental retardation or absence of severe mental retardation. Alcohol consumption during pregnancy may be capable of causing both a shift toward lower intellectual ability and cases of severe mental retardation in the form of fetal alcohol syndrome, depending on the dose. The consequences of inappropriately categorizing or failing to categorize can be viewed as forms of misclassification.

A commonly encountered decision in selecting a disease endpoint is the optimal level of aggregation or disaggregation, sometimes referred to as lumping versus splitting. The decision should be based on the entity that is most plausibly linked to exposure, reflecting an understanding of the pathophysiology of the disease generally and the specific etiologic process that is hypothesized to link exposure to the disease. There are unlimited opportunities for disaggregation, with subdivisions of disease commonly based on severity (e.g., obesity), age at occurrence (e.g., premenopausal versus postmenopausal breast cancer), exact anatomic location (e.g., brain tumors), microscopic characteristics (e.g., histologic type of gastric cancer), clinical course (e.g., Alzheimer's disease), molecular traits (e.g., cytogenetic types of leukemia), or prognosis (e.g., aggressiveness of prostate cancer). For any given disease, experts are continually deriving new ways in which the disease might be subdivided, particularly through the use of refined biological markers. There are a number of laudable but distinctive goals for such refined groupings, including identification of subsets for selecting appropriate treatment, assessing prognosis, or evaluating etiology. The goals of the epidemiologic study must be matched to the classification system to identify the optimal level of aggregation. There is no generic answer to the lumping versus splitting dilemma; it depends on the goal.

In principle, errors of excessive subdivision should only affect statistical power. That is, subdividing on irrelevant features of the disease, such as the day of the week on which it was diagnosed or the clinician's zodiac sign, would not lead to a loss of validity but only a loss of precision. It would be as though a random number was assigned to each event and they were grouped on the basis of the numerical assignment. By definition, selection based on an attribute that is unrelated to etiology constitutes a random sample. The loss of precision is not a small concern, however, given that imprecision and random error are frequently major barriers to distinguishing the signal from the noise. In studies of genetic susceptibility markers, for example, imprecision resulting from an interest in effect modification places severe burdens on study size (Greenland, 1983) and can result in a degree of imprecision that renders studies virtually uninformative. If greater aggregation is biologically appropriate, more informative studies can be conducted.

Errors of excessive aggregation adversely affect validity (Rothman, 1986). The motivation to lump is often an increase in statistical power or lack of awareness of the opportunity for disaggregation. If, in fact, the correct choice is made to aggregate potential subgroups, then precision is enhanced without sacrificing validity. In the above example, if we had foolishly divided the cases based on the clinician's zodiac sign, and some clever researcher was wise enough to reaggregate them, the precision of the study's results would be enhanced. The risk of lumping is as follows: if the subset of disease that is affected by an exposure is lumped with other subsets of disease that are unrelated to exposure, inclusion of those irrelevant cases is a form of misclassification that produces a diluted measure of association. The addition of irrelevant cases is identical to what would be produced by adding non-cases, an infusion of subjects with the exposure prevalence characteristic of the study base.

Assume that two diseases, for example, Hodgkin's disease and non-Hodgkin's lymphoma are entirely distinctive in their etiology. When we create a disease entity called lymphoma by aggregating the two, and conduct research to address the etiology of this condition, relative to studies of Hodgkin's disease alone or non-Hodgkin's lymphoma alone, the study suffers from misclassification. For purposes of studying Hodgkin's disease, infusing cases of non-Hodgkin's lymphoma is tantamount to infusing healthy persons who were incorrectly diagnosed, and conversely, if our purpose were to examine the etiology of non-Hodgkin's lymphoma. We can create entities such as lymphoma or even cancer or all illness and try to study the etiology of such diffuse entities. We can accurately measure and quantify the association between exposure and various diseases, reflecting a mixture of the subsets that are truly influenced by exposure and those that are not. In one sense, the misclassification is semantic in that the association between a given exposure and the inappropriately broad set of diseases is accurately measured. A more informative basis for inferring etiology however, would be the quantification of the association for the subset that is etiologically related to exposure and a documentation of the absence of association for the subset that is not related to exposure. If we are unaware of the heterogeneity among cases, what may be measured is a very small association that falls below the level of the study's resolution and is therefore simply not detected at all.

DIFFERENTIAL AND NONDIFFERENTIAL DISEASE MISCLASSIFICATION

In addition to the special substantive issues that apply to disease misclassification and its consequences, there are a number of methodological issues that need to be appreciated to assess the consequences of different patterns of misclassification. A key distinction is between subtypes of disease misclassification that are invariant with respect to exposure (non-differential misclassification of disease) versus those that differ as a function of exposure status (differential misclassification of disease).

The result of nondifferential disease misclassification depends on the type of design (cohort versus case–control), whether the error is due to disease under-ascertainment (false negatives) or overascertainment (false positives), and the measure of association (ratio or difference). The general principle is that non-differential misclassification in a dichotomous variable tends to produce bias towards the null (Rothman, 1986). Whatever the value would have been without misclassification, whether above or below the null value, nondifferential mis-classification in a dichotomous variable will most often bias the effect estimate by moving it closer to the null value (Kleinbaum et al., 1982). If the association is truly inverse, then the bias will be upward toward the null, and if the association is positive, then the bias will be downward toward the null. While this rule applies to many of the circumstances in which disease misclassification occurs, there are also some important exceptions to the rule in which no bias is expected to occur on average (Poole, 1985). Situations in which bias is absent should be identified and even sought out if the investigator or evaluator of the data has such an opportunity.

The consequences of erroneous assessment of disease depend on the study design. In a case–control study, the process by which potential cases are identified needs to be examined (Brenner & Savitz, 1990). Underascertainment of disease, if non-differential with respect to exposure, is tantamount to randomly sampling cases. In other words, a disease assessment mechanism that has a sensitivity of 80% is functionally equivalent to having decided to randomly sample 80% of eligible cases. The exposure prevalence among cases should not be altered due to underascertainment, though precision will be reduced due to the unnecessary loss of otherwise eligible cases. On the other hand, if undiagnosed cases remain under consideration as eligible potential controls past the time of disease onset, they will introduce selection bias since they have the exposure prevalence expected of cases and should have been removed from the study base once their disease began. Only under the null hypothesis, when exposure prevalence is identical among cases and the study base, will no bias result. Alternatively, if those cases who were erroneously not identified (and thus excluded) can be identified and omitted from the study base from which controls are sampled, then this bias can be averted. Inclusion of cases in the study base from which controls are to be sampled after their disease has begun will yield a biased sample. For reasonably rare diseases, however, the proportion of false negative cases among the pool of controls should have a negligible quantitative impact on the results.

In contrast, in a case–control study, disease overascertainment (imperfect specificity) will mix true cases with a potentially sizable number of misdiagnosed (false positive) cases, particularly if the disease is reasonably rare. Thus, the identified case group will have a blend of the exposure prevalence among true cases and the exposure prevalence among erroneously diagnosed false positive cases. This mixing will yield a bias towards the null, giving the observed case group an exposure prevalence between that of true cases and that of a random sample of the study base, represented by the false positives. Only when there is no association between exposure and disease, whereby cases would have the same exposure prevalence as the study base, will no bias result. Given the risk of overwhelming true cases with false positives when disease is rare, it is important in case–control studies to seek the maximum level of specificity even at the expense of some loss in sensitivity (Brenner & Savitz, 1990). Therefore, comparing results for varying levels of disease sensitivity and specificity (see Section below, "Examine results across levels of diagnostic certainty") suggests that the most valid estimates will be obtained for the most restrictive, stringent disease definitions. Given that only ratio measures of effect (odds ratios) can be assessed in case–control studies, all of the comments about bias due to nondifferential misclassification refer to the odds ratio.

In contrast, nondifferential underascertainment of disease in cohort studies does not produce a bias in ratio measures of effect (risk ratios, odds ratios) (Poole, 1985; Rothman & Greenland, 1998). Assume that the disease identification mechanism, applied identically among exposed and unexposed subjects, successfully identifies 80% of the cases that are truly present. The absolute rate of disease will be 0.80 times its true value in both the exposed and unexposed groups. For ratio measures of effect, the sampling fractions cancel out, such that there is no bias—0.80 times the disease rate among exposed subjects divided by 0.80 times the disease rate among unexposed subjects produces an unbiased estimate of the risk ratio. Note the minimal assumptions required for this to be true: only disease underascertainment is present and it is identical in magnitude for exposed and unexposed subjects. If these constraints can be met, either in the study design or by stratification in the analysis, then unbiased measures of relative risk can be generated. In this situation, however, the measure of rate difference will be biased, proportionately smaller by the amount of underascertainment. For a given sampling fraction, for example, 0.80, the rate difference will be 0.80 times its true value: 0.80 times the rate in the exposed minus 0.80 times the rate in the unexposed equals 0.80 times the true difference.

For non-differential disease overascertainment, the consequences are the opposite with respect to ratio and difference measures, i.e., bias in ratio measures but not in difference measures of effect. In contrast to underascertainment, in which a constant fraction of the true cases are assumed to be missed, overascertainment is not proportionate to the number of true cases but instead to the size of the study base or denominator. That is, the observed disease incidence is the sum of the true disease incidence and the incidence of overascertainment, with the total number of false positive cases a function of the frequency of overascertainment and the size of the study base. If the disease incidence due to overascertainment is identical for exposed and unexposed subjects, the effect is an addition of the same constant to the true incidence in both groups. For ratio measures of effect (rate ratios, odds ratios), the addition of a constant to the numerator and denominator will yield an estimate that is biased towards the null. On the other hand, for measures of effect based on differences (risk or rate difference), the extra incidence due to false positive diagnoses will cancel out. Assume that the true incidence of disease is 10 per 1000 per year among the exposed and 5 per 1000 per year among the unexposed for a rate ratio of 2.0 (10/1000 / 5/1000) and a rate difference of 5 per 1000 per year (10/1000 − 5/1000). If the overascertainment due to false positive diagnoses were 2 per 1000 per year among both the exposed and unexposed, the rate ratio would be biased toward the null as follows: Among the exposed, the observed incidence rate would be 12 per 1000 (10/1000 true positives plus 2/1000 false positives) and among the unexposed, the observed incidence rate would be 7 per 1000 (5/1000 true positives plus 2/1000 false positives) for a rate ratio of 1.7 (12/1000 / 7/1000), biased toward the null. In general, the ratio of X plus a constant divided by Y plus a constant is closer to 1.0 than X divided by Y (bias in ratio measures toward the null), so that the overascertainment always yields a bias toward the null. The rate difference however, would not be affected: the observed rate difference of 12/1000–7/1000 = 5/1000 is the same as the true rate difference, 10/1000–5/1000 = 5/1000. In general, X plus a constant minus Y plus a constant is the same as the difference between X and Y (no bias in rate difference). If we are aware that non-differential disease overascertainment is present, then difference measures would have an advantage over ratio measures in avoiding bias.

When disease overascertainment or underascertainment differs according to exposure status (differential misclassification), the direction and magnitude of bias can still be predicted based on the direction and magnitude of error by determining which groups will be spuriously large and which groups will be spuriously small. If disease ascertainment is less complete among the unexposed, for example, then a bias towards a falsely elevated measure of association results. If disease overascertainment occurs preferentially among the unexposed, then the measure of effect will be biased downward. Any errors that inflate the rate of disease among the exposed or reduce the rate of disease among the unexposed will bias the measure of effect upwards, and errors that reduce the rate of disease among the exposed or inflate the rate of disease among the unexposed will bias the measure of effect downwards. Note that the null value does not provide a meaningful benchmark in assessing the effects of differential misclassification. The predicted direction of bias cannot be generalized as moving toward the null or away from the null given that the movement of the effect estimate due to misclassification is defined solely by its absolute direction, up or down. The true measure of effect, the one that would be obtained in the absence of disease misclassification, is artificially increased or decreased, and may cross the null value.

With this background on the consequences of disease misclassification, the challenge is to make practical use of the principles to assess the potential for bias and to develop methods for minimizing or eliminating bias. First, we have to determine the situation that is operating in a specific study to know which principle to invoke. Identification of the study design should be straightforward, defined solely by whether sampling is outcome-dependent (case–control design) or not (cohort design) (Morgenstern & Thomas, 1993). Determining whether disease underascertainment, overascertainment, or both are present is not so easily achieved, requiring careful scrutiny of methods and results. The following discussion provides some strategies for evaluating the type and amount of disease misclassification, as well as methods for seeking to ensure that a given study has a known type of error that can be more readily managed. If the form of disease misclassification can be defined or constrained to one type, the impact on the results is at least predictable if not correctable. When both false positive and false negative errors are present in a dichotomous outcome and those errors are nondifferential with respect to exposure, regardless of the design or measure of effect, bias toward the null will result.

ASSESSING WHETHER MISCLASSIFICATION IS DIFFERENTIAL BY EXPOSURE

In evaluating the influence of possible disease misclassification, careful consideration must be given to whether the errors are likely to differ as a function of the exposure of interest. Misclassification of disease that is differential by exposure directly distorts the measure of effect, and therefore even relatively modest differences are capable of generating spurious increases or decreases in the estimated measures of effect. Non-differential misclassification of disease may produce no bias, but may also result in bias toward the null.

An understanding of the processes that generate erroneous assignment of disease status provides the basis for judging whether the source of error is likely to be independent of exposure. If the misclassification results from clerical errors, for example, then the critical question concerns the potential for such clerical errors being somehow influenced by exposure status. Certainly if the clerk is aware of the person's exposure status, the potential for differential error is enhanced whether by conscious tendencies to assign disease status taking exposure into account or by unconscious proclivities. The basis for differences can be quite subtle. For example, does the medical record quality and clarity differ for exposed and unexposed subjects, making one group more prone to error than another? If, for example, exposure information is also obtained from medical records and better records are more likely to mention the exposure of interest, those same higher quality records that note exposure may also be more likely to comprehensively identify disease.

Exposures may directly or indirectly affect the likelihood of seeking medical attention and thereby the opportunity to be diagnosed. Health behaviors such as tobacco and alcohol use have a number of psychological and sociological correlates as well as direct biologic effects on health. If, for example, heavy alcohol users are less likely to seek medical care for health conditions that do not always come to medical attention, e.g., colon polyps or infertility, then whatever the true incidence of disease among drinkers and nondrinkers, drinkers will be less likely to be diagnosed with those conditions. Disease misclassification will be differential, with more undiagnosed cases among drinkers than nondrinkers, and whatever the true relative risk may be between heavy alcohol use and the health outcome, the measured relative risk will be biased downward.

Other exposures of interest sometimes serve as a marker or signal of more regular or intensive medical care and thus provide a greater opportunity for diagnosis of subclinical disease. For example, among the variety of contraceptive methods that are commonly used, oral contraceptives are unique in requiring a regular schedule of visits to a physician for renewal of the prescription. Intrauterine devices, diaphragms, and condoms do not require regular office visits. As a by-product of obtaining regular medical examinations, blood pressure screening will be more frequent for women using oral contraceptives than for women who use other methods of contraception. Asymptomatic hypertension is therefore almost certain to be found proportionately more often among oral contraceptive users than among women using other methods of contraception or no contraception, under the realistic assumption that there is much undetected hypertension in the population that is diagnosed only if medical care is sought for other purposes. The extent of underdiagnosis is presumably reduced among women who take oral contraceptives relative to women who use other forms of contraception. Unless the intensified surveillance of women using oral contraceptives is taken into account, the association between oral contraceptive use and hypertension will be spuriously elevated.

For some well-established risk factors for disease, the association between exposure and disease may be so familiar as to become a marker for greater scrutiny or even function as a diagnostic criterion. An extreme case is in the diagnosis of certain occupational pulmonary diseases, such as silicosis or asbestosis, in which a history of exposure to the presumed agent (silica or asbestos) is required, along with radiographic findings and pattern of symptoms. Exposure history literally is a component of the definition of disease. In the complex diagnostic process that begins with a patient presenting to a physician, the entire avenue of exploration, request for diagnostic tests, interpretation of those tests, elicitation of information on symptoms, and final diagnosis would be affected by the reported history of occupational exposure. A person employed as a clerk and one employed as an insulation worker would travel down different diagnostic paths when presenting with pulmonary symptoms, and accurate determination of whether or not the person has asbestosis would undoubtedly be affected by the presumed history of asbestos exposure.

More subtle forms of exposure-driven diagnosis can also result in differential disease misclassification, typically creating a spuriously strong association if the exposure increases the probability of more accurate or complete diagnosis. Tobacco use is a firmly established, major cause of a variety of diseases, including cancer of the lung and bladder, coronary heart disease, and chronic obstructive pulmonary disease. While several of these diseases have unambiguous diagnoses, such as advanced lung cancer, there are others such as chronic bronchitis or angina that can involve a certain amount of discretionary judgment on the part of the physician. Integration of the complete array of relevant data to reach a final diagnosis is likely to include consideration of the patient's smoking history. This can be viewed as good medical practice that takes advantage of epidemiologic insights since the probabilities of one diagnosis or another are truly altered by the smoking history. Incorporation of the exposure history into the diagnostic evaluation however, may well result in a more complete assessment or even overdiagnosis of diseases known to be related to tobacco among patients with a smoking history. In some instances, the greater reluctance to diagnose a nonsmoker as having bronchitis and the greater willingness to diagnose a smoker as having bronchitis may help make the diagnoses more accurate, but such exposure-driven judgments also have the potential to introduce disease misclassification that is differential in relation to smoking history.

Another way in which differential disease misclassification may arise is as a natural consequence of the exposure of interest rather than as a result of the behavior of the affected individual or the predilections of the person making the diagnosis. The exposure may alter our ability to accurately diagnose the disease. In examining the causes of spontaneous abortion, for example, we have to contend with ambiguity of diagnosis, particularly in the first few weeks of pregnancy. Early spontaneous abortion may not be recognized at all or misinterpreted as a heavy menstrual period, and conversely, a late, heavy menstrual period may be misinterpreted as a spontaneous abortion. If we are interested in examining the influence of menstrual cycle regularity or other menstrual bleeding characteristics on the risk of spontaneous abortion, a problem arises. Our ability to make accurate diagnoses will be greatest for women who have regular menstrual cycles, which may be viewed as the unexposed group, and the exposed women with irregular menstrual cycles will be less accurately diagnosed. The solution to such a problem may reside in a diagnostic method such as evaluation of hormone metabolites in urine (Wilcox et al., 1988), thus freeing the diagnosis from the influence of menstrual cycle regularity. Such an approach to diagnosis eliminates the association between the exposure of interest and the accuracy of disease diagnosis.

The many opportunities for differential misclassification should be considered comprehensively, addressing all the ways in which exposure could directly or indirectly affect the accuracy of disease classification. Of course, if there is little or no disease misclassification at all, then there is little or no differential misclassification. The greater the absolute magnitude of error, all other things being equal, the greater the potential for that error to be differential across exposure groups. If the sensitivity and specificity of classification are both 98%, then there is little room for exposure to influence it, whereas if sensitivity and specificity are 80% or 50%, there is abundant opportunity for important variation in the accuracy of disease classification among exposure groups to arise.

All the events that lie between the occurrence of the underlying biologic phenomenon of interest and identification as a case of disease in a particular study must be examined. The cascade of events typically includes symptom recognition, seeking of medical care, diagnostic evaluation, assignment of a diagnosis, notation in some database, and ascertainment from that data base, or sometimes a diagnostic process designed specifically for the study. For assessing under-ascertainment, it may be helpful to work backwards from the diagnosed cases of disease, asking, "What had to happen for me to know of their disease?" Moving all the way back to the development of the underlying pathophysiology should help to reveal, at each step, how the recognized case made it into the study and how others who had made it through the preceding steps could have been lost. For each such source of loss, we ask whether the probability of its occurrence would have been likely to differ in relation to exposure. The role of exposure in this process must be examined broadly, in that it may influence each one of those steps through biological, behavioral, or social processes.

EVALUATION OF DISEASE MISCLASSIFICATION

In this section, a variety of options for examining, understanding, and in some cases mitigating the adverse consequences of disease misclassification are considered. None even approximates the avoidance of misclassification altogether, of course, but for many reasons that may include ethical constraints, lack of control over clinical evaluations, or resource limitations, disease misclassification is inevitable to some extent. Given results from a completed study, what can be done to determine whether there is bias due to disease misclassification or to eliminate bias that may be present?

Examine Results Across Levels of Diagnostic Certainty

The certainty of disease diagnoses can often be categorized at least in ordinal if not quantitative terms, such as definite, probable, and possible. These levels may be assigned based on established systems for tabulating clinical and laboratory findings, or formulated specifically for application in a given study. What is postulated in assigning such labels is that if the absolute truth were known, those classified as definite would contain the highest proportion of persons with the disease present, those labeled as probable the next highest, and those called possible having the lowest proportion of truly diseased persons. The only inference is ordinal, such that these three groups might contain 100%, 80%, and 60% who truly have disease or 50%, 30%, and 10%. Although it would be more desirable to be able to attach precise quantitative probabilities to these categories, even information on the *relative* degree of certainty has value in interpreting study results. The improved sensitivity in going from possible to probable to definite is virtually certain to be accompanied by a loss in specificity, i.e., increasing numbers of persons erroneously excluded (false negatives).

As noted previously, the greater concern in misclassification of relatively rare diseases is usually with false positives, since even a modest loss in specificity can result in overwhelming the few true positives with many false positives. Sensitivity is critical for enhancing precision, since false negative cases are not contributing to the pool of identified cases, but the infusion of a handful of false negatives into a large group of true negatives would have little impact on measures of effect. Given those considerations, bias in measures of association should be least when using the most stringent, restrictive case definitions and greatest for the more uncertain, inclusive categories. Because specificity is presumably highest for the most restrictive definition, when a gradient in measures of effect across levels of diagnostic certainty is found, the most valid result is likely to be for the most definite cases—whether those show the strongest or weakest measure of association.

If, in fact, the most certain cases yield the most valid results, one might question the value of considering the other categories at all. In other words, why not just set up a highly restrictive case definition at the outset and accept the loss of some true cases in order to weed out a greater proportion of the non-cases? First, the opportunity to examine a gradient in certainty of classification is informative. The contrast between results for more versus less certain cases generates a spectrum of information that is helpful in assessing the magnitude and impact of disease misclassification. Observing a risk ratio of 2.0 for definite cases in isolation may be less informative than observing a risk ratio of 2.0 for definite cases, 1.5 for probable cases, and 1.2 for possible cases. The opportunity to assess pattern of risk in relation to diagnostic certainty is an incentive to retain strata of cases that are less certain. Nevertheless, if resource limitations force us to commit to only one case definition, then the more restrictive one would generally be preferred. Second, our initial assessment of certainty of diagnosis may be in error, in which case we would lose precision and not gain validity by restricting cases to the highest level of diagnostic certainty. Observing relative risks around 2.0 for definite, probable, and possible cases may suggest that all three categories are equally likely to contain true positive cases, even if we do not know exactly what the proportion is. If, in fact, there were empirical evidence that the groups were similar with regard to their patterns of risk, aggregating them would be a reasonable strategy for enhancing precision with little or no loss in validity.

Many physiologic parameters have no true threshold for abnormal, so that the more restrictive and extreme the cutpoint, the more likely it is that persons labeled as abnormal will suffer clinical consequences. This phenomenon is clearly illustrated in that case of considering semen parameters related to male infertility, in which the cutpoints for normality are rather arbitrary relative to the clinical consequences for fertility. In fact, as the abnormal semen parameters are defined with increasingly restrictive criteria, the certainty that there is a clinically important functional abnormality present is enhanced. For example, when sperm concentration reaches 0 per ml, conception will be impossible, when it is very low, e.g., < 5 million per ml, conception is very unlikely, etc. In a study of infertility patients treated in the Netherlands (Tielemans et al., 2002), the investigators considered three case definitions of increasing restrictiveness, using a combination of sperm concentration, motility, and morphology as characterized in the table footnote (Table 9.1). As more stringent standards were applied to define sperm abnormality, the association with cigarette smoking became stronger but also less precise. This pattern is consistent with a true effect of tobacco use on semen parameters, but one that is diluted by misclassification using more liberal disease definitions. The restricted study population referred to in the table excluded those who were least likely to be aware of the cause of their infertility as described in detail in the manuscript.

An important potential drawback to this approach is the possibility that a strategy intended to establish levels of diagnostic certainty might instead reflect fundamentally different disease subsets that have different etiologies. For example, definite cases with a key symptom required to label them as certain may actually have a different condition than those lacking that symptom and labeled possible. Severity, often used to establish certainty, may also be associated with qualitative differences in etiology, as illustrated earlier in this chapter for mental retardation. Severe mental retardation is diagnosed with greater certainty than mild mental retardation, but may well also represent a fundamentally different entity with a different pathogenesis and different determinants. If a study were conducted that found a given exposure was associated with a risk ratio of 2.0 for severe mental retardation and 1.5 for mild mental retardation, it would not necessarily correspond to more disease misclassification among those individuals labeled as having mild mental retardation. Both results could be perfectly valid, reflecting differing magnitudes of association with different health outcomes. The judgment about whether the groups identified as more or less certain to have the disease reflect the same entity with differing quality or different entities has to be made based on substantive knowledge about the exposures and diseases under investigation. The study results

TABLE 9.1. Estimated Odds Ratios for Abnormal Semen Parameters and Male Cigarette Smoking in the Total Study Population and the Restricted Population, the Netherlands, 1995–1996*

	Total Population					Restricted Population				
	NO.†	OR	95% CI	OR	95% CI	NO.	OR	95% CI	OR	95% CI
Case Definition A‡										
Male smoking	153	1.25	0.88, 1.79	1.34	0.90, 2.00	51	1.98	0.96, 4.11	2.07	0.95, 4.51
Female smoking	137			0.86	0.58, 1.29	41			0.90	0.42, 1.93
Case Definition B§										
Male smoking	75	1.69	1.11, 2.57	1.97	1.20, 3.24	23	2.30	1.00, 5.27	2.99	1.17, 7.67
Female smoking	58			0.73	0.44, 1.21	13			0.51	0.19, 1.38
Case Definition C¶										
Male smoking	20	1.92	0.98, 3.74	2.62	1.22, 5.61	7	2.45	0.77, 7.81	4.58	1.20, 17.47
Female smoking	12			0.50	0.22, 1.14	1			0.09	0.01, 0.87

*Smoking by the male partner was entered alone and simultaneously with female smoking into logistic regression models.

†Number of cases with the particular risk factor.

‡Sperm concentration below 20×10^6/ml, less than 50% spermatozoa with forward progression and also less than 25% spermatozoa with rapid progression, less than 14% spermatozoa with normal forms, or abnormal values for more than one parameter.

§Sperm concentration below 5×10^6/ml, less than 10% spermatozoa with forward progression, less than 5% spermatozoa with normal forms, or abnormal values for more than one parameter.

¶Azoospermia

OR, odds ratio (calculations based on the control group with the following characteristics: sperm concentration of 20×10^6/ml or more, 50% or more spermatozoa with forward progression of 25% or more spermatozoa with rapid progression, and 14% or more spermatozoa with normal forms); CI, confidence interval.

Tielemans et al., 2002.

alone will not make it clear which is operative if the magnitude of association differs across groups.

Evaluate Alternate Methods of Disease Grouping

The constitution of disease groups is subject to varying definition, sometimes based on pathologic characteristics, sometimes based on clinical manifestations or disease course, and increasingly based on molecular analyses. Designing epidemiologic research requires making decisions about what constitutes a meaningful disease entity for study, and that question depends in part on the exposure of interest. If our interest is in the effect of heat waves on mortality, for example, all cause mortality may be the appropriate entity to consider if the mechanism is one in which persons whose health is compromised for any reason are more susceptible. On the other hand, we may believe that only a subset of diseases will mediate an effect of heat on mortality, perhaps heart or respiratory disease only if we believe that the isolated effect is one of cardiopulmonary stress, and heat would not be expected to increase risk of death due to injury or infection. The rationale for considering and choosing the optimal disease entity is a focus on what set of conditions may reasonably be expected to be influenced by the exposure under study. As we zero in on heart disease deaths, omitting deaths that are not thought to be plausibly related to heat, the adverse effects of high temperature should become increasingly clear. When we study all deaths from a wide range of factors not likely to be related to the heat wave, such as cancer, motor vehicle injury, and infant deaths from congenital anomalies, the inclusion of those entities not truly related to heat will generate a correct measure of the impact of heat on total mortality but the strength of association (relative risk) will be reduced even though in principle the risk difference would not be affected.

Selection of the proper disease entity depends on our understanding of the etiologic process. There is almost always some degree of uncertainty regarding the etiologic mechanism that might link a particular exposure and disease outcome, even for extensively researched topics. Furthermore, different hypothesized etiologic mechanisms often lead to different expectations regarding the disease subset that is likely to be causally related to the exposure under study. The optimal grouping of diseases to evaluate as the study outcome measure is the complete aggregation that is plausibly related to the exposure, including cases that could be affected and excluding cases that are not potentially affected. Exclusion of relevant cases leads to loss of power or precision, and inclusion of cases of disease that are not potentially related to the exposure of interest in the analysis biases the measure of the relationship between exposure and disease as a form of misclassification. The additional cases of disease that are not plausibly related to the exposure represent false positives relative to the exposure–disease relationship under study, and have the same impact as any other source of false positives on the results.

If benzene exposure truly caused only one form of leukemia, acute myeloid leukemia, as some have argued (Wong, 1995), then studies of benzene and leukemia that include other forms, such as chronic myeloid leukemia and acute lymphocytic leukemia would be expected to yield weaker ratio measures of association. That weaker measure would accurately reflect the impact of benzene on total leukemia, but would reflect a smaller magnitude than would be found for acute myeloid leukemia alone. Those cases of other forms of leukemia would act analogously to false positive cases of acute myeloid leukemia, diluting the measured association. Under the hypothesis of an effect limited to acute myeloid leukemia, the exposure pattern of cases of other types of leukemia would be identical to those of persons free of disease. On the other hand, if multiple types of leukemia are in fact affected by benzene, as suggested in a recent review (Savitz & Andrews, 1997) and a report from a large cohort study (Hayes et al., 1997), then restricting an already rare disease, leukemia, to the subset of acute myeloid leukemia, is wasteful. Relative to studying all leukemias, there would be a substantial loss of precision, and may not be a gain in specificity of association with benzene exposure.

Often we are faced with uncertainty and reasonable arguments that would support more than one approach to disease grouping. Rather than arbitrarily adopting one strategy, the best approach may be to examine the results under several scenarios and consider what impact misclassification would be likely to have had under those alternative assumptions. If, in fact, there is a causal association with at least some subset of disease, then the analysis that is restricted to that subset will show a stronger exposure–disease association than analyses that are more inclusive. If there is reasonable doubt about whether etiologically distinctive subsets of disease may be present, there is an incentive to present and evaluate results for those subsets. Should the subsets all yield similar measures of effect, then one might infer that nothing was gained and the exposure has similar consequences for all the subgroups of disease. On the other hand, generating data for disease subsets is the only means for discovering that some subsets are affected by the exposure whereas others are not.

For example, we hypothesized that among all cases of preterm delivery, distinctive clinical presentations may correspond to different etiologic mechanisms: some occur following spontaneous onset of labor, some following spontaneous rupture of the chorioamniotic membranes, and some result from medical interventions in response to health complications of the mother or fetus that require early delivery, such as severe pre-eclampsia or fetal distress (Savitz et al., 1991). If this is a valid basis for dividing cases to study etiology, then associations with subsets of cases will be stronger than for the aggregation of all preterm delivery cases. At present, the empirical evidence regarding such heterogeneity is mixed, with some risk factors distinctive by subtype whereas other potential causes of preterm birth appear to be associated with two or all three subgroups (Lang et al., 1996; Berkowitz et al., 1998).

Some diseases are aggregations of subgroups, in a sense demanding consideration of subtypes of a naturally heterogeneous entity. Brain cancer is defined solely by the anatomic location of the tumor, with a wide range of histologic types with varying prognosis and quite possibly varying etiology. In a rather sophisticated examination of the issue of magnetic field exposure and brain cancer in a Canadian case–control study, Villeneuve et al. (2002) hypothesized that the exposure acts as a tumor promoter and would thus show the strongest association for the most aggressive subtypes of brain cancer. Subsets of brain cancer were examined empirically (Table 9.2) and there was clear heterogeneity in pat-

TABLE 9.2. The Risk of Brain Cancer According to the Highest Average Level of Occupational Magnetic Field Exposure Ever Received by Histological Type. Canadian National Enhance Cancer Surveillance System, Male Participants, 1994–1997

HIGHEST AVERAGE OCCUPATIONAL EXPOSURE MAGNETIC FIELDS EVER RECEIVED	CASES	CONTROLS	ODDS RATIO*	95% CI	ODDS RATIO†	95% CI
All Brain Cancers						
$<0.3\ \mu T$‡	410	420	1.0		1.0	
$\geq 0.3\ \mu T$	133	123	1.11	0.84–1.48	1.12	0.83–1.51
$\geq 0.6\ \mu T$	42	29	1.38	0.79–2.42	1.33	0.75–2.36
Astrocytomas						
$<0.3\ \mu T$	163	160	1.0		1.0	
$\geq 0.3\ \mu T$	51	54	0.93	0.60–1.44	0.93	0.59–1.47
$\geq 0.6\ \mu T$	12	16	0.61	0.26–1.49	0.59	0.24–1.45
Glioblastoma Multiforme						
$<0.3\ \mu T$	143	156	1.0		1.0	
$\geq 0.3\ \mu T$	55	42	1.50	0.91–2.46	1.48	0.89–2.47
$\geq 0.6\ \mu T$	18	6	5.50	1.22–24.8	5.36	1.16–24.78
Other						
$<0.3\ \mu T$	92	94	1.0		1.0	
$\geq 0.3\ \mu T$	23	21	1.11	0.59–2.10	1.10	0.58–2.09
$\geq 0.6\ \mu T$	9	7	1.50	0.53–4.21	1.58	0.56–4.50

*Unadjusted odds ratio obtained from the conditional logistic model.

†The odds ratio was adjusted for occupational exposure to ionizing radiation and vinyl chloride.

‡Referent group.

Villeneuve et al., 2002.

terns of association across tumor groupings. A modest association was found for brain cancer in the aggregate (relative risks of 1.3–1.4 in the highest exposure category), with markedly stronger associations for the more aggressive subtype, glioblastoma multiforme, with relative risks over 5.0. Whether this pattern reflects a causal effect or not, the heterogeneity in risk across subtypes provides informative suggestions and helps to focus additional research that addresses the same hypothesis or actually refine the hypothesis about whether and how magnetic fields might affect brain cancer.

As in many suggested approaches to epidemiologic data analysis, there is no analysis that can discern the underlying truth. Hypotheses are proposed, results are generated, and then interpretations are made, with greater information provided when informative disease subsets can be isolated, and considered. Several caveats to this approach must be noted however. Alternative grouping schemes need to have a logical basis in order for the results to be interpretable. A plausible theoretical foundation is needed for each approach to grouping that is then examined in order for the association to have any broader meaning and to advance understanding of disease etiology. To note that an arbitrarily chosen subset of cases, such as those who came to the clinic on Tuesdays, shows a stronger relationship to disease than cases in the aggregate, is of little help in evaluating misclassification and understanding the causal process. Through random processes, there will always be disease subsets more and less strongly related to exposure, but to be worthy of evaluation, finding such heterogeneity or even the absence of heterogeneity that might have been expected under some plausible hypothesis should advance knowledge. In fact, random error becomes a much greater problem for case subgroups than for the disease group in the aggregate, simply due to a diminution of the numbers of cases in the analysis. Arbitrary, excessive splitting of cases for analysis has the danger of generating false leads based solely on random error. Nonetheless, except when imprecision is extreme, it would often be preferable to have a less precise result for the subgroup of cases that is truly affected by the exposure than to have a more precise result for a broader aggregation of cases, some of which are affected by the exposure and some of which are not.

Verify Diagnostic Accuracy for Subset of Study Participants

Empirical evidence on the accuracy of disease ascertainment for a subset of study participants is very useful in judging the extent to which the study results may have been distorted by misclassification. As noted above, subjecting persons who are thought to have the disease to a more thorough diagnostic evaluation is often feasible since there are a relatively modest number of such persons to examine. Even if it is not feasible to verify all diagnoses in this manner, a sufficient number can be evaluated to estimate the proportion of identified cases that are false positives. Ideally, a sufficient number of exposed and unexposed cases can be evaluated to determine whether the proportion who are erroneously labeled as diseased is associated with or independent of exposure status (i.e., whether disease misclassification is differential or non-differential).

On the other hand, assuming disease is relatively rare, there are many persons presumptively identified as disease-free, and subjecting each one to definitive diagnostic evaluation to correct false negatives is generally not feasible or necessary. Instead, some sample of individuals identified as free of disease can be evaluated with more definitive diagnostic tests to verify the absence of disease. Often, the challenge is to screen a sufficient number of presumptive non-cases to identify any false negatives or know that a sufficient number have been evaluated, even if no missed cases of disease are found.

With quantitative estimates of the frequency of disease misclassification, an estimate of the magnitude of association in the absence of those errors can be made through simple algebra (Kleinbaum et al., 1982). Within an exposure stratum, for example, a certain proportion of those labeled as having the disease represent false positives and the correction for that false positive proportion is to deplete the cell by that amount. If there were 100 persons classified as having disease, and the false positive proportion were 8%, then 8 persons would be moved to the no disease cell, leaving 92. If there were also some fraction of those labeled disease-free who represent false negatives, then some number of persons would need to be shifted from the no disease to the disease cell. Assuming that there were originally 900 persons classified as free of disease and that 2% are false negatives, then 18 persons would move across cells. The net change in the proportion with disease would be from $100/1000 = 0.10$ to $110/1000 = 0.11$. A comparable adjustment would be made in the other exposure strata to produce adjusted measures of the rate ratio. More sophisticated methods are available that account for the imprecision in the correction terms, and incorporate the precision of that estimate in the variability of the adjusted measures (Rothman & Greenland, 1998, pp. 353–355). Additional refinements would incorporate misclassification of exposure and adjustment for confounding factors, making the algebra much more complex.

This approach was applied to the evaluation of chronic obstructive pulmonary disease in the Nurses Health Study (Barr et al., 2002). In such large cohort studies, direct confirmation is infeasible due to the geographic dispersion of participants and the lengthy interval over which diagnoses occur. Using self-reported information from the questionnaire, women were classified as definite, probable, or possible cases, depending on the amount of detail that they were able to provide to document the diagnosis of chronic obstructive pulmonary disease. A random sample of 422 women who reported the disease was initially selected, and medical records were obtained for 376 women to allow for the direct confirmation of physician-diagnosed chronic obstructive pulmonary disease. The propor-

tion confirmed in this manner was 78%, with a greater proportion of those assigned as definite confirmed than among those classified initially as probable or
possible (Table 9.3). Note that this reflects the opportunity to examine and confirm (or refute) self-reported diagnoses, but does not allow for assessment of false
negative reports, i.e., women who would be considered to have chronic obstructive pulmonary disease based on medical record review but who did not report
it on the questionnaire.

Assess Number of Erroneous Diagnoses to Change the Results

A simpler evaluation of the potential impact of misclassification addresses the
number of errors of a given type that would be required to shift results by some
specified amount. By focusing on the absolute number of such shifted cases, both
the magnitude and precision of the observed pattern are addressed in this exercise. Having identified a positive association between exposure and disease, we
might ask how many false positive cases among exposed subjects would have
been required to produce a spurious association of that magnitude if there really
were no association, or how many false negatives would have been required
among unexposed study participants to produce such a pattern spuriously. Alternatively, with a finding of no association, we might ask how many missed
cases among the exposed or false positive cases among the unexposed would
have been required to have produced a spurious absence of association if the true
relative risk were 1.5 or 2.0 or some other value of interest based on previous
literature.

The pattern of misclassification in such an assessment is often considered to
be completely differential with respect to exposure, i.e., that all false positives
occur among exposed subjects or all false negatives occur among the unexposed,
which is often unrealistic. Even where tendencies exist to enhance the form of
disease misclassification across exposure groups, it would rarely be so complete,
making the worst case scenarios highly improbable ones. Also, even though the
result that is derived is quantitative, i.e., a given number of errors made, it can
only be examined intuitively for its plausibility: Does it seem plausible that a
given number of false positive or false negative diagnoses could have occurred?
In general, it would seem more plausible for a small number of cases to be in
error than a large number, but little more can be said based on such an evaluation. More complex scenarios of false positive and false negative diagnoses distributed across exposure strata would tend to be more realistic and thus more
useful than extreme scenarios.

This strategy was applied in an examination of the potential for detection bias
to produce a spurious positive association between estrogen use and endometrial
cancer (Hulka et al., 1980), examining a scenario that is more complicated than
a simple count of false positive or negatives. The debate was based on the pre-

TABLE 9.3. Proportion of Cases Confirmed* Among Participants with a Self-Reported Physician Diagnosis of Chronic Obstructive Pulmonary Disease in the Nurses' Health Study, United States, 1976–2000

	Self-report of COPD		Method of Confirmation‡			
CRITERION†	RECORDS OBTAINED (NO.)	CASES CONFIRMED IN MEDICAL RECORD (%)	PULMONARY FUNCTION TEST RESULT (%)	CHEST RADIOGRAPH OR COMPUTED TOMOGRAPHY (%)	PHYSICIAN NOTATION (%)	FEV_1 % PREDICTED§ (MEAN (STANDARD DEVIATION))
Definite	73	86	81	51	60	45 (18)
Probable	218	80	71	50	64	50 (19)
Possible	273	78	67	48	67	50 (19)

*Confirmed using medical records and uniform diagnostic criteria.

‡All three elements were not available for some participants.

§Among participants with pulmonary function test reports.

COPD, chronic obstructive pulmonary disease; FEV_1, forced expiratory volume in 1 second.

Barr et al., 2002.

vious suggestion that inferred positive associations between estrogen use and endometrial cancer were largely attributable to estrogen causing vaginal bleeding, which led to more intensive diagnostic surveillance and detection of otherwise subclinical cancers. In a case–control study, this would manifest itself as a spuriously high proportion of cases who had experienced bleeding compared to controls, and was cited as the rationale for choosing controls who had themselves experienced vaginal bleeding and would thus have been carefully scrutinized for the presence of endometrial cancer.

Hulka et al. (1980) conducted a number of relevant analyses, including a simulation of the potential magnitude of such a bias, if present. In a hypothetical population of 100,000 women age 50 and older, an estimate was made of the proportion of women with asymptomatic cancer (the pool in which selective detection could occur), the proportion of women using estrogen, and the number of diagnosed endometrial cancer cases (who would be enrolled in a study). As shown in Figure 9.1, only the women who fall into the intersection of those three groups contribute to the bias, i.e., asymptomatic cancer, estrogen user, diagnosed cases. In this scenario, there would be only 5 such cases. Their inclusion would yield a relative risk of 3.9 comparing estrogen users to nonusers, and their exclusion (eliminating the hypothesized detection bias) would yield a relative risk of 3.7. Under a set of reasonable assumptions, the hypothesized bias is therefore negligible in magnitude.

Create Subgroups with Accurate Ascertainment or Non-Differential Underascertainment

For a number of reasons, accurate ascertainment of disease may be unattainable for the entire study population. There may be subgroups within the study population, however, in which disease ascertainment is accurate. Some diseases are largely asymptomatic, for example carcinoma *in situ* of the cervix, but among women who obtain annual Pap smear screening the diagnosis is likely to be virtually complete. Valid results can therefore be obtained within the subset of the population in which ascertainment is complete, in this instance among women who obtain annual screening. The potential disadvantage of this approach is that the marker of completeness of ascertainment may well be a marker of other factors that affect the occurrence of disease. That is, the attributes required to have complete diagnosis may also be true modifiers of the effect of interest. If obtaining regular Pap smear screening acts as a modifier of the risk factor under investigation, then the stratum-specific result among those obtaining Pap smears would be valid, but the result may apply only to women who obtain annual Pap smear screening.

This strategy is applicable to studies in which a common but often subclinical disease outcome is of interest, such as adenomatous polyps of the colon

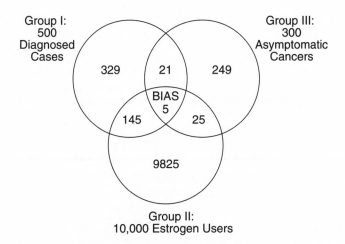

Group I:
500
Diagnosed
Cases

Group III:
300
Asymptomatic
Cancers

329   21   249

BIAS
5

145   25

9825

Group II:
10,000 Estrogen Users

FIGURE 9.1. Detection bias and endometrial cancer: diagnosed cases and asymptomatic cases. Assuming a hypothetical population of 100,000 women age ≥50 years, three groups are formed: Group I = the 5-year cumulative incidence of diagnosed cancer; Group II = the 5-year period prevalence of estrogen use; Group III = the 5-year period prevalence of asymptomatic cancer (Hulka et al., 1980).

NOTES TO FIGURE 9.1

1. Incidence of diagnosed endometrial cancer = 1/1000/year* × 5 years × 100,000 women = 500 diagnosed cases (Group I).
2. 5-year period prevalence of estrogen use = 10%† of 100,000 women = 10,000 women having used estrogen (Group II).
3. 5-year period prevalence of asymptomatic cancers = 3/1000 (27,28) × 100,000 women = 300 asymptomatic cancers (Group III).
4. 30% of diagnosed cases used estrogen = 0.30 × 500 = 150.
5. 10%† of asymptomatic cases used etrogen = 0.10 × 300 = 30.
6. 20%‡ of estrogen users with previously asymptomatic cancer bled and became diagnosed cases = 0.20 × 30 = 5.
7. 6% of non-estrogen-using diagnosed cases were asymptomatic = 0.06 × 350 = 21.

(Smith-Warner et al., 2002). In a case–control study conducted within a large colonoscopy trial in Minneapolis, cases were defined as those individuals screened and found to be positive for adenomatous polyps, and controls were defined as a sample of individuals screened and found to be negative. Essentially, the experience of having undergone a colonoscopy defines a stratum in which polyp status is more accurately defined than for an unscreened population. As the authors recognized, however, restricting the source of controls in this manner may address the problem of disease misclassification through underdiagnosis, but introduces a potential problem with selection bias in that the study base has been implicitly sampled through having received a colonoscopy.

The selection to be screened may well be a source of distortion in the distribution of the exposure of interest, dietary intake of fruits and vegetables and thereby bias measures of association. For that reason, another control group was selected from the general population using drivers' license records, referred to as community controls. As shown in Table 9.4, the two control groups yielded generally similar results for both men and women, subject to some imprecision. For vegetable intake among men, results for the community controls tended to show stronger inverse gradients than the colonoscopy-negative controls. Except for juice intake among women, associations were generally absent or weak. Inclusion of the two control groups, one of which was diagnosed accurately to be free of polyps, allows evaluation of the impact, if any, of incomplete diagnosis and selection bias, but only relative to each other and not relative to a true "gold standard" that is free of either potential bias.

Even if a stratum cannot be created in which disease ascertainment is accurate, perhaps subgroups can be isolated in which there is only non-differential underascertainment and an absence of false positives. In such a study, ratio measures of association will be nearly unbiased (Rothman & Greenland, 1998). Ensuring the absence of overascertainment is essential for this approach to be effective. By creating strata with varying degrees of underascertainment, information is also generated for examining a dose-response gradient in potential for bias due to differential underascertainment. That is, if we can define strata of low, moderate, and high degrees of underascertainment, examining measures of association across those strata may help to indicate whether bias is present.

Attempts to create strata with accurate disease ascertainment or non-differential underascertainment will result either in finding that the exposure–disease association does or does not differ in relation to the presumed indicator of the magnitude of non-differential disease underascertainment. When the estimated measure of association differs, then as long as the basis for stratification is valid, the more accurate measure comes from the stratum that is free of overascertainment or influenced solely by non-differential underascertainment. When the results are similar across strata, then there are several possible explanations. The effort to isolate the subset that is affected only by non-differential underascertainment may have been unsuccessful, i.e., all strata continue to suffer from such bias. Alternatively, there may have been no bias due to disease misclassification in the first place so that stratification failed to generate the expected pattern.

Restrict Inference to Disease Outcome That Can Be Ascertained Accurately

Many, perhaps most, diseases have a spectrum of severity, with the probability of manifesting symptoms and being detected increasing as the severity of the condition increases. Prostate cancer in older men, for example, is extremely common and usually asymptomatic, but the form of the disease that is more aggressive and metastasizes to bone results in clinical symptoms that more often lead

TABLE 9.4. Multivariate-Adjusted Odds Ratios* for Colorectal Adenomas by Quintile of Fruit and Vegetable Intake for Women and Men, Minnesota Cancer Prevention Research Unit Case-Control Study, 1991–1994

FOOD GROUP QUINTILE	Mean Intake (Servings/week)		Cases vs. Colonoscopy-Negative Controls				Cases vs. Community Controls			
			Women		Men		Women		Men	
	WOMEN	MEN	OR	95% CI	OR	95% CI	OR	95% CI	OR	95% CI
Fruits										
1	3.3	2.1	1.00		1.00		1.00		1.00	
2	7.4	5.9	0.95	0.52, 1.72	0.79	0.46, 1.36	0.65	0.34, 1.25	0.73	0.43, 1.23
3	11.2	9.6	0.91	0.50, 1.63	1.06	0.61, 1.84	0.78	0.40, 1.52	1.00	0.59, 1.68
4	15.8	14.7	1.10	0.59, 2.05	0.79	0.44, 1.43	0.61	0.30, 1.20	0.62	0.36, 1.06
5	27.5	26.9	1.34	0.66, 2.69	0.66	0.35, 1.24	0.68	0.32, 1.43	0.75	0.41, 1.35
p trend				0.54		0.16		0.29		0.44
Vegetables										
1	10.1	8.8	1.00		1.00		1.00		1.00	
2	17.6	15.1	1.12	0.62, 2.01	1.29	0.75, 2.23	1.08	0.56, 2.07	0.67	0.39, 1.13
3	23.8	20.2	1.16	0.62, 2.16	1.11	0.64, 1.93	0.86	0.44, 1.68	0.73	0.43, 1.26
4	31.6	27.1	2.26	1.23, 4.14	1.30	0.72, 2.34	1.34	0.69, 2.59	0.59	0.34, 1.03
5	51.4	44.7	1.70	0.87, 3.34	0.90	0.48, 1.69	1.40	0.67, 2.92	0.55	0.30, 0.98
p trend				0.10		0.69		0.24		0.16

(continued)

TABLE 9.4. Multivariate-Adjusted Odds Ratios* for Colorectal Adenomas by Quintile of Fruit and Vegetable Intake for Women and Men, Minnesota Cancer Prevention Research Unit Case-Control Study, 1991–1994 (continued)

FOOD GROUP QUINTILE	Mean Intake (Servings/week)		Cases vs. Colonoscopy-Negative Controls				Cases vs. Community Controls			
			Women		Men		Women		Men	
	WOMEN	MEN	OR	95% CI	OR	95% CI	OR	95% CI	OR	95% CI
Juice										
1	0.5	0.5	1.00		1.00		1.00		1.00	
2	2.2	1.9	0.81	0.48, 1.39	1.53	0.86, 2.73	0.97	0.53, 1.78	1.16	0.67, 2.01
3	4.8	4.2	0.72	0.41, 1.27	1.24	0.73, 2.10	0.80	0.43, 1.51	0.83	0.51, 1.35
4	7.7	7.4	0.61	0.34, 1.09	0.88	0.52, 1.51	0.56	0.31, 1.03	0.75	0.45, 1.26
5	14.2	15.1	0.50	0.27, 0.92	0.98	0.55, 1.73	0.56	0.30, 1.06	0.97	0.56, 1.67
p trend				0.02		0.97		0.04		0.58
Total Fruits and Vegetables										
1	18.4	16.5	1.00		1.00		1.00		1.00	
2	31.8	26.8	0.76	0.42, 1.38	0.80	0.46, 1.38	0.61	0.32, 1.18	0.76	0.45, 1.30
3	41.8	36.1	1.06	0.59, 1.92	1.05	0.60, 1.83	1.01	0.52, 1.94	0.95	0.56, 1.61
4	53.8	48.5	1.48	0.79, 2.78	0.82	0.44, 1.51	0.71	0.36, 1.38	0.46	0.27, 0.80
5	82.8	75.9	0.96	0.47, 1.96	0.61	0.31, 1.22	0.76	0.34, 1.66	0.60	0.32, 1.12
p trend				0.79		0.40		0.86		0.20

*Adjusted for age (continuous), energy intake (continuous), fat intake (continuous), body mass index (continuous), smoking status (never, current, former), alcohol status (nondrinker, former drinker, current drinkers consuming <1 drink/week, current drinkers consuming ≥1 drink/week), nonsteroidal antiinflammatory use (yes, no), multivitamin use (yes, no), and hormone replacement therapy use (yes, no in women only).

OR, odds ratio; CI, confidence interval.

Smith-Warner et al., 2002.

to an accurate diagnosis. Endometriosis, in which there is endometrial tissue located at abnormal anatomic locations in the abdominal cavity, is quite common and largely undetected, but the form of the disease that is more extensive appears to be more likely to produce symptoms that lead to diagnosis. Some of the confusion is semantic, i.e., whether disease is truly present when the requisite biologic changes have occurred but there are no overt symptoms and such symptoms may never arise. For studying etiology, however, the biologic entity itself is often of primary interest, so that variability in symptom occurrence, recognition, care-seeking, and ultimately disease diagnosis represent opportunities for misclassification. An accurate diagnosis often requires many steps, as discussed above, but the probability of all those events occurring is often highest when the disease is most severe in terms of stage or scope.

The most informative approach to the study of diseases with a spectrum of severity is to comprehensively identify all cases across the spectrum of disease, even the least severe, in order to determine empirically whether risk factors differ for more versus less severe variants of the condition. When comprehensive diagnosis is infeasible due to the invasiveness or expense of the methods for definitive diagnosis, e.g., laparoscopic surgery to diagnose endometriosis, compromise in the study design is required. Shifting interest to the study of severe endometriosis or aggressive prostate cancer is one strategy for conducting a valid study that is capable of comprehensive ascertainment, accepting the consequent inability to examine potential influences on less severe variants of the disease. That is, a more readily studied endpoint is substituted for the less feasibly studied one.

In a case–control study of prostate cancer, analyses were divided based on case aggressiveness to evaluate the potential implications of both selection bias (incomplete ascertainment of cases) as well as true biologic differences in etiology for more versus less aggressive tumors (Vogt et al., 2002). This multicenter case–control study was conducted in the late 1980s in Atlanta, Detroit, and 10 counties in New Jersey. Controls were chosen through random-digit dialing for men under age 65 and through the Health Care Financing Administration records for men age 65 and older. Among a much larger pool of participants, 209 cases and 228 controls had blood specimens analyzed for lycopenes and other specific types of carotenoids, antioxidants found in fruits and vegetables. For lycopenes (Table 9.5), the inverse association with prostate cancer risk was much more pronounced among aggressive cases as compared to nonaggressive cases (as defined in the footnote to the table), with odds ratios of 0.37 versus 0.79 in the highest compared to lowest quartile. For the other categories of carotenoids, however, differences were not striking or consistent in direction. Nevertheless, these data are helpful in considering the potential for a bias due to incomplete ascertainment of non-aggressive prostate cancer cases.

The spectrum of severity may be based on the actual size of an anatomic change, e.g., tumor size, the exact location of the pathologic alteration, e.g.,

TABLE 9.5. Prostate Cancer Odds Ratios for All Cases and for Nonaggressive and Aggressive Cases from a U.S. Multicenter Case-Control Study, 1986–1989

| | | Quartile of Serum Carotenoid | | | | | | | |
| | 1 (low)† | | 2 | | 3 | | 4 (high) | | TEST FOR TREND, |
	RANGE	ODDS RATIO (REFERENCE)‡	RANGE	ODDS RATIO	RANGE	ODDS RATIO	RANGE	ODDS RATIO	P VALUE
α-Carotene (μg/dl)	0.0–1.4		1.5–3.2		3.3–4.7		4.8–29.4		
All cases		1.00		1.40		1.29		1.24	0.60
Nonaggressive cases§		1.00		1.08		1.30		0.95	0.91
Aggressive cases		1.00		1.65		1.01		1.91	0.17
β-Carotene (μg/dl)	0.3–8.2		8.3–14.8		14.9–23.1		23.2–117.5		
All cases		1.00		1.56		1.54		1.64	0.22
Nonaggressive cases		1.00		1.16		1.48		1.54	0.20
Aggressive cases		1.00		1.57		1.34		1.61	0.41
β-Cryptoxanthin (μg/dl)	0.3–4.9		5.0–7.1		7.2–11.1		11.2–44.3		
All cases		1.00		1.39		1.29		0.98	0.65
Nonaggressive cases		1.00		1.09		1.27		0.93	0.82
Aggressive cases		1.00		2.03		1.57		1.22	0.84

Lutein/zeaxanthin (μg/dl)	3.6–14.1	14.2–19.6	19.7–26.6	26.7–80.8	
All cases	1.00	1.11	1.03	1.51	0.17
Nonaggressive cases	1.00	1.04	1.35	1.32	0.36
Aggressive cases	1.00	0.91	0.57	1.73	0.10
Lycopene (μg/dl)	0.5–10.7	10.8–17.1	17.2–24.7	24.8–57.4	
All cases	1.00	0.97	0.74	0.65	0.09
Nonaggressive cases	1.00	1.05	0.72	0.79	0.36
Aggressive cases	1.00	0.93	0.79	0.37	0.04

†Quartile cutpoints were based on the distribution for each exposure among controls.

‡All models were adjusted for age, race, study center, and month of blood draw.

§Among cases, distributions by stage and grade, respectively, were as follows: 146 localized, 23 regional, and 21 distant; 75 well differentiated, 70 moderately differentiated, 38 poorly differentiated, and one undifferentiated. Stage and grade were combined to form categories of disease aggressiveness. After the exclusion of 33 subjects because of missing information on grade and/or stage, "nonaggressive" disease included 111 cases with well- or moderately differentiated grade and localized stage. "Aggressive" disease included 65 cases with poorly differentiated to undifferentiated grade and/or regional to distant stage. This system of categorization seeks to distinguish between disease that is more versus less likely to progress and become fatal (Gann et al., Cancer Res 1999;59:1225–30).

Vogt et al., 2002.

whether it results in recognizable symptoms, or other features of the disease process. It is quite possible that these peculiarities of size and location are of no etiologic significance and represent random variations in a single disease entity that extends into the range in which misclassification is more common. If that is true, a study of diagnosable disease should yield information that is applicable to undiagnosable disease under the assumption that the diagnosable fraction represents incomplete underascertainment of the total spectrum of disease that is present. If the subsets of disease that are and are not recognizable have different etiologies, then of course, the study of recognizable disease will still be valid for the endpoint it examines, and a strong case can be made that the more severe version of the disease is the one that is more important to understand and ultimately prevent.

Pregnancy loss illustrates these issues nicely, since there is a spectrum of severity, ranging from very early loss that is unrecognizable other than through daily hormone assays, to the medically and emotionally severe outcome of a fetal loss in the second trimester of pregnancy. Reliance on clinically recognized or medically treated miscarriage is vulnerable to incomplete ascertainment relative to the universe of pregnancy losses, in that women will vary in recognizing symptoms of pregnancy and pregnancy loss and may or may not seek medical care in response to an uncomplicated pregnancy loss. On average, the more advanced the pregnancy at the time of the loss, the more likely it is to result in recognizing symptoms and seeking medical care. Study of risk factors for pregnancy loss using medical records for case identification (Savitz et al., 1994) is capable of considering only a part of the spectrum of pregnancy loss. Early losses (before 6 weeks) are subject to grossly incomplete ascertainment, and a rising proportion of losses will be identified through medical care up to approximately 12–15 weeks' gestation, at which time the ascertainment is thought to become virtually complete. A study based on medically treated spontaneous abortion may be excellent for pregnancies that survived to 14–20 weeks' gestation, acceptable for pregnancies that reached 10–14 weeks' gestation, and completely inadequate for pregnancies that ended prior to 10 weeks' gestation.

INTEGRATED ASSESSMENT OF POTENTIAL FOR BIAS DUE TO DISEASE MISCLASSIFICATION

The first requirement in evaluating the implications of disease misclassification is to articulate clearly the nature of the error and its consequences. This, in turn, requires a clear articulation of the sequence of biological, behavioral, and medical care events required to become a recognized case in a given study. With that in hand, hypotheses regarding the process through which disease overascertainment or disease underascertainment or both may have occurred can be specified.

In speculating about these errors, special attention needs to be given to whether the error is likely to be related to or independent of exposure, since the consequences differ greatly. Several of the most plausible scenarios of error should be specified, without trying to be exhaustive in including those that are very unlikely to have had a material effect on the results.

Next, the consequences of each of those pathways of error in disease ascertainment should be considered first in qualitative terms, with appropriate consideration of the study design. That is, the predicted direction of bias should be specified, recognizing that this can vary for ratio versus difference measures, and may or may not be absolute in direction (upward or downward) or operate relative to the null value (bias toward or away from the null). The product of this effort is a statement about the direction of bias that would result from each of the mechanisms for disease misclassification.

Finally, and most challenging, is the need to quantify the magnitude of potential bias. To do so formally requires quantifying the amount of misclassification that is likely to have occurred, or more feasibly, considering a range of potential errors and their consequences on the study results in the form of a sensitivity analysis. With a limited number of the most plausible scenarios, and a few alternative estimates of the magnitude of misclassification, it is possible to derive a sense of whether disease misclassification may have had a major effect on the final results. If only some scenarios lead to the suggestion of a large effect, then those scenarios should be examined further and others should be noted as unlikely to have produced substantial error and dropped from further consideration. For those that remain of concern, further empirical evaluation or validation studies might be considered, or opportunities to do further research on the topic that overcomes that source of potential bias would be sought.

Data analysis can help to address whether bias due to disease misclassification has occurred. A number of strategies were suggested to isolate subsets of subjects or disease with less misclassification. Creating a gradient of diagnostic certainty allows evaluation of the pattern of results for more definite compared to less certain cases. There are often questions about the optimal extent of disease aggregation (lumping versus splitting), and in light of such uncertainty, measures of association based on alternate grouping schemes can be informative. The overriding goal should be to focus on the disease entity most plausibly related to the exposure(s) of interest. Verification of the accuracy of disease classification in a subgroup, if not feasible for the entire population, can help to assess what results would have been produced had this refinement been applied to the entire study population. Closely related is an examination of the number of classification errors required to change the results by a given amount or to yield measures of the association of interest. Given that nondifferential disease underascertainment generally produces unbiased ratio measures of effect, opportunities can be sought to create strata in which nondifferential disease underascertainment is the only form of error. Finally, when misclassification makes it impossible to study the full spectrum of a disease entity, including the subset that is highly susceptible to misclassification, the interest can sometimes be shifted to a subset of the disease that is more tractable, i.e., the more severe and therefore more accurately diagnosed cases. Some degree of disease misclassification is inherent in epidemiologic studies, but through careful evaluation of the source and manifestation of the problems, the consequences can be mitigated or at least understood for accurate interpretation of the study results.

REFERENCES

Barr RG, Herbstman J, Speizer FE, Camargo CA Jr. Validation of self-reported chronic obstructive pulmonary disease in a cohort study of nurses. Am J Epidemiol 2002;155: 965–971.

Berkowitz GS, Blackmore-Prince C, Lapinski RH, Savitz DA. Risk factors for preterm birth subtypes. Epidemiology 1998;9:279–285.

Brenner H, Savitz DA. The effects of sensitivity and specificity of case selection on validity, sample size, precision, and power in hospital-based case-control studies. Am J Epidemiol 1990;132:181–192.

Greenland S. Tests for interaction in epidemiologic studies: a review and a study of power. Stat Med 1983;2:243–251.

Hayes RJ, RB, Yin S-N, Dosemeci M, Li G-L, Wacholder S, Travis LB, Li C-Y, Rothman N, Hoover RN, Linet MS. Benzene and the dose-related incidence of hematologic neoplasms in China. J Natl Cancer Inst 1997;89:1065–1071.

Hulka BS, Grimson RC, Greenberg RG, Kaufman DG, Fowler WC Jr, Hogue CJR, Berger GS, Pulliam CC. "Alternative" controls in a case-control study of endometrial cancer and exogenous estrogen. Am J Epidemiol 1980;112:376–387.

Kleinbaum DG, Kupper LL, Morgenstern H. Epidemiologic research: principles and quantitative methods. Belmont, CA: Lifetime Learning Publications, 1982.

Lang JM, Lieberman E, Cohen A. A comparison of risk factors for preterm labor and term small-for-gestational-age birth. Epidemiology 1996;7:369–376.

Marchbanks PA, Peterson HB, Rubin GL, Wingo PA, and the Cancer and Steroid Hormone Study Group Research on infertility: definition makes a difference. Am J Epidemiol 1989;130:259–267.

Morgenstern H, Thomas D. Principles of study design in environmental epidemiology. Environ Health Perspect 1993;101 (Suppl 4):23–38.

Poole C. Exception to the rule about nondifferential misclassification (abstract). Am J Epidemiol 1985;122:508.

Rose G. Sick individuals and sick populations. Int J Epidemiol 1985;14:32–38.

Rothman KJ. Modern epidemiology. Boston: Little, Brown and Company, 1986.

Rothman KJ, Greenland S. Modern epidemiology, Second edition. Philadelphia: Lippincott-Raven Publishers, 1998.

Rothman KJ, Greenland S. Modern epidemiology, Second edition. Philadelphia: Lippincott-Raven Publishers, 1998:353–355.

Savitz DA, Andrews KW. Review of epidemiologic evidence on benzene and lymphatic and hematopoietic cancers. Am J Ind Med 1997;31:287–295.

Savitz DA, Blackmore CA, Thorp JM. Epidemiology of preterm delivery: etiologic heterogeneity. Am J Obstet Gynecol 1991;164:467–471.

Savitz DA, Brett KM, Evans LE, Bowes W. Medically treated miscarriage among Black and White women in Alamance County, North Carolina, 1988–1991. Am J Epidemiol 1994;139:1100–1106.

Schwartz J. Low-level lead exposure and children's IQ: a metaanalysis and search for a threshold. Environ Res 1994;66:42–55.

Smith-Warner SA, Elmer PJ, Fosdick L, Randall B, Bostick RM, Grandits G, Grambsch P, Louis TA, Wood JR, Potter JD. Fruits, vegetables, and adenomatous polyps. The Minnesota Cancer Prevention Research Unit case-control study. Am J Epidemiol 2002;155:1104–1113.

Tielemans E, Burdorf A, te Velde E, Weber R, van Kooij R, Heederik D. Sources of bias in studies among infertility clinics. Am J Epidemiol 2002;156:86–92.

Villeneuve PJ, Johnson KC, Mao Y, Canadian Cancer Registries Epidemiology Research Group. Brain cancer and occupational exposure to magnetic fields among men: results from a Canadian population-based case–control study. Int J Epidemiol 2002;31:210–217.

Vogt TM, Mayne ST, Graubard BI, Swanson CA, Sowell AL, Schoenberg JB, Swanson GM, Greenberg RS, Hoover RN, Hayes RB, Ziegler RG. Serum lycopene, other serum carotenoids, and risk of prostate cancer in US Blacks and Whites. Am J Epidemiol 2002;155:1023–1032.

Wilcox AJ, Weinberg C, O'Connor J, et al. Incidence of early loss of pregnancy. N Engl J Med 1988;319:188–194.

Wong O. Risk of acute myeloid leukemia and multiple myeloma in workers exposed to benzene. Occup Environ Med 1995;52:380–384.

10

RANDOM ERROR

Previous chapters considered the role of systematic error or bias in the evaluation of epidemiologic evidence. In each case, specific phenomena were considered which would predictably result in erroneous estimates of effect, and the discussion was focused on evaluating whether the underlying conditions that would lead to the bias were present. Hypotheses of bias constitute candidate explanations, ideally specific and testable, for why the observed results might not reflect the true causal relation or lack of relation between exposure and disease. Random error is different in character, despite the fact that it also generates estimates of effect that deviate from the correct measurement. The key difference is that random error, by definition, does not operate through measurable, testable causal pathways, making it a more elusive concept. We can ask why a coin does not land as heads or tails exactly 50% of the time in a series of trials. Perhaps the subtle differences in the way it was flipped or the wind speed and direction happened to favor heads or tails slightly. Although there is a physical process involving movement and gravity that could in principle lead to a predictable result on any given trial or series of trials, we ascribe the deviation of a series of outcomes from the expected 50/50 split as random error.

The two pathways that lead to statistically predictable patterns of random error are sampling and random allocation. Sampling black and white balls from an urn, there will be a predictable pattern of deviation from the true ratio in a series of selections. Similarly, we can describe in statistical terms a distribution of outcomes from a series of random allocations to two groups and how probable it is that a sample will deviate from some known true value by a given amount. In simple experiments, the probability of obtaining a sample that deviates from the population by a given amount or more can be calculated, e.g., the probability of obtaining 5 or more heads in 7 coin flips. Without working out the precise physics that leads to the toss of heads on any given flip of the coin, we can predict the pattern. Similarly, when we randomly assign exposure using a perfectly unbiased allocation procedure, giving some rats the active agent and some the placebo, we can calculate the probability of all 10 rats who get the active agent being less prone to disease and all 10 rats who get the placebo being susceptible to disease, generating a false impression that the agent is more beneficial than it truly is. Why our unbiased algorithm for assignment went wrong and when it will go wrong are unknown but we can calculate the probability that it did. Thus, the pattern of deviation can be predicted but the effect of random error on any given result cannot be predicted logically in either direction or magnitude no matter how much it is scrutinized or how well the statistical properties of sampling distribution are understood. Random error is therefore a source of uncertainty that allows for the possibility that our measured results deviate from the correct result, but it cannot be put forward as a deterministic explanation for a given research finding to be tested or measured directly. Going from the simple sampling or randomized allocation mechanisms noted above to the complexity of an observational epidemiologic study, the statistical principles that guide our interpretation of random error apply qualitatively, at best (Greenland, 1990). Because of random error, the true causal parameter will never be identical to the observed estimate, even in the absence of systematic biases. Random error characterizes the uncertainty or unexplained variability in such estimates relative to their true value.

The direction of deviation between the true and measured effect distorted by random error is equally likely to be positive or negative; that is, random error is equally likely to produce higher or lower estimates relative to the true value. Where errors in measurement of exposure or disease result in distorted estimates of effect, we can predict the impact of those errors to some extent by examining the degree and pattern of misclassification. There is also a random element in how any given systematic bias operates, such that the translation of a well-understood source of misclassification, selection bias, or confounding into the precise error that results in a given study has a probabilistic aspect to it. Nevertheless, the etiology of those sources of bias can be traced and sometimes corrected, in contrast to random error, which cannot.

Despite the inability to describe what causes random error to be present or to define the pathways by which it operates in a given study, we have some advantages in evaluating its impact relative to systematic error. First, we can presume that small deviations between the true and measured values are more probable than large deviations, and with some assumptions, we can even estimate the probability that deviations of differing magnitudes between the measured and true values will occur. Second, as the study size becomes larger, the probability of a deviation of at least a given magnitude decreases, in contrast to all the other forms of bias that have been discussed. If there is bias from non-response or confounding, increasing study size will not make it go away. None of these attributes actually define the underlying phenomenon that generates random error, but they do suggest ways to evaluate and minimize its possible influence on the results of epidemiologic research.

SEQUENTIAL APPROACH TO CONSIDERING RANDOM AND SYSTEMATIC ERROR

One of the common practices pertaining to addressing random error in evaluating epidemiologic research findings, often applied in other scientific disciplines as well, is to give the consideration of random error undue prominence. This often takes the form of postponing discussion of potential bias until there is firm statistical evidence for an association (Hill, 1965), presuming the other biases are only operative or important when *(1)* a positive association is found, and *(2)* that association is not attributed to random error. Both implications are erroneous.

First, there is no reason whatsoever to limit consideration of random error to situations in which a positive (or negative) association *has* been observed. Random error produces distortion that depends on study size and in no way on the magnitude of measured association: null, positive, and inverse associations are equally susceptible to distortion by random error. Ostensibly null findings warrant just as much scrutiny for the contribution of random error as positive associations do. A wide confidence interval, reflecting susceptibility to substantial random error, is just as problematic whether the point estimate is near the null or not—in either case, we are uncertain to a substantial degree about the true value for the measurement.

Second, random error does not automatically deserve primacy over consideration of systematic error as study results are scrutinized. Approaches that first scan results for statistical significance or confidence intervals that exclude the null value reflect an implicit decision that random error must be somehow disproven as a candidate explanation *before* considering confounding, measurement error, or selection bias. In the extreme case, only results that are found to be statistically significant are examined for systematic error, suggesting that not only is random error more important but also that systematic biases are incapable of generating results that are spuriously close to the null or at least not significantly different from the null. Perhaps the focus on associations that deviate from the null is motivated in part by looking for interesting findings (i.e., non-null results) at the expense of focusing on the comprehensive, critical evaluation of all the scientifically important findings. Surely, if the results are worth generating, given all the effort that requires, they are worthy of evaluation in a comprehensive, systematic manner.

The credibility of the findings is a function of freedom from both systematic and random error. Practically, we do need to focus our effort on the major sources of distortion that operate, and in small studies, random error may well be at the top of the list, whereas in larger studies, various forms of systematic error will likely predominate. Perhaps the availability of a refined statistical framework for examining random error that is far better developed and more widely applied than those for other forms of error may tempt epidemiologists to give special attention to this concern, like looking for lost keys where the light is brightest. Instead, we need to look for the lost keys in the location where they were most likely lost.

SPECIAL CONSIDERATIONS IN EVALUATING RANDOM ERROR IN OBSERVATIONAL STUDIES

Observational studies make the conventional tools for evaluation of random error far more tenuous than in experimental studies (Greenland, 1990). There are two considerations that make the application of classical frequentist statistics less applicable to observational research: First, there is generally not a formal sampling of participants from a defined roster, except in some instances in recruiting cohorts or selecting controls in case–control studies. More often, the choice of study setting and participants is based on a variety of scientific and logistical decisions that do not resemble a random sampling procedure. Second, whereas in experiments, the exposure or treatment is randomly assigned (as in laboratory studies on animals or in randomized controlled trials in humans), in observational studies, exposure occurs through a diverse and often ill-defined implicit allocation method.

The frequentist statistical framework for measuring and describing random error is based on sampling theory and the probability of obtaining deviant samples or deviant allocation through purely random processes. The random sampling involved in the allocation of the exposure or treatment is critical because one can formally consider the universe of other ways in which the units could have been sampled or assigned. That is, if we allocate 20 rats or 20 people to one of two treatments, 10 per group, we can formally delineate all the ways treatment could be distributed across those participants. Given random allocation, one can ask the critical question of how probable is it, under some assumption about the truth, that a perfectly unbiased method of assigning treatment has generated results that deviate by specified amounts from that assumed, true value. We are not considering a biased method in assigning treatment but a perfectly valid one that will still yield groups that are not perfectly balanced in regard to baseline risk, and will occasionally generate assignments that are substantially deviant from equal baseline risk. Sampling theory is used to quantify the probability of obtaining deviant samples of any given magnitude.

Even in the case of a randomized trial, however, a focus solely or primarily on random error is justified only when other critical features of the study have been properly designed and managed. Characteristics of the study such as biased assessment of outcomes by participants or researchers, control for other determinants of outcome that happen to be unequally distributed, and compliance with study protocols need to be considered alongside the possibility that a perfectly random procedure for allocation went awry. Nevertheless, in a carefully designed trial, those other issues may be put to rest with greater confidence than in an observational study, giving greater *relative* importance to the role of random error.

In the case of observational studies, the model of random allocation and a distribution of potential imbalances in that allocation as the basis for the interpretation of statistical results is simply not applicable (Greenland, 1990). That is, the framework for generating estimates of variability due to random sampling cannot be justified based on a random sampling or random assignment process. It is difficult to develop a compelling rationale for treating exposures that result from societal forces or individual choice as though they were randomly assigned, and thus the interpretation of results that are predicated on such allocation must be less formal, at a minimum. There are elements of chance in observational studies, of course, such as selection of the study setting and time period. Such qualitative elements of randomness however, fall far short of a justification for direct application of the technology that was generated for experiments in which the exposure of interest is randomly allocated. The concept of random error still applies to observational epidemiologic studies, in that we believe that random forces will prevent us from measuring precisely the causal association of interest, but its origins and thus its statistical properties are poorly defined. Nonetheless, like random error in experimental studies, the scatter introduced by random error in observational studies is presumed to be symmetrical, and big studies suffer less from the problem than small studies. Thus, in observational studies, there is a desire to quantify the role of random error, despite recognition that we cannot do so precisely.

We thus have a dilemma in which it is recognized that random error contributes to observational studies but the dominant statistical framework was constructed for other types of research. It is not surprising that epidemiologists have turned to that approach as a means of addressing random error, nor is it surprising that the lack of direct applicability of the framework is often neglected. The recommended approach, subject to much-needed improvement, is to apply the tools that are built on the random sampling paradigm in a flexible manner so as to inform judgments about the potential impact of random error on the study findings, while recognizing that the product is at best a guideline or clue to interpretation. As discussed in the section, "Interpretation of Confidence Intervals," confidence intervals should not be used to define boundaries or dichotomize results as compatible or incompatible with other findings, but to broadly characterize the study's precision and convey some notion of how influential random error may have been (Poole, 2001). Probability values, used on a continuous scale and cautiously interpreted may also have value for the same purpose (Weinberg, 2001). What is indefensible in observational studies, and questionable even in experimental ones, is a rigid, categorical interpretation of the results epitomized by statistical significance testing or equivalently, examination of confidence interval boundaries. The evidence itself is not categorical: random error does not act in an all-or-none fashion, the underlying assumptions for statistical testing are not met, and any attempt to claim that the study results are "due to chance" or "not due to chance" is unwarranted.

STATISTICAL SIGNIFICANCE TESTING

Despite eloquent arguments against relying on a comparison of observed p-values to some critical threshold, typically 0.05 or 0.01 (Rothman, 1978; Poole, 1987, 2001; Greenland, 1990), epidemiologic study results, like those of most other sciences, continue to be commonly presented and interpreted (some have said degraded) using this benchmark. Sophisticated statisticians and most epidemiologists appreciate that systematic error is often as serious (or more serious) a threat to study validity as random error, and they recognize in principle that rigid, simplistic interpretation of statistical tests is not a valid or useful approach to the assessment of study findings. In fact, it was recently suggested that in practice, epidemiologists generally have the good sense to consider a constellation of statistical, methodological, and biological factors as they interpret their data (Goodman, 2001). Nevertheless, despite many admonitions, the first question typically asked by those who are interested in the interpretation of epidemiologic findings continues to be, "Were the results statistically significant?" Students of epidemiology seem to understand the arguments against statistical significance testing, yet many are seduced by the shorthand, "Is it significant?" as an appealing substitute for thinking more comprehensively about the evidence.

The reasons for the persistence of this bad habit are worthy of some consideration. One motive is a laudable effort to restrain the temptation of an excessively exuberant investigator to overinterpret each association as important. There is good reason to believe, however, that statistical testing actually encourages rather than discourages overinterpretation (Goodman, 1999a,b; Poole,

2001). The desire for a simple approach to categorize study findings as *positive* (statistically significant) or *negative* (not statistically significant) is understandable, since the alternative is much less tidy.

The parallel approach to systematic error, in which we would categorize results as *susceptible to misclassification* versus *immune from misclassification* or *prone to selection bias* versus *free of selection bias* would be no less absurd. It is obvious that such methodologic issues do not occur in an all-or-none manner, nor is the probability that they are present zero or one. Particularly when studies generate many findings, it is tempting to find some approach to help whittle down the results into a more manageable short list of those that really deserve scrutiny. The alternative to arbitrary dichotomization of findings is to scrutinize each and every result for the information it provides to advance knowledge on one narrowly defined hypothesis (Cole, 1979). If there is a narrowing of focus to selected findings it should be based on the magnitude of prior interest and the quality of information generated by the study.

Unfortunately, as pervasive as statistical testing remains in epidemiology (Savitz et al., 1994), the concepts of statistical testing are more entrenched in other branches of research; communication with colleagues, as well as lawyers and policy makers, often places unrelenting pressure on epidemiologists to generate and use statistical tests in the interpretation of their findings. Just as it is a challenge to substitute a more valid, but complex, interpretation of results for communication *among* epidemiologists, it is a challenge to explain to those outside the discipline what is required to make meaningful inferences in epidemiology. The argument that "everyone else does it" is specious, but unfortunately many epidemiologists are not so secure as to be comfortable in deviating from the (inappropriate) norms of our colleagues working in more advanced scientific disciplines.

Results of statistical tests are often posed and interpreted as asking whether the results are *likely to have occurred by chance alone*. More formally, we estimate the probability of having obtained results as or more extremely divergent from the null as those observed, under the assumption that the null hypothesis is true. Then we ask whether the calculated p-value falls below the critical value, typically 0.05, and if it does, we declare the results unlikely to have arisen by chance alone if the null hypothesis is true. If we cannot conclude that the results are unlikely to have arisen by chance alone—i.e., they do not pass this screening—a conclusion is drawn that the results *could* have arisen by chance alone even if the null hypothesis is true. It is then inferred that no meaningful association is present—i.e., what has been observed as a deviation from the null reflects random error, and therefore there is no need for discussion of other potential biases that might have yielded this association. If the result passes the screening and is found to be statistically significant, then an association may be declared as *established* and further examined for contributing biases or the possibility of applying a causal interpretation. There are a series of important problems with this conventional strategy built around statistical significance testing that are detrimental to valid interpretation of epidemiologic study results.

The premises for generating probability values themselves, even without considering their use to dichotomize findings, are highly contrived. The precise question that is asked for which p-values are the answer is as follows: Assuming that the null hypothesis is correct (e.g., the relative risk is 1.0), what is the probability of obtaining results as extreme or more extreme as the one which was observed? The null hypothesis is assumed to be correct, not tested; it is the compatibility of the data with the null hypothesis that is evaluated, not the legitimacy of the null hypothesis itself. Since we are truly interested in how likely it is that the null hypothesis or some other hypothesis is correct, there are approaches to more directly evaluate the strength of support the data provide for or against particular hypotheses (Goodman, 1999a,b). Though the decision-making framework leads us to reject or not reject the null hypothesis, the only concrete information we typically have available is how probable the data are assuming the null hypothesis to be true, not the probability of the hypothesis being true given the data obtained.

As noted previously, observational epidemiology studies lack a random sampling or random allocation element that would justify the calculation and conventional interpretation of p-values (Greenland, 1990). The premise for estimating the probability of a given set of results under the null hypothesis is based on sampling theory, where one can imagine repeating the assignment of exposure over and over, generating a distribution of results from those random assignments, and comparing the results that were obtained with the distribution of results that would have been obtained if the allocation were made over and over. Without that anchor, the p-values themselves are less relevant and certainly not so reliable as to make sharp distinctions.

The p-value that is generated is subjected to one more important, arbitrary simplification by testing it against some set value, typically 0.05 or 0.01, with the results then dichotomized as *statistically significant* or *not statistically significant*. The observed data are declared compatible with the null and the null hypothesis is not rejected or they are found to be incompatible with the null and the null hypothesis is rejected. The null hypothesis is designated the sole benchmark of interest, and rather than assessing the degree of compatibility of the data with the null hypothesis (or some other hypothesis of interest), a decision is made to reject or fail to reject the null hypothesis. The decisiveness, formality, simplicity, and ostensibly scientific character of this rule holds great appeal to epidemiologists and other scientists, but we should always look skeptically when dichotomies are created from information that logically must fall along a continuum. It seems far more plausible that results provide varying degrees of support for varying hypotheses, one of which is the null, but that information is lost, not gained, in forcing a dichotomous decision. We do not really need to decide anything from a given study, in the sense of choosing a drug or making a policy judgment, and there is no reason to pretend that such a dichotomous decision hangs in the balance. In practice, epidemiologists and other scientists integrate the statistical considerations with a wide array of other aspects of the evidence to judge the overall state of the science on any given topic (Goodman, 2001). Even if we were somehow called upon to "get off the fence" and decide the truth (as statistical testing would imply), rigid adherence to formal statistical tests would be a terrible strategy for doing so.

Our original goal of examining and describing the extent to which random error may have distorted study results and finding a means of quantifying the superiority of large studies over small studies has been diverted (not solved) by the framework of p-values and especially statistical significance testing. Whether the measured value is the null or some value other than the null, we are interested in assessing and quantifying the role of random error. A preferable way of quantifying random error for any estimate that is generated, including the null value, is through construction of confidence intervals, which can help to avoid dichotomizing results and characterize the improved precision as study size increases.

The primacy given to statistical significance testing gives an undue emphasis to the importance of random over systematic error, and although often touted as a way of ensuring conservatism in the interpretation of results, the practice may actually encourage overinterpretation of positive findings (Goodman, 1999a). In observational studies, the additional sources of error make attainment of statistical significance a weak benchmark for identifying causal associations. Testing does not discriminate findings that are *real*, and thus potentially causal, versus findings that are *likely to be due to chance*. Given all the work that is required to develop and conduct epidemiologic studies, consuming substantial financial and human resources, it is terribly wasteful not to fully appreciate what the study results can tell us and degrade the findings into a statistical test.

MULTIPLE COMPARISONS AND RELATED ISSUES

The concern with random error has also been applied to the interpretation of the array of results within a given study or even more broadly, to a broader universe of results from the same data collection effort or generated by the same investigator. Here the concern as typically raised is not with the evaluation of precision in a specific measure of association, which is the focus in generating a confidence interval, but rather with using the broader array of results to help judge a specific findings.

When examining an array of results, one can ask about the probability that a specified number of those findings will appear to be statistically significantly different from the null value. That is, a conventional critical p-value of 0.05 applies to a single observed result, but if one is interested in maintaining this critical value for an array of results, for example 10 measures of association, then the critical p-value for each of those measures must be smaller to ensure that the critical p-value for the aggregate of findings remains 0.05, i.e., that there is a 5% probability of one p-value of less than 0.05 if all the null hypotheses are true. A formula that provides the basis for calculating the actual critical p-value for one or more statistically significant results is $1 - (1 - \text{alpha})^n$ where alpha is the critical p-value for each measure, typically 0.05, and n is the number of such calculations that are made. Taking this experiment-wise error into account using the Bonferroni correction is intended to be and is, of course, conservative. Fewer findings will be declared statistically significant, but of course there is also a tremendous loss of statistical power that results from making the critical p-values more stringent. The formal statistical hypothesis that is addressed is how likely is it that we would observe an array of findings that is as extreme or more extreme than the array we obtained under the assumption that all associations being explored are truly null? We assume that there are no associations present in the whole array of data, just as we assume the individual null hypothesis is true to generate a p-value for an individual finding.

Consideration of an array of findings is most often used to ask whether a given result from a study that attains some critical p-value is nevertheless likely to have arisen by chance. Consideration of the number of such calculations made in the course of analyzing data from the study is used to address the question, "How many statistically significant measures of association would we expect even if none are truly present?" Assuming that the universal null hypothesis is correct, and that there are truly no associations present in the data, the number of statistically significant results that are generated will increase as the number of associations that are examined increases. From this perspective, a result that emerges from examination of many results is more likely to be a *false positive* finding than a result that is generated in isolation or from a small array of results. According to the formal technology of generating p-values and assigning statistical significance, this is certain to be true.

Despite the technical accuracy of this line of reasoning, there are a number of serious problems with attempts to use the concept of multiple testing, as conventionally applied, to interpret individual study results (Savitz & Olshan, 1995). The relevant constellation of results that defines the universe of interest is arbitrarily defined, sometimes consisting of other results reported in a given publication, but it could just as legitimately be based on the results generated from that data collection effort or by that investigator. Each measure of effect that is generated addresses a different substantive question, and lumping those results together simply because the same data collection effort produced them all makes no logical sense. It would be no less arbitrary to group all the results of a given investigator, all those in a given issue of a journal, or those generated on subjects in the same city (Rothman, 1990). Should the context include all past and future uses of the data set, accounting for analyses not yet done?

By shifting the frame of reference from the individual comparison to a set of comparisons from the same study or data set, it follows that the threat of random error in a given measure of association is somehow affected by other past and future analyses of the data. Independent of the process of generating the data, it is implied that the very act of generating additional measures of association bears upon the interpretation of the one of interest. Short of data fabrication, nothing that is done with the data set will affect a given result; so how can the data "know" what else you've done with them? Given the expense of conducting epidemiologic studies, and the desire to generate relevant information on an array of scientifically important issues, pressure to constrain exploitation of data could only be harmful and inefficient. Each result, even if many are generated, needs to be scrutinized and challenged on its own merits (Cole, 1979). All the usual concerns with potential bias apply, and random error is certainly among those concerns. The amount of random error in a given measure of association is a function of study size, however, not of other analyses done with the data.

On a slightly more abstract level, but also motivated by a concern with multiple comparisons, the question may be raised as to how the hypothesis originated. In particular, was it conceived before the data were analyzed (a priori hypothesis) or after the data were analyzed (post hoc hypothesis)? Under this line of reasoning, independent of the quality of the data and the background state of knowledge based on previous epidemiologic studies and other lines of relevant research, results addressing hypotheses that were postulated before the conduct of data analyses are viewed as more credible than those that emerged later. The sequence of hypothesis formulation and data analysis is seen as critical to interpretation of study results, but on closer consideration this makes no sense. Such an argument assigns an almost mystical property to the data—the numbers are somehow thought to "know" when the idea arose and deserve to be discounted more if the idea arose later rather than earlier. A given result does not "know" when the idea arose and its validity and precision are not affected by such issues (Poole, 1988; Cole, 1993). Undoubtedly, questions conceived prior to the study will often tend to be based on more extensive background literature and will often lead to more refined efforts at data collection. Where prior hypotheses lead to more careful measurement of the exposure of interest and optimized designs to address the study question, those improvements should translate into more credible findings. Evaluating the totality of evidence after the study certainly must include ancillary support from previous studies, and strong prior evidence will often be associated with formulation of a priori hypotheses and associated with more conclusive cumulative findings when the study is completed. However, it is solely the quality of the evidence that determines its value, not the timing of data analysis or the mental processes of the investigator.

In practice, many who interpret epidemiologic data continue to put a great deal of stock in the multiple comparisons issue. Arguments are made that a result should be given more credence because it came from an a priori hypothesis or less credence because it did not. Sometimes investigators will be careful to point out that they had a question in mind at the inception of the study, or to make special note of what the primary basis was for the study having been funded. Reviewers of manuscripts sometimes ask for specification of the primary purpose of the study, particularly when presenting results that address issues other than the one that justified initial funding of the research. At best, these are indirect clues to suggest that the investigators may have been more thorough in assessing the relevant background literature on the primary topic before the study as compared to secondary interests. Perhaps that effort helped them to refine data collection or to choose a study population that was especially well-suited to address the study question. The only consequence of interest is in how the data were affected, and it is the quality of the data that should be scrutinized rather than the investigators' knowledge and when it arose. If all that foresight and planning failed to result in a suitable study design, there should be no extra points awarded for trying and if they were just lucky in having ideal data for an unanticipated study question, then no points should be deducted for lack of foresight.

Analogous arguments are commonly made that a result should be given less credence because it came from an ex post facto hypothesis, sometimes referred to as data dredging or fishing. Such criticisms are without merit, other than perhaps to focus attention to the possibility of substantive concerns. If a particular finding has little context in the literature, then even with the addition of new supporting evidence, the cumulative level of support is likely to remain modest. If an issue was not anticipated in advance, this may result in lower quality data to address the question, with inferior exposure or disease measurement or lack of data on relevant potential confounders. Any such problems warrant close examination and criticism. What does not warrant scrutiny is how many analyses were done, what other uses have been made of the data, or how and when the analysis plans came about.

Where selective analyses and reporting of findings become important is in the dissemination of findings through presentations at research meetings and especially in the published literature. Often, the primary hypothesis is of sufficient importance that investigators will be motivated to publish the results regardless of the outcome, whether confirming or refuting previous literature. On the other hand, secondary hypotheses may well be dismissed quickly if the results are not interesting (i.e., not positive), and thus the body of published literature is not only incomplete but is a biased sample from the work that has been done (Dickersin et al., 1987; Chalmers, 1990). If data are dredged not simply to glean all that can be obtained from the data but to find positive results (at its worst, to skim off statistically significant findings), then the available literature will provide a poor reflection of the true state of knowledge. At the level of the individual investigator, results-based publication constitutes a disservice to science, and decisions by editors to favor positive over null findings would exacerbate the difficulty in getting the scientific literature to accurately reflect the truth.

Techniques have recently been proposed and are becoming more widespread that make beneficial use of the array of findings from a study to improve each of the estimates that are generated (Greenland & Robins, 1991; Greenland & Poole, 1994). The goal is to take advantage of information from the constellation of results to make more informed guesses regarding the direction and amount of random error and thereby produce a set of revised estimates that are probabilistically, in the aggregate, going to be closer to their true values. Estimates are modified through empirical Bayes or Bayesian shrinkage; the most extreme and imprecise estimates in an array of results are likely to have random error that inflated the estimates, just as those far below the null value are likely to suffer from random error that reduced the estimates. By using this information on likely direction and magnitude of random error, obtainable only from the constellation of findings, outliers can be shrunk in light of presumed random error toward more probable estimates of the magnitude of association. Instead of simply giving less attention to extreme, imprecise results informally, the findings from other analyses of the data help to produce a better estimate. The nature of random error, which will tend to generate some erroneously high and some erroneously low measures of association is exploited to make extremely high and low imprecise values less extreme since it is almost certain that random error has introduced distortion that contributes to their being outliers. A better guess of their values, free of random error, is that they would be closer to the null on average.

INTERPRETATION OF CONFIDENCE INTERVALS

Random error is always present to some extent and generates error in estimating measures of effect. Furthermore, larger studies suffer less distortion from random error than smaller studies. Thus, some method is needed to quantify the amount of random error that is present. Though the underlying rationale for constructing confidence intervals is based on the same sampling theory as p-values, they are useful for characterizing the precision in a much more general way. The statistical framework is used to help make an assessment of the role of random error, but it is advisable to step back from the formal underpinnings and not attempt to make fine distinctions about values within or outside the interval, to screen results as including or excluding the null value, or to let the confidence interval dominate the basis for drawing conclusions.

Starting with a known true value for the measure of interest, the confidence interval is the set of values for which the p-value will be greater than 0.05 (for a 95% confidence interval) in a test of whether the data deviate from the true value. That is, assuming the point estimate is the correct value, all those values up to the boundary of the interval would genreate p-values of 0.05 or greater if tested using the given study size. Obviously, as the study size gets larger, the array of values that would generate $p > 0.05$ becomes smaller and smaller, and thus the confidence interval becomes narrower and narrower. A consequence of the manner in which the interval is constructed is that the true value for the parameter of interest will be contained in such intervals in a specified proportion of cases, 95% if that is the chosen coverage. Confidence intervals, despite being based on many of the same unrealistic assumptions as p-values and statistical tests, are much more useful for quantifying random error, so long as they are not merely used as substitutes for statistical tests. If one uses the formal statistical properties of confidence intervals, the bounds of the interval can be interpreted as two-tailed statistical tests of the null hypothesis—if the lower bound of a 95% confidence interval exceeds the null value, then the p-value is less than 0.05. If the interpretation of the confidence interval is solely based on whether that interval includes or excludes the null value, then it functions as a statistical test and suffers from all the drawbacks associated with an arbitrary dichotomization of the data. Instead, confidence intervals should be used as *interval estimates* of the measure of interest, conveying a sense of the precision of that estimate.

Only marginally better is the use of confidence intervals to define bounds of compatibility, i.e., interpreting the interval as a range within the true value is likely to lie. In this view, the confidence interval is treated as a step function (Poole, 1987), with values inside the interval presumed to be equally likely and values outside the interval equally unlikely. In reality, the point estimate and values near it are far better estimates of the true value based on the data than values further away but still within the interval. Similarly, values toward the extremes of the interval and values just outside the interval are not meaningfully different from one another either. A slight variant of the exclusionary interpretation of confidence intervals is to compare confidence intervals from two or more studies to assess whether they overlap. If they do overlap, the interpretation is that the results are *statistically compatible* and if they do not, the results are believed to be *statistically different* from one another. If the goal is to test the statistical difference in two estimates, or an estimate and a presumed true value, there are more direct ways to do so. In fact, if such a difference is of particular interest, the point estimate of that difference can be calculated and a confidence interval constructed around the estimated difference.

Confidence intervals are useful to convey a sense of the random variation in the data, with a quantitative but informal interpretation of the precision of that estimate. Values toward the center of the interval are more compatible with the observed results than values toward the periphery, and the boundary point itself is rather improbable and unworthy of special focus. The p-value function is a description of the random error that is present, and the bounds of the confidence interval help to describe how peaked or flat the p-value function is around the point estimate. In a large study, the p-value function will be highly peaked, with the most probable values very close to the point estimate, whereas in a small study, it will be flatter, with fairly probable values extending more widely above and below the point estimate. The confidence interval, while ill-suited to making fine distinctions near the extremes of the interval, is nonetheless very useful for providing a rough indication of precision.

The information provided by the confidence interval can be used to compare the precision of different studies, again not focusing on the exact values but more generally on the width of the interval. A simple measure, the confidence limit ratio (Poole, 2001) has very attractive features for characterizing precision and making comparisons across studies. Two studies with point estimates of a relative risk of 2.0, one with a 95% confidence interval of 1.1 to 3.3, and the other with a confidence interval of 0.9 to 4.3 (confidence limit ratios of 3.3/1.1 = 3.0 and 4.4/0.9 = 4.8) are different but not substantially different in their precision. A study with a confidence interval of 0.4 to 9.6 (confidence limit ratio = 9.6/0.4 = 24) is well worth distinguishing as less precise, perhaps so imprecise as to render any inferences meaningless

Confidence intervals are helpful in comparing results from one study to results from others, not formally testing them but assessing whether they are close to or far from the point estimate, taking the imprecision of that point estimate and overlap of intervals into account. Broadly characterizing the extent of overlap in confidence interval coverage (not dichotomizing as overlapping versus non-overlapping) can be helpful in describing the similarity or differences in study findings. For example, a study with a relative risk of 1.0 and a confidence interval of 0.4 to 2.0 is fairly compatible with a study yielding a relative risk of 1.5 with a confidence interval of 0.8 to 3.0. Two larger studies with narrower confidence intervals but the same point estimates—for example, a relative risk of 1.0, with a confidence interval of 0.8–1.2, and a relative risk of 1.5, with a confidence interval of 1.1–2.2—would be interpreted as more distinctly different from one another. Beyond the formal comparisons across studies, confidence intervals allow for a rapid assessment of the magnitude of imprecision, especially to describe whether it is at a level that calls into serious question the information value of the study. Studies with cells of 2 or 3 observations, which tend to generate extremely imprecise estimates and confidence limit ratios of 10 or more, can quickly be spotted and appropriately discounted. This informal interpretation of confidence intervals, aided by calculation and examination of the confidence interval ratio, is a valuable guide to imprecision.

INTEGRATED ASSESSMENT OF RANDOM ERROR

Random error contributes to the uncertainty in estimated measures of effect and therefore warrants close scrutiny as a contributor to the deviation between the results of epidemiologic studies and the true causal effect of exposure on disease. Because the framework for quantification is so much more fully developed and familiar than that for other forms of error, however, it may be given undue prominence. Furthermore, a well-justified concern with the role of random error is often translated into an inappropriate method for interpreting study results. The central role given to the statistical null hypothesis is not warranted. The technology of experiments has been transferred directly to observational studies, yet it is not directly applicable because of the lack of randomization in exposure assignment. What we would like from an examination of random error is a clear characterization of the imprecision in study results, not a test of whether the data or more extreme data are unlikely to have been observed assuming the null hypothesis is true. A simple goal of taking imprecision into account in the interpretation of study results is often made convoluted and difficult to apply for the intended purpose.

In evaluating random error, the most conventional approach is to test statistical significance, either openly or covertly through the calculation and presentation of confidence intervals. These intervals are then used to dichotomize results based on whether the null value is included within or excluded from the confidence interval (Savitz et al., 1994). The focus should be on the extent to which random error may have distorted the study's results, rather than compatibility of the data with the null hypothesis. Random error can bias results in either direction, and it is of interest for measurements at or near the null, as well as measurements more deviant from the null. There is no basis for dichotomizing random error as *important* or *not important* but instead the goal should be to quantify its potential impact on the study's findings.

Confidence intervals are more useful than p-values or statistical tests for quantifying the impact of random error. Confidence intervals should not be interpreted as statistical tests or bounds defining compatible and incompatible results, but rather for their width or narrowness, indicating how imprecise or precise the estimates are. Informal use of confidence intervals assists in comparing results across studies for general compatibility, assessing the extent to which random error is a major or minor problem in a given study, quantifying the benefits of increased study size, and conveying information about the role of random versus various forms of systematic error. For these purposes, a simple measure like the confidence limit ratio of the upper to the lower bound is a useful adjunct to the position of the interval itself.

A series of more advanced approaches have become popular recently that can use information on an array of study findings to make more informed estimates about the direction and magnitude of random error, and thereby produce improved estimates that are likely to be closer to the value that would have been obtained in the absence of random error (Greenland & Robins, 1991). Instead of the usual situation in which the influence of random error is assumed to be symmetric (on the appropriate scale) around the observed value, consideration of a distribution of results can suggest that certain values are deviantly high or low, likely to be due in part to random processes. Therefore, the better estimate is not the original (naive) estimate but one that is shrunk by some amount in the direction of the null value. Such approaches go beyond quantifying random error and begin to compensate for it to produce improved estimates, reflecting significant progress in refining epidemiologic data analysis. Efforts to incorporate other random elements such as those that are part of misclassification are being developed, as well as more comprehensive approaches to the integration of random and systematic error.

REFERENCES

Chalmers I. Underreporting research is scientific misconduct. JAMA 1990;263:1405–1408.

Cole P. The evolving case-control study. J Chron Dis 1979;32:15–27.

Cole P. The hypothesis generating machine. Epidemiology 1993;4:271–273.

Dickersin K, Chan S, Chalmers TC, Sacks HS, Smith H Jr. Publication bias and clinical trials. Control Clin Trials 1987;8:343–353.

Goodman SN. Towards evidence-based medical statistics. I. The P-value fallacy. Ann Intern Med 1999a;130:995–1004.

Goodman SN. Towards evidence-based medical statistics. II. The Bayes factor. Ann Intern Med 1999b;130:1005–1013.

Goodman SN. Of P-values and Bayes: a modest proposal. Epidemiology 2001;21:295–297.

Greenland S. Randomization, statistics, and causal inference. Epidemiology 1990;1:421–429.

Greenland S, Poole C. Empirical-Bayes and semi-Bayes approaches to occupational and environmental hazard surveillance. Arch Environ Health 1994;49:9–16.

Greenland S, Robins JM. Empirical-Bayes adjustments for multiple comparisons are sometimes useful. Epidemiology 1991;2:244–251.

Hill AB. The environment and disease: association or causation? Proc Roy Soc Med 1965;58:295–300.

Poole C. Beyond the confidence interval. Am J Public Health 1987;77:195–199.

Poole C. Induction does not exist in epidemiology, either. In Rothman KJ (ed), Causal Inference. Chestnut Hill, MA: Epidemiology Resources Inc., 1988:153–162.

Poole C. Low P-values or narrow confidence intervals: which are more durable? Epidemiology 2001;12:291–294.

Rothman KJ. A show of confidence. N Engl J Med 1978;299:1362–1363.

Rothman KJ. No adjustments are needed for multiple comparisons. Epidemiology 1990;1:43–46.

Savitz DA, Olshan AF. Multiple comparisons and related issues in the interpretation of epidemiologic data. Am J Epidemiol 1995;142:904–908.

Savitz DA, Tolo K-A, Poole C. Statistical significance testing in the American Journal of Epidemiology, 1970 to 1990. Am J Epidemiol 1994;139:1047–1052.

Weinberg CR. It's time to rehabilitate the P-value. Epidemiology 2001;12:288–290.

11

INTEGRATION OF EVIDENCE ACROSS STUDIES

As in other sciences, results from a single epidemiologic study are rarely if ever sufficient to draw firm conclusions. No matter how much care is taken to avoid biases and ensure adequate precision, idiosyncrasies inherent to any study render its results fallible. If nothing else, the chosen study population may demonstrate a different exposure—disease relation than other populations would show, so that the bounds of inference would need to be tested. Furthermore, limitations in methods ranging from subtle methodologic pitfalls to mundane clerical errors or programming mistakes render conclusions even for the study population itself subject to error. Therefore, rather than seeking a single, perfect study to provide clear information on the phenomenon of interest, the full array of pertinent results from a series of imperfect studies needs to be considered in order to accurately summarize the state of knowledge and draw conclusions.

Multiple studies provide an opportunity to evaluate *patterns* of results to draw firmer conclusions. Not only can the hypothesis of a causal relation between exposure and disease be examined using the full array of information, but hypotheses regarding study biases can be evaluated as well. The concept of *replication* reflects a narrow, incomplete subset of the issues that can be fruitfully evaluated across a series of studies that address the same causal relationship. As often applied, the search for replicability refers to a series of methodologically similar studies which enables the reviewer to examine the role of random error in accounting for different findings across those studies. Given that research designs and study methods inevitably differ in epidemiology, however, the question is not simply, "Are the studies consistent with one another?" but rather, "What is the summary of evidence provided by this series of studies?" A series of studies yielding inconsistent results may well provide strong support for a causal inference when the methodologic features of those studies are scrutinized and the subset of studies that support an association are methodologically stronger, while those that fail to find an association are weaker. Similarly, consistent evidence of an association may not support a causal relation if all the studies share the same bias that is likely to generate spurious indications of a positive association. In order to draw conclusions, the methods and results must be considered in relation to one another, both within and across studies.

CONSIDERATION OF RANDOM ERROR AND BIAS

There has been a dramatic rise in interest and methodology for the formal, quantitative integration of evidence across studies, generally referred to as meta-analysis (Petitti, 1994; Greenland, 1987, 1998). In the biomedical literature, much of the motivation comes from a desire to integrate evidence across a series of small clinical trials. The perceived problem that these tools were intended to address is the inability of individual trials to have sufficient statistical power to detect small benefits, whereas if the evidence could be integrated across studies, statistical power would be enhanced. If subjected to formal tests of statistical significance, which is the norm in assessing the outcome of a clinical trial, many individual trials are too small to detect clinically important benefits as statistically significant. When such non-significant tendencies are observed across repeated studies, there is an interest in assessing what the evidence says when aggregated. Note that the intended benefits were focused on reducing random error through aggregation of results, implicitly or explicitly assuming that the individual studies are otherwise compatible with regard to methods and freedom from other potential study biases.

The value of this effort to synthesize rather than merely describe the array of results presumes an emphasis on statistical hypothesis testing. A rigid interpretation of statistical testing can and does lead to situations in which a series of small studies, all pointing in the same direction, for example, a small benefit of treatment, would lead to the conclusion that each of the studies found no effect (based on significance testing). If the evidence from that same series of studies were combined, and summarized with a pooled estimate of effect, evidence of a statistically significant benefit would generate a very different conclusion than the studies taken one at a time. Obviously, if a series of small studies shows similar benefit, those who are less bound by adherence to statistical testing may well infer that the treatment appears to confer a benefit without the need to assess the statistical significance of the array of results. Those who wish to compare the array of results to a critical p-value, however, are able to do so. In fact, as discussed below in the section on "Interpreting Consistency and Inconsistency," the consistency across studies with at least slightly different methods and the potential for different biases might actually provide greater confidence of a true benefit. Identically designed and conducted studies may share identical biases and show similar effects across the studies due to those shared errors.

As discussed in Chapter 10, in well-designed and well-executed randomized trials, the focus on random error as the primary source of erroneous inferences may be justified. That is, if the principles of masked, objective assessment of outcome are followed, and an effective randomization procedures is employed to ensure that baseline risk does not differ across exposure groups, the major threat to generating valid results is a failure of the random allocation mechanism to yield groups of baseline comparability. Generating a p-value addresses the probability that the random allocation mechanism has generated an aberrant sample under the assumption that there is no true difference between the groups. Thus, repetition of the experiment under identical conditions can be used to address and reduce the possibility that there is no benefit of treatment but the allocation of exposure by groups has, by chance, generated such a pattern of results. A series of small, identical randomized trials will yield a distribution of results, and the integration of results across those trials would provide the best estimate of the true effect. In the series of small studies, the randomization itself may not be effective, although the deviation in results from such randomization should be symmetrical around the true value. Integration of information across the studies should help to identify the true value around which the findings from individual studies cluster.

The randomized trial paradigm and assumptions have been articulated because the direct application of this reasoning to observational studies is often problematic, sometimes severely so. Just as the framework of statistical hypothesis testing has limited applicability to a single epidemiologic study, the framework of synthetic meta-analysis has limited applicability to a set of observational studies.

Observational studies are rarely if ever true replications of one another. The populations in which the studies are conducted differ, and thus the presence of potential effect-modifiers differs as well. The tools of measurement are rarely identical, even for relatively simple constructs such as assessment of tobacco use or occupation. Exact methods of selecting and recruiting subjects differ, and the extent and pattern of nonparticipation varies. Susceptibility to confounding will differ whenever the underlying mechanism of exposure assignment differs. Thus, the opportunity to simply integrate results across a series of methodologically identical studies does not exist in observational epidemiology. Glossing over these differing features of study design and conduct, and pretending that only random error accounts for variability among studies is more likely to generate misleading than helpful inferences.

Closely related to this concern is the central role assigned to statistical power and random error in the interpretation of study results. The fundamental goal of integrating results is to draw more valid conclusions by taking advantage of the evidence from having several studies of a given topic rather than a single large study. While enhanced precision from the larger number of subjects accrued in multiple studies is an asset, the more valuable source of insight is often the opportunity to understand the influence of design features on study results. This can only be achieved by having multiple studies of differing character and scrutinizing the pattern that emerges, not suppressing it through a single synthetic estimate. Imagine two situations, one with a single study of 5000 cases of disease in a cohort of 1,000,000 persons, and the other a series of 10 studies with 500 cases each from cohorts of 100,000 persons. The single, extremely precise study would offer limited opportunity to learn from the methodologic choices that were made since a single protocol would have been followed. Differing approaches to measurement of exposure and disease, control of confounding, and modification of the estimated effect by covariates would be limited because of the lack of diversity in study methods. In contrast, the variation in methodologic decisions among the 10 studies would provide an opportunity to assess the pattern of results in relation to methods. With variability in attributes across studies (viewed as a limitation or barrier to deriving a single estimate), one can gain an understanding of how those study features influence the results (an advantage in evaluating hypotheses of bias and causality).

DATA POOLING AND COORDINATED COMPARATIVE ANALYSIS

Pooling is the ultimate aggregation of evidence from multiple studies addressing the same topic in a similar manner. In this instance, it is not just the final results that are synthesized, but the raw data that are merged in the analysis. This procedure obviously requires data from each of the component studies rather than relying on published information. Furthermore, it requires a certain minimum degree of compatibility across studies in the structure of the data (study design and measurements). The ideal situation for data pooling, of course, is when a true multicenter study has been conducted, where identical research protocols were followed to assure that the data would be identical in all respects. Sometimes the equivalent of a multicenter study with a common protocol results from a systematic effort by a consortium of investigators or a funding agency to ensure such compatibility.

In pooling data across studies that were not designed to be so fully compatible, some compromises or assumptions are necessary to allow the integration of results. In fact, such efforts should be viewed with appropriate skepticism as to whether a single estimate from the aggregation of studies is the most informative way to understand the evidence that the set of studies are providing. The only goal of pooling is to reduce random error by merging multiple studies. The logic behind this approach is straightforward: if a series of studies are indistinguishable with regard to methods, then any differences among their results is presumably due to random error. It is as though one large study was done and the results had been arbitrarily subdivided, losing precision in such a division with no compensating gains in validity. Under those conditions, nothing could be learned from examining the variability among the studies about the influence of study design and conduct on results. The most succinct presentation of results, and the one that would most accurately describe the role of random error, would be a pooled estimate. In practice, it is very rare for epidemiologic studies to be so comparable in design and conduct that the differences among them are uninformative.

An evaluation of the role of residential magnetic field exposure and the risk of childhood leukemia (Greenland et al., 2000) provides a useful illustration of the value and limitations of the approach. A series of studies largely from the United States and Western Europe had evaluated the hypothesis that prolonged residential exposure to elevated levels of magnetic fields from outside power lines and electrical wiring in the home might lead to an increased risk of leukemia in children. Many methodologic concerns within each of the studies and the irregular pattern of results rendered the findings inconclusive regarding a causal relation between magnetic field exposure and cancer (NRC, 1997; Portier and Wolfe, 1998). Although there were many concerns, only one of those issues, random error, could be addressed by data pooling. In this instance, the most informative results might come from studying the occupants of homes with the very highest levels of magnetic fields, but such homes were rare in each of the studies (Table 11.1). Thus, enhancing precision for the higher dose portion of the dose–response curve was a perfectly valid, if narrow, goal.

Only a handful of cases and controls had been identified in each of the studies whose home measurements were above 0.2 microTesla, and even fewer above 0.3 microTesla, with the vast majority of homes between 0.05 and 0.2 microTesla (Table 11.1). To generate improved estimates of the dose–response function relating measured magnetic fields to childhood leukemia risk, Greenland et al. (2000) obtained raw data from all the investigators who had conducted relevant studies of this topic and pooled the data to generate dose–response estimates across a wide exposure range. The results are most interesting: no indication of increasing leukemia risk with increasing exposure was found for the range below 0.2 microTesla, whereas above that level, a clear (though still imprecise) indication was found of increasing risk with increasing exposure (Fig. 11.1). Risk estimates for exposure in the range of 0.3 to 0.6 microTesla, which no individ-

TABLE 11.1. Study-Specific Distributions of Magnetic-Field Data, Pooled Analysis of Magnetic Fields, Wire Codes, and Childhood Leukemia

FIRST AUTHOR†	Magnetic-Field Category (μT)						TOTAL	NO MEASURE*
	≤ 0.1	$> 0.1\text{-}\leq 0.2$	$> 0.2\text{-}\leq 0.3$	$> 0.3\text{-}\leq 0.4$	$> 0.4\text{-}\leq 0.5$	> 0.5		
Cases								
Coghill	48	5	2	0	1	0	56	0
Dockerty	72	9	3	1	1	1	87	34
Feychting	30	1	1	2	0	4	38	0
Linet	403	152	41	20	13	9	638	46
London	110	30	5	9	4	4	162	68
McBride	174	77	32	11	1	2	297	102
Michaelis	150	17	3	3	3	0	176	0
Olsen	829	1	0	0	0	3	833	0
Savitz	24	7	2	3	0	0	36	62
Tomenius	129	16	5	0	0	3	153	0
Tynes	146	2	0	0	0	0	148	0
Verkasalo	30	1	0	0	1	0	32	3
Controls								
Coghill	47	9	0	0	0	0	56	0
Dockerty	68	13	1	0	0	0	82	39
Feychting	488	26	18	10	2	10	554	0
Linet	407	144	41	17	5	6	620	69
London	99	28	6	2	2	6	143	89
McBride	194	96	28	5	3	3	329	70
Michaelis	372	29	7	4	0	2	414	0
Olsen	1658	3	2	2	0	1	1666	0
Savitz	155	28	10	3	2	0	198	67
Tomenius	546	119	24	4	2	3	698	21
Tynes	1941	25	7	5	4	22	2004	0
Verkasalo	300	9	6	4	0	1	320	30

*No measure for a residence at or before time of diagnosis (cases) or corresponding index date (for controls).

†See Greenland et al. (2000) for citations to original reports.

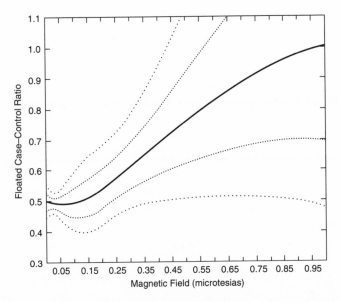

FIGURE 11.1. Floated case–control ratios from 3-degree-of-freedom quadratic-logistic spline model fit to pooled magnetic field data, with adjustment for study, age, and sex. Inner dotted lines are pointwise 80% confidence limits; outer dotted lines are pointwise 99% confidence limits (Greenland et al., 2000).

ual study could address, were the most supportive of a positive relation between magnetic fields and leukemia. Note that the myriad limitations in the design of individual studies, including potential response bias, exposure misclassification, and confounding were not resolved through data pooling, but the sparseness of the data in a range of the dose–response curve in which random error was a profound limitation was overcome to some extent.

A technique that is often better suited to maximizing the information from a series of broadly comparable studies, which also requires access to the raw data or at least to highly cooperative collaborators willing to undertake additional analyses, is comparative analysis. In this approach, rather than integrating all the data into the same analysis, parallel analyses are conducted using the most comparable statistical techniques possible. That is, instead of the usual situation in which different eligibility criteria are employed, different exposure categories are created, different potential confounders are controlled, etc., the investigative team imposes identical decision rules on all the studies that are to be included. Applying identical decision rules and analytic methods removes those factors as candidate explanations for inconsistent results and sharpens the focus on factors that remain different across studies such as the range of exposure observed or selective non-response.

The basic design and the data collection methods are not amenable to modification at the point of conducting comparative analysis, of course, except for those that can be changed by imposing restrictions on the available data (e.g., more stringent eligibility criteria). The series of decisions that proceed from the raw data to the final results are under the control of the investigators conducting the comparative analysis. Methodologically, the extent to which the choices made account for differences in the results can be evaluated empirically. When multiple studies address the same issue in a similar manner and yield incompatible results, the possibility of artifactual differences resulting from the details of analytic methods needs to be entertained. Comparative analysis addresses this hypothesized basis for differences in results directly, and either pinpoints the source of disparity or demonstrates that such methodologic decisions were not responsible for disparate findings. The opportunity to align the studies on a common scale of exposure and response yields an improved understanding of the evidence generated by the series of studies.

Lubin and Boice (1997) conducted such an analysis to summarize the evidence on residential radon and lung cancer. A series of eight pertinent case–control studies had been conducted, but both the range of radon exposure evaluated and the analytic approaches differed, in some cases, substantially, across studies. They found that the radon dose range being addressed across the series of studies differed markedly (Fig. 11.2), and the results could be reconciled, in part, by more formally taking the dose range into account. Each study had focused on the internal comparison of higher and lower exposure groups within their study settings, yet the absolute radon exposure levels that the studies addressed were quite distinctive, with the highest dose group ranging from approximately 150 Bq/m^3 to approximately 450 Bq/m^3. If in fact the studies in a lower dose range found no increase in risk with higher exposure, and those in the higher dose range did find such a pattern, it would be difficult to declare the studies inconsistent in a sense. They would be internally inconsistent but consistent relative to one another.

In this instance, the results were largely compatible when put on a common scale, with a combined relative risk estimate for a dose of 150 Bq/m^3 of 1.14 (Table 11.2). Even the combination of evidence across residential and occupational exposures from miner studies, where the doses are typically much higher, showed compatible findings when put on a common dose scale. Few exposures permit the quantification of dose to reconcile study findings, but this example clearly illustrates the need to go beyond the notion of consistent or inconsistent in gleaning the maximum information from a set of studies.

SYNTHETIC AND EXPLORATORY META-ANALYSIS

Instead of data pooling, which is logistically difficult due to the need to obtain raw data and conduct new analyses, epidemiologists have increasingly turned to

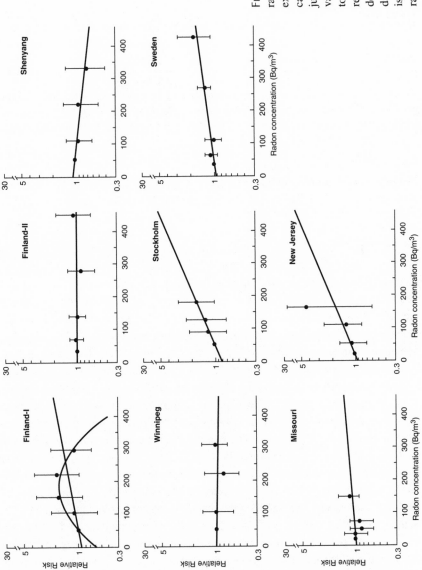

FIGURE 11.2. Relative risks (RRs) for radon concentration categories and fitted exposure–response models for each case–control study. Fitted lines are adjusted to pass through the quantitative value for the baseline category. Models fit to the logarithm of the RRs are linear with respect to radon. There was a significant departure from linearity in the Finland-I data, and also shown is the model which is linear and quadratic with respect to radon (Lubin & Boice, 1997, page 53).

TABLE 11.2. Estimates of the Relative Risk at 150 Bq/m³ and the 95% Confidence Interval for Each Study and for All Studies Combined, Meta-Analysis of Epidemiologic Studies of Residential Radon and Lung Cancer

STUDY	RR*	95% CI	REPORTED IN ORIGINAL PAPER[†]
Finland-I[‡]	1.30	1.09–1.55	NA
Finland-II	1.01	0.94–1.09	1.02
New Jersey	1.83	1.15–2.90	1.77
Shenyang	0.84	0.78–0.91	0.92[§]
Winnipeg	0.96	0.86–1.08	0.97
Stockholm	1.83	1.34–2.50	1.79
Sweden	1.20	1.13–1.27	1.15
Missouri	1.12	0.92–1.36	NA
Combined[¶]	1.14	1.01–1.30	

*Values shown are estimated RR at 150 Bq/m³, i.e., exp($b \times 150$), where b was the estimate of β obtained from a weighted linear regression fitting the model $\log(RR) = \beta(x - x_0)$, where x_0 is the quantitative value for the lowest radon category and x is the category-specific radon level.

†RR at 150 Bq/m³, based on or computed from exposure-response relationship provided in original reports. Exposure response was not available (NA) in Finland-I and Missouri studies.

‡For Finland-I, there was a significant departure from linearity ($P = 0.03$). The estimated RR for 150 Bq/m³ under a linear-quadratic model was 1.71.

§Taken from results in pooled analysis (18).

¶Combined estimate and CI based on a random effects model. Fixed effects estimate was 1.11 (95% CI = 1.07–1.15).

RR, relative risk; CI, confidence interval.

Lubin & Boice, 1997.

meta-analysis as a quantitative approach to integrating information from a set of published studies on the same topic. In meta-analysis, the unit of observation is the individual study and statistical tools are applied to the array of study results in order to extract the most objective, useful information possible about the phenomenon of interest. The methods and results of the included studies are analyzed to draw inferences from the body of relevant literature. The tools of meta-analysis have been described in detail elsewhere (Petitti, 1994; Greenland, 1998).

In synthetic meta-analysis, the goals are comparable to those of data pooling. The large number of observations acquired by integrating multiple studies are used to derive a more precise measure of effect than could be obtained from any of the individual studies. The goal is to generate a precision-weighted average result from across the series of studies, as illustrated in Table 11.2 for the estimated relative risk of 1.14 (95% confidence interval = 1.01–1.30) for lung cancer from exposure to 150 Bq/m³ in the meta-analysis of Lubin and Boice (1997). Statistical methods are available that take the variability among studies into account and derive a common point and interval estimate. Obviously, by taking into account all the data that comprise the individual studies, the overall estimate is markedly more precise than any of the original studies taken in isolation. Cynics suggest that the main goal of meta-analysis is to take a series of studies that demonstrate an effect that is not statistically significant and combine the studies to derive a summary estimate that is statistically significant, or worse yet, to take a series of imprecise and invalid results and generate a highly precise invalid result.

One of the challenges in conducting such meta-analyses is to ensure that the studies that are included are sufficiently compatible methodologically to make the exercise of synthesizing a common estimate an informative process. The algebraic technology will appear to work even when the studies being combined are fundamentally incompatible with respect to the methods used to generate the data. In practice, studies always differ from one another in potentially important features such as study locale, response proportion, and control of confounding, so that the decision to derive a summary estimate should be viewed at best as an exercise, in the same spirit as a sensitivity analyses. The question that is addressed by a meta-analysis is as follows: If none of the differing features of study methods affected the results, what would be the best estimate of effect from this set of studies? The value and credibility of that answer depends largely on the credibility of the premises.

An alternative approach to synthetic meta-analysis focused on the derivation of a single, pooled estimate, is to apply the statistical tools of meta-analysis to examine and better understand the sources of heterogeneity across the component studies. By focusing on the variability in results as the object of study, we can identify and quantify the influences of study methods and potential biases on study findings, rather than assume that such methodologic features are unimportant. The variability in study features, which are viewed as a nuisance when seeking a summary estimate, is the raw material for exploratory meta-analysis (Greenland, 1998).

In exploratory meta-analysis, the structural features of the study, such as location, time period, population source, and the measures of study conduct such as response proportion, masking of interviewers, and amount of missing information, are treated as potential determinants (independent variables) of the study results. Through exploratory meta-analysis, the manner in which study methods influence study results can be quantified, perhaps the most important goal in evaluating a body of epidemiologic literature. In parallel with the approach to examining methods and results within a single study, the focus of previous chapters, the same rationale applies to the examination of methods and results across studies. Just as the insights from such analyses of potential biases within a study help to assess the credibility of its findings, the pattern of results across a series of studies helps to more fully understand the constellation of findings and its meaning.

Sometimes, systematic examination of the pattern of results across studies yields a clear pattern in which methodologic quality is predictive of the results.

That is, studies that are better on average tend to show stronger (or weaker) measures of association, suggesting where the truth may lie among existing results or what might be expected by extrapolating to studies that are even better than the studies conducted thus far. For example, if higher response proportions were independently predictive of stronger associations, one would infer, all other things being equal, that a stronger association would be expected if non-response could be eliminated altogether. The studies with the higher response proportion are presumably yielding more valid results, all other things equal, and thus the observation that these studies yield stronger associations supports an association being truly present and stronger in magnitude than was observed even in the study with the best response thus far. The opposite pattern, higher response proportions predicting weaker association, would suggest that no association or only a weak one is present. Heterogeneity of results across studies is being explained in a manner that indicates both which results among completed studies are more likely to be valid and the basis for projecting what would be found if the methodologic limitation could be circumvented altogether. In meta-regression, such independent effects of predictors can be examined with adjustment for other features of the study that might be correlated with response proportions. With a sufficient number of observations, multiple influences on study findings can be isolated from one another.

Interpretation of the patterns revealed by exploratory meta-analysis is not always straightforward, of course, just as the corresponding relation between methods and results is not simple within individual studies. For example, one might observe that studies conducted in Europe tend to yield different results (stronger or weaker associations) than those conducted in North America. Neither group is necessarily more valid, but this pattern would encourage closer scrutiny of issues such as the methods of diagnosis, available tools for selecting controls in case–control studies, cultural attitudes toward the exposure of interest, or even the very nature of the exposure, which may well differ by geographic region. Sometimes there are time trends in which results of studies differ systematically as a function of the calendar period of study conduct, again subject to a variety of possible explanations. Even when features of the studies that do not correspond directly to indices of quality are predictive of results, much progress has been made beyond simply noting that the studies are inconsistent. The product of examining these attributes is refinement of the hypotheses that might explain inconsistent results in the literature.

The requirements for the application of exploratory meta-analysis are substantial, and often not met for topics of interest. The key feature is having a sufficient number of studies to conduct regression analyses that can examine and isolate multiple determinants of interest. The number of available studies determines in part the feasibility of conducting meta-regression with multiple predictors, just as the number of individual subjects does so in regression analyses of individual studies (Greenland, 1998). A second requirement is sufficient variability in potential influences on study results for informative evaluation, as in any regression analysis. If all studies of a given topic use a population-based case–control design, the influence of design on results cannot be examined. The alternative to exploratory meta-analysis, which is not without its advocates, is a careful narrative review and description of the relationship between study methods and results, without a formal statistical analysis of that pattern. The traditional detailed review of the literature without quantitative analysis may lend itself to closer scrutiny of individual study methods and their results. In addition, narrative reviews avoid the potential for the appearance of exaggerated certainty resulting from the meta-analysis. Ostensibly precise, quantitative information can be misleading if the assumptions that went into its generation are not kept firmly in mind. On the other hand, without statistical tools, it is difficult if not impossible to isolate multiple determinants from one another and discern patterns clearly. The reasons for a multivariate approach to examining influences on results across studies is identical to the rationale for multivariate analysis in studies of individuals: without it, there is no way to understand how multiple influences operate, independent of and in relation to one another.

INTERPRETING CONSISTENCY AND INCONSISTENCY

Among the most complex issues in the interpretation of a body of scientific literature is the meaning of consistency and inconsistency in results across studies. For those unwilling or unable to grapple with the details, a sweeping pronouncement of consistent implies that the phenomenon is understood and all the studies are pointing in the same (correct) direction. On the other hand, inconsistency among studies may be interpreted as lack of support for the hypothesis, an indication that the truth is unknown, or evidence that all the studies are subject to error. The reality in either case is more complex. Examined in detail, a series of studies addressing the same question will always show some inconsistencies, regardless of the truth and the quality of the individual studies.

The search for consistency may derive from the expectations of laboratory experiments in which replication is expected to yield identical results, subject only to random error, if the phenomenon is operating as hypothesized. When different researchers in different laboratories apply the same experimental conditions, and they observe similar results, it suggests that the original finding is valid. The ability to consistently generate a predicted result across settings strongly supports the hypothesized phenomenon. In contrast, inconsistency across laboratories, for example, or across technicians within a laboratory suggests some error has been made in the experiment or that some essential element of the phenomenon has not yet been identified. If the originally reported phenomenon cannot be replicated despite multiple attempts to do so, then the original study is appropriately assumed to be in error. Certainly, epidemiologists seek confirmation, but pure replication is never feasible in observational epidemiology in that the conditions (populations, study methods) inevitably differ across studies.

Inconsistent Findings

As commonly applied, the criticism that studies are inconsistent has several implications, all of them interpreted as suggesting that the hypothesized association is not present: (*1*) No association is present, but random error or unmeasured biases have generated the appearance of an association in some but not all studies. (*2*) No conclusions whatsoever can be drawn from the set of studies regarding the presence or absence of an association. (*3*) The literature is methodologically weak and pervasive methodologic problems are the source of the disparate study findings. An equally tenable explanation is that the studies vary in quality and that the strongest of the studies correctly identify the presence of an association and the methodologically weaker ones do not, or vice versa. Unfortunately, the observation of inconsistent results per se, without information on the characteristics of the studies that generated the results and the nature of the inconsistency, conveys very little information about the quality of the literature, whether inferences are warranted, and what those inferences should be. Inconsistencies across studies can arise for so many reasons that without further scrutiny the observation has little meaning.

Random error alone inevitably produces inconsistency in the exact measures of effect across studies. If the overall association is strong, then such deviations may not detract from the overall appearance of consistency. For example, if a series of studies of tobacco use and lung cancer generate risk ratios of 7.0, 8.2, and 10.0, we may legitimately interpret the results as consistent. In contrast, in a range of associations much closer to the null value, or truly null associations, fluctuation of equal magnitude might well convey the impression of inconsistency. Risk ratios of 0.8, 1.1, and 1.5 could well be viewed as inconsistent, with one positive and two negative studies, yet the studies may be estimating the same parameter, differing only due to random error. When the precision of one or more of the studies is limited, the potential for random error to create the impression of inconsistency is enhanced. While the pursuit of substantive explanations for inconsistent findings is worth undertaking, the less intellectually satisfying but often plausible explanation of random error should also be seriously entertained. Results that fluctuate within a relatively modest range do not suggest that the studies are flawed, but rather may simply suggest that the true measure of the association is somewhere toward the middle of the observed range and the scatter reflects random error. Conversely, substantial variability in findings across studies should not immediately be assumed to result from random error, but random error should be included among the candidate contributors, particularly when confidence intervals are wide.

Those who compile study results will sometimes tally the proportion of the studies that generate positive or negative associations, or count the number of studies that produce statistically significant associations. While there are ways to infer whether the count of studies deviates from the expectation under the null (Poole, 1997), it is far preferable to examine the actual measures of effect and associated confidence intervals. To count the proportion of studies with relative risks above or below the null sacrifices all information on the magnitude of effect and variation among the studies generating positive and inverse associations. A focus on how many were statistically significant hopelessly confounds magnitude of effect with precision. A series of studies with identical findings, for example, all yielding risk ratios of 1.5, could well yield inconsistent findings with regard to statistical significance due to varying study size alone. Variability in study size is one easily understood basis for inconsistency due to its affect on precision. As suggested in Chapter 10, statistical significance is of little value in interpreting the results of individual studies, and the problems with using it are compounded if applied to evaluating the consistency of a series of studies.

Another mechanism by which a series of methodologically sound studies could yield inconsistent results is if the response to the agent in question truly differs across populations, i.e., there is effect measure modification. For example, in a series of studies of alcohol and breast cancer, one might find positive associations among premenopausal but not postmenopausal women, with both sets of findings consistent and valid. Some studies may include all or a preponderance of postmenopausal women and others predominantly premenopausal women. If the effect of alcohol varies by menopausal status, then the summary findings of those studies will differ as well. Whereas the understanding of breast cancer has evolved to the point that there is recognition of the potential for distinctive risk factors among premenopausal and postmenopausal women, for many other diseases the distinctiveness of risk factors in subgroups of the population is far less clear. Where sources of true heterogeneity are present, and the studies vary in the proportions of participants in those heterogeneous groups, the results will inevitably be inconsistent. All studies however may well be accurate in describing an effect that occurs only or to a greater extent in one subpopulation.

This differing pattern of impact across populations is one illustration of effect modification. In the above example, it is based on menopausal status. Analogous heterogeneity of results might occur as a function of baseline risk. For example, in studies of alcohol and breast cancer, Asian-American women, who generally have lower risk, might have a different vulnerability to the effects of alcohol compared to European-American women, who generally have higher risk. The prevalence of concomitant risk factors might modify the effect of the one of interest. If the frequency of delayed childbearing, which confers an increased risk of breast cancer, differed across study populations and modified the effect of alcohol, the results would be heterogeneous across populations that differed in their childbearing practices.

Where strong interaction is present, the potential for substantial heterogeneity in study results is enhanced. For example, in studies examining the effect of alcohol intake on oral cancers, the prevalence of tobacco use in the population will markedly influence the effect of alcohol. Because of the strong interaction between alcohol and tobacco in the etiology of oral cancer, the effect of alcohol intake will be stronger where tobacco use is greatest. If there were complete interaction, in which alcohol was influential *only* in the presence of tobacco use, alcohol would have no effect in a tobacco-free population, and a very strong effect in a population consisting of all smokers. Even with less extreme interaction and less extreme differences in the prevalence of tobacco use, there will be some degree of inconsistency across studies in the observed effects of alcohol use on oral cancer. If we were aware of this interaction, of course, we would examine the effects of alcohol within strata of tobacco use and determine whether there is consistency within those homogeneous risk strata. On the other hand, if unaware of the interaction and differing prevalence of tobacco use, we would simply observe a series of inconsistent findings.

There is growing interest in genetic markers of susceptibility, particularly in studies of cancer and other chronic diseases (Perera & Santella, 1993; Tockman et al., 1993; Khoury, 1998). These markers reflect differences among individuals in the manner in which they metabolize exogenous exposures, and should help to explain why some individuals and not others respond to exposure to the same agent. If the proportion that is genetically susceptible varies across populations, then the measured and actual effect of the exogenous agent will vary as well. These molecular markers of susceptibility are not conceptually different from markers like menopausal status, ethnicity, or tobacco use, although the measurement technology differs. All provide explanations for why a specific agent may have real but inconsistent effects across populations.

Until this point, we have considered only inconsistent results among a set of perfectly designed and conducted studies that differ from one another solely due to random error or true differences in the effect. Introducing methodological limitations and biases offers an additional set of potential explanations for inconsistent results. By definition, biases introduce error in the measure of effect. Among an array of studies of a particular topic, if the extent and mix of biases varies across studies, results will vary as well. That is, if some studies are free of a particular form of bias and other studies are plagued to a substantial degree by that bias, then results will be inconsistent across those sets of studies. Susceptibility to bias needs to be examined on a study-by-study basis, and considered among the candidate explanations for inconsistent results. In particular, if there is a pattern in which the findings from studies that are most susceptible to

a potentially important bias differ from those of studies that are least susceptible, then the results will be inconsistent but highly informative. The studies that
are least susceptible to the bias would provide a more accurate measure of the
association.

In order to make an assessment of the role of bias in generating inconsistent
results, the study methods must be carefully scrutinized, putting results aside.
Depending on preconceptions about the true effect, there may be a temptation to
view those studies that generate positive or null results as methodologically superior because they yielded the right answer. In fact, biases can distort results in
either direction, so that unless truth is known in advance, the results themselves
give little insight regarding the potential for bias in the study. Knowing that a
set of studies contains mixed positive and null findings tells us nothing about
which of them is more likely to be correct or whether all are valid or all are in
error. In particular, there is no logical reason to conclude from such an array of
results that the null findings are most likely to be correct, by default—mixed
findings do not provide evidence to support the hypothesis of no effect. The demand on the interpreter of such evidence is to assess which are the stronger and
weaker studies and examine the patterns of results in relation to those methodologic attributes.

Consistent Findings

There are basically two ways to generate a series of consistent findings: they may
be consistently right or consistently wrong. When an array of studies generates
consistent findings, a reasonable inference might be that despite an array of potential biases in the individual studies, the problems are not so severe as to prevent the data from pointing in the direction of the truth. Hypothesized biases
within an individual study cannot be confirmed or refuted, but it may be possible to define a gradation of susceptibility to such biases across a series of studies. If a series of studies with differing strengths and limitations, and thus varying vulnerability to bias, all generate broadly comparable measures of association,
one might infer that the studies are all of sufficient quality to have accurately approximated the association of interest.

Unfortunately, it is also possible for a series of studies to generate consistently
incorrect findings. There are often similarities across studies in the design or
methods of conduct that could yield similarly erroneous results. For example, in
studies of a stigmatized behavior, such as cocaine use, in relation to pregnancy
outcome, there may be such severe underreporting as to yield null results across
a series of studies. On the other hand, cocaine use is strongly associated with
other adverse behaviors and circumstances that could confound the results, including tobacco and alcohol use and sexually transmitted infection. These tendencies may well hold across a wide range of populations. Thus, the observation

of a consistent association with adverse pregnancy outcome (Holzman & Paneth, 1994) may well be a result of consistent confounding. Perhaps the key difference between asking whether a single study has yielded an erroneous result and whether a series of studies has consistently done so is that in the latter case, the search is for attributes *common* to the studies.

The credibility assigned to consistent results, often implicit rather than explicit, is that the studies compensate for one another's weaknesses. The possibility of substantial bias resulting from a methodologic flaw in a single study is countered by evidence from other studies that do not suffer from this weakness yet show the same result. This manner in which studies can compensate for one another's weaknesses is central to the interpretation of a series of studies, and therefore warrants closer examination.

Compensating Strengths Across Studies

Replication in Epidemiology. Aside from reducing random error, in the tradition of confirmation, the major benefit to conducting multiple studies of the same topic is the opportunity to assess the pattern of results across diverse studies that are conducted in different settings and populations using methods that differ from one another. One of Bradford-Hill's criteria for causality was consistency (Hill, 1965), but it needs further elaboration to be useful. Consistency of results can sometimes demonstrate that features of the study setting and methods that are expected to be inconsequential under a causal hypothesis do not in fact affect the study results. Such study features as questionnaire design, interviewer training and interview methods, and techniques of data analysis preclude one study from being identical to another, yet identification of an etiologic relationship should not be highly dependent on such methodologic details. When study findings are consistent across studies that differ only in such details of implementation, such as the wording of the questionnaire or a particular instruction given to the interviewers, the association is less likely to be the result of some idiosyncrasy in one study or another.

When results across such similar studies are not consistent with one another, the inference is that random error or methodologic biases have influenced at least some of the results. Under a causal hypothesis, we would expect the findings to be robust to minor differences in study technique and differ primarily due to random error. Conceptually, there are aspects of random error that go beyond the conventional view of random error arising from statistical variation in randomized assignments. There is a random element in the choice of interviewers to be hired for the study, the sequence in which the questions are asked, and many other details of data collection and analysis that are likely to have at least subtle effects on the results. One very mundane problem that undoubtedly affects isolated studies is simple programmer error. Given how often coding or analytic errors are uncovered and corrected, surely there are times that they escape detection. These inadvertent sources of erroneous results are highly unlikely to occur across multiple studies, just as a biased or dishonest data collector can distort results from a single study, but is not plausible that a series of studies on the same topic would all suffer from such misfortune. The problems will increase the dispersion of study findings, creating the potential for unexplained inconsistencies.

Sometimes, under a causal hypothesis, some features of the study setting and methods *should* influence the results, and if that does not occur, the consistent evidence may argue *against* a causal association. One of the key ways in which this can occur is a function of dose. Where markedly different doses evaluated across studies yield similar measures of association, the consistency may run counter to a causal explanation. For example, oral contraceptives have changed markedly in the estrogen content over the years, with notably lower doses at present compared to in the past. If we observed identical associations between oral contraceptive use and thromboembolism for those past high doses and the present low doses, as a form of consistency, we would be advised to call into question whether we have accurately captured an effect of the oral contraceptives or some selective factor associated with oral contraceptive users. That is, consistency despite critical differences may suggest that a shared bias accounts for the results.

When trying to evaluate the role of a specific potential bias, an array of studies offers the opportunity to examine the relationship between vulnerability to those biases and the pattern of results. A single study always has the potential for spurious findings due to its methods, both design and conduct. While close scrutiny of that study is helpful in assessing the likelihood, direction, and magnitude of potential bias, there are real limits in the strength of inference that can be made from a single result in evaluating hypotheses of bias or causality. The vulnerability to bias may be assessed in qualitative terms in an individual study, but not with any anchor of certainty. In contrast, a series of studies that clearly differ in their susceptibility to bias, ranging from highly vulnerable to virtually immune, offers an opportunity to examine whether the gradient of susceptibility corresponds to a gradient of results. If there is a clear pattern across studies, for example, in which higher quality of exposure assessment corresponds to stronger associations, then it may be inferred that a true association is present that is diluted, to varying degrees, from exposure misclassification. On the other hand, if the series of studies with differing quality of exposure assessment were invariant in their results, a causal association would seem less likely to be present and explanations of some consistent bias should be entertained.

Evolution of Epidemiologic Research. The ideal manner in which a series of studies should evolve is to build sequentially upon those that precede them, with the new ones addressing specific deficiencies in those that precede them. Ideally, each subsequent study would combine all the strengths of its predecessors and remedy at least one limitation of the prior studies. In such a system for the evolution of the literature, each study would address a non-causal explanation for an observed association and either reveal that the previous studies had been in error because they had not been quite so thorough, or demonstrate that the hypothesized source of bias was not influential. If the improvement resulted in a major shift in the findings, the new study would suggest that the previous studies were deficient and suffered from a critical bias that had been identified and eliminated. While discovering that a potentially important refinement had no impact may seem like a disappointment, such an observation could be of profound importance in addressing and eliminating a non-causal explanation. Assume, for example, a key potential confounder was neglected in a series of studies, and the next study provided precise measurement and tight control for that potential confounding factor, but the study results do not differ from those that came before. It might be inferred that all the previous studies were also free from confounding, though this could not be addressed directly within those studies. In this simple view of how studies evolve, exonerating a potential bias in one study negates the possibility of that bias in the studies that came before, since the improvements are cumulative.

We now move from this ideal model, in which studies build perfectly and logically on one another through cumulative improvements, to a more realistic one in which studies are stronger in some respects than previous ones, but are often weaker in other respects. For logistical reasons, making one refinement tends to incur sacrifices along other dimensions. Applying a demanding, detailed measurement protocol to diminish the potential for information bias may well reduce the response proportions and increase the potential for selection bias, for example. Choosing a population that is at high risk for the disease and thus yields good precision may incur some cost in terms of susceptibility to confounding. Conducting a study that is extremely large may sacrifice rigor in the assessment of exposure or disease. In epidemiology, as in life, there's no "free lunch."

The critical question is whether, when a series of studies with differing strengths and weaknesses are conducted and consistent results are found, an inference can be made that none of the apparent deficiencies distorted the results and all are pointing in the correct direction. If one study is susceptible to confounding, another to bias in control selection, and yet another to exposure measurement error, but all yield the same measure of effect, can one infer that none of the hypothetical problems are of great importance? This question is different from the situation in which a series of studies share the same deficiency, and may yield consistent but biased results due to common unidentified problems. It also differs from the situation in which one or more studies are free of all major threats to validity.

There are two reasons that a series of studies with differing strengths and weaknesses may yield consistent results: either the disparate deficiencies all yield errors of the same nature to produce consistently erroneous results or the deficiencies are all modest in their impact and the studies yield consistently valid results. The distinction between these two possibilities requires a judgment based on the credibility of the two scenarios, specific to the substantive and methodologic issues under consideration. Generally, it is unlikely that a series of studies with differing methodological strengths and weaknesses would yield similar results through different biases acting to influence findings in a similar manner. Faced with such a pattern, the more plausible inference would be that the potential biases did not distort the results substantially and, thus, the series of studies are individually and collectively quantifying the causal association between exposure and disease accurately.

It is also possible that despite the recognition of potential biases that were resolved in one or more of the studies, all the studies might share a remaining limitation that has not been identified or is known but cannot readily be overcome. For example, many exposures simply cannot be randomized for ethical or logistical reasons, and thus no matter how much study designs vary, all address exposure that is incurred due to circumstances outside the investigator's control. While the studies may vary with regard to some potential remediable biases being present or absent, all may continue to share an insurmountable, important limitation. Consistency across such studies suggests that the weaknesses that vary across studies are unlikely to account for spurious results but any deficiency that the studies have in common may still do so. Only the variation in methodologic strengths and weaknesses across existing studies can be examined, not the possible effects of improvements not yet undertaken.

INTEGRATED ASSESSMENT FROM COMBINING EVIDENCE ACROSS STUDIES

Several conclusions can be drawn from this discussion of consistency and inconsistency in aggregation of results across a series of epidemiologic studies. First, without considering study quality and specific methodologic features of the studies, there is little value in simply assessing the pattern of results. To dichotomize studies as positive or null and examine whether a preponderance fall in one category or another yields no credible insights about the literature. This is the case whether those studies are consistent or inconsistent with one another, though traditionally a series of studies that generate similar results are viewed as correct whereas inconsistent results are viewed as inconclusive or weak. If consistent, it needs to be asked as if the studies share a methodologic deficiency. When such a flaw common to the studies cannot be detected, and there is not a clear case for different errors producing bias in the same direction across the studies, then it is more reasonable to infer that they are likely to be valid.

If inconsistent, there is a need to first consider whether there are specific reasons to expect the results to differ across studies—for example, the study populations differ in the prevalence of an important effect modifier. Evaluation of the patterns continues with the examination of gradients of quality and specific methodologic strengths and weaknesses among the studies. Such an evaluation, with or without the tools of meta-analysis, yields hypotheses regarding the operation of biases. Which of the results are most likely to be valid depends on the estimated effect of those different biases and a judgment about what the findings would have been in the absence of the consequential biases. Among the completed studies may well be one or more that have those desirable attributes.

The process for scrutinizing inconsistent findings helps to define the boundaries of current knowledge. By evaluating the methodologic details of studies and their results, judgments can be made about the most important candidate explanations for the inconsistency. Those are precisely the study design, conduct, and analysis features that would help to resolve the controversy. One may also infer that some potential sources of bias do not seem to be of consequence, and therefore in assessing the tradeoffs inherent in designing and conducting research, other threats to validity may be given greater attention even at the expense of the bias now believed to have been ameliorated. This evaluation of the evidence generates not just an accurate assessment of the state of knowledge, but also some indication of its certainty and the requirements for further research to enhance its certainty.

This evaluation process involves judgments about the impact that hypothesized biases are likely to have had on the results. Several approaches can be used to make such judgments. Evidence from other studies that were free of such limitations suggests whether there was any effect. Assessment of the direction of bias and potential magnitude based on differing scenarios, or sensitivity analyses, combined with information on the plausibility of those scenarios generates useful information. Methodological literature, in the form of theoretical or quantitative consideration of biases or empirical evaluations of bias is critical.

Careful evaluation of results across a series of studies is highly informative, even when it does not provide definitive conclusions. Juxtaposing results from studies with differing strengths and limitations, with careful consideration of the relationship between design features and results, is essential both in drawing the most accurate conclusions possible at a given point in time and in planning how to advance the literature. Substantive understanding of the phenomenon integrated with appreciation of the relation of study design features to potential biases is required. While far more subtle and challenging than the simple search for consistency or its absence, it is also far more informative.

REFERENCES

Bradford-Hill AB. The environment and disease: association or causation? Proc Royal Soc Med 1965;58:295–300.

Greenland S. Quantitative methods in the review of epidemiologic literature. Epidemiol Rev 1987;9:1–30.

Greenland S. Can meta-analysis be salvaged? Am J Epidemiol 1994;140:783–787.

Greenland S. Meta-analysis. In Rothman KJ, Greenland S, Modern epidemiology. Philadelphia: Lippincott-Raven Publishers, 1998;643–673.

Greenland S, Sheppard AR, Kaune WT, Poole C, Kelsh. A pooled analysis of magnetic fields, wire codes, and childhood leukemia. Epidemiology 2000;11:624–634.

Holzman C, Paneth N. Maternal cocaine use during pregnancy and perinatal outcomes. Epidemiol Rev 1994;16:315–334.

Khoury MJ. Genetic epidemiology. In Rothman KJ, Greenland S, Modern epidemiology. Philadelphia: Lippincott-Raven Publishers, 1998;609–621.

Lubin JH, Boice JD Jr. Lung cancer risk from residential radon: meta-analysis of eight epidemiologic studies. J Natl Cancer Inst 1997;89:49–57.

National Research Council. Possible health effects of exposure to residential electric and magnetic fields. Committee on the Possible Effects of Electromagnetic Fields on Biological Systems, Board on Radiation Effects Research, Commission on Life Sciences, National Research Council. Washington, DC: National Academy Press, 1997.

Perera FP, Santella R. Carcinogenesis. In Schulte PA, Perera FP (eds), Molecular epidemiology: principles and practices. San Diego: Academic Press, Inc., 1993;277–300.

Petitti DB. Meta-analysis, decision analysis, and cost-effectiveness analysis in medicine. New York: Oxford University Press, 1994.

Poole C. One study, one vote: ballot courting in epidemiologic meta-analysis. Am J Epidemiol 1997;145:S85.

Portier CJ, Wolfe MS, eds. Assessment of health effects from exposure to power-line frequency electric and magnetic fields. Working group report. In: US Department of Health and Human Services, National Institute of Environmental Health Sciences, National Institutes of Health publication no. 98-3981, 1998.

Tockman MS, Gupta PK, Pressman NJ, Mulshine JL. Biomarkers of pulmonary disease. In Schulte PA, Perera FP (eds), Molecular epidemiology: principles and practices. San Diego: Academic Press, Inc., 1993;443–468.

12

CHARACTERIZATION OF CONCLUSIONS

The final product of the evaluation of epidemiologic evidence is some form of conclusion about what the research tells us. The audiences for that interpretation are quite varied, ranging from researchers seeking to identify the next frontier to be explored to policy makers who would like to incorporate the information appropriately into their decisions. This inference goes beyond the delineation of potential biases, or evidence for and against a causal association, and inevitably extends beyond the bounds of objective criteria into the realm of judgment that should begin with logical integration. While the refinements in evaluating evidence presented in the preceding chapters are intended to take broad questions about the evidence—"How strong is it?"—and make them much more specific and testable—"How likely is it that the exposure–confounder relationship is strong enough to fully explain the observed association?"—there is nevertheless a need for informed speculation as narrower questions are integrated into a broader judgment. Even if the elements required to reach a judgment are clearly defined and the evidence regarding each of those components is objectively presented, knowledgeable people will still come to different conclusions at the end because of the manner in which they combine the threads of evidence.

A constant challenge in the interpretation of evidence, especially problematic in trying to present a true bottom line, is the desire to provide clarity, whether or not the evidence warrants a clear statement. Many of those who wish to make use of the knowledge encourage or may even demand such clarity, including policy makers, attorneys, journalists, or the general public, as well as scientists. At a given point in the evolution of our understanding, the only justifiable assessment may be a murky, complex one that includes alternate scenarios and some probability that each is correct. Explaining such a state of affairs is often tedious to those who are only mildly interested and may demand a rather sophisticated understanding of epidemiologic methods to be fully understood. Thus, there will often be pressure to provide a simpler inference, placing the evidence on some scale of adjectives such as *suggestive, strong,* or *weak.* For example, the International Agency for Research on Cancer has a well-developed system for classifying carcinogens into such categories as *probable* and *possible* (Vainio, 1992). A common question from reporters or the lay public to the technical expert that seeks to cut through the often complex and seemingly wishy-washy conclusions is "What would you do?" as a result of the new information. The idea is that good scientists prefer to remain noncommittal and focus on the points of uncertainty, but that they nevertheless have the ability as human beings to wisely integrate the evidence so that their personal application of the information reflects such wisdom. Behavioral decisions of the scientist, like those of anyone else, will typically go well beyond the assessment of the epidemiologic evidence and incorporate other lines of research and even the personal values that affect life decisions, realms that even the most expert epidemiologist is not uniquely qualified to address in a generalizable manner.

Researchers who wish to justify their grant application or argue why their publication is useful may have the opposite temptation, seeking out or even exaggerating the uncertainty to make their contribution seem more important. No one is free of incentives and values when it comes to the distractions from objectivity in the interpretation of evidence. While much attention is focused on those with a direct financial interest, such as private corporations or the opposing parties in legal conflicts, the sources of personal bias are much broader. A topic as seemingly neutral as whether coronary heart disease has continued to decline in the 1990s (Rosamond et al., 1998) raises great concern not just from researchers who have found conflicting results, but from those who believe that more radical changes are needed in social systems to effect benefit, from those who administer programs intended to reduce coronary heart disease, and from those who wish to defend or criticize the cost of medications associated with the prevention and treatment of these diseases. No one is neutral. In this chapter, the basis for drawing conclusions from epidemiologic data is discussed, and a range of purposes and audiences with interest in those epidemiologic conclusions is considered.

APPLICATIONS OF EPIDEMIOLOGY

In order to enjoy the benefits of epidemiologic research in applications to public health policy, clinical medicine, or individual decision-making, inferences must be drawn. Providing results from individual studies or even results with discussion of their validity is insufficient. Addressing issues of disease patterns and causation in populations is not an academic exercise but fundamentally a search for insights that will provide benefit to public health decisions, broadly defined. As evidence moves from the purely scientific arena to the realm of decisions, there is a temptation to move from what is truly a continuum of certainty to a dichotomy. It is often asked whether the epidemiologic evidence does or does not justify a particular action, since the decision itself is truly dichotomous even though the evidence that supports one approach or another is not. By characterizing the epidemiologic evidence more fully, not just as sufficient or insufficient, decision-makers will be armed with the information they need to incorporate the epidemiologic insights more accurately. The evidence will often be less tidy, but by being more faithful to the true state of affairs, the ultimate decisions should be wiser.

One temptation to be avoided is the assertion that the epidemiologic evidence has not advanced to the point of making a useful contribution to policy decisions at all; for example, because it is inconclusive, we ask that it not be used in setting policy or that no policy be made. Either approach is undesirable. Any information is better than no information in applications to decision-making, so long as the quality of the available evidence is accurately portrayed and properly used. Even relatively weak epidemiologic studies may at least put some bounds on the possibilities—for example, demonstrating that the relative risk is unlikely to be above 50 or 100. Similarly, the suggestion that there may be a hazard associated with a given exposure, even if based on one or two studies of limited quality, should not be neglected altogether, nor should the policy decision be unduly influenced by preliminary, fallible data. Weak evidence may well be of very limited value in discriminating among viable policy options, but limited evidence would generally be expected to be of limited (not zero) value. The consequence of assigning the epidemiologic evidence a weight of zero is simply to increase the weight assigned to other lines of evidence used to make the decision, both other scientific approaches to the issue and nonscientific concerns.

The argument that decisions be suspended altogether until good evidence has accumulated is also unrealistic, in that no action is just one of many courses of action, and is no less a decision than other courses of action. Policy makers will continue to set policy, regulate environmental pollutants, evaluate drugs for efficacy and safety, and recommend dietary guidelines with explicit or implicit scientific input. Individuals will continue to choose the foods they eat, purchase and use medications, engage in sexual activity, and drive automobiles with or without conclusive epidemiologic evidence. Because public health issues for which epidemiologic evidence is relevant pervade society, many decisions made collectively and individually could benefit from epidemiologic insights, even those that are based on evolving information.

Epidemiologic evidence remains forever inconclusive in the sense that scientific certainty is an elusive goal. The potential for erroneous conclusions can be successively narrowed through increasingly refined studies, but there is no point at which the potential for bias has been completely eliminated. Instead, the lines of evidence bearing on a public health decision, with epidemiologic data providing one of the critical streams of information, reach a point where the practical benefits of further epidemiologic information and refinement are limited. For well-studied issues such as the health hazards of asbestos or benefits of using seat belts, epidemiology has offered much if not all that it can for informing the basic policy decision—asbestos exposure should be minimized; seat belt use should be maximized. Further refining the risk estimates or extending the information to previously unstudied subgroups is not without value, but the evidence has accumulated to the point that major shifts in policy resulting from that new knowledge are highly unlikely. (The effectiveness of interventions, for example, may still benefit from epidemiologic scrutiny; perhaps refining the understanding of dose–response functions for asbestos or the benefits of seat belt use in conjunction with air bags could help to further refine policy.)

An example of a situation in which each bit of epidemiologic evidence is beneficial to policy decisions is drinking water safety. The balancing of risks and benefits in regard to drinking water treatment in the United States must incorporate the well-established risk of waterborne infection associated with inadequate treatment, the potential adverse effects of low levels of chlorination by-products on cancer and reproductive health, and myriad economic and engineering considerations associated with alternate approaches to providing drinking water to the public (Savitz & Moe, 1997). Decisions about changing from chlorination to other methods of treatment (e.g., ozonation), as well as decisions regarding specific methods of drinking water chlorination, are based on a precarious balance of epidemiologic, toxicologic, economic, and other considerations, including public perception. Shifts in any of those considerations may well lead to a modification of policy. For example, if the threat of waterborne infection were found to be greater than previously thought, or if the chlorination levels required to reduce the threat of waterborne infection were found to be greater than expected, support for increased levels of chlorine treatment would be strengthened despite the present ambiguous indications regarding adverse health effects of chlorination by-products. If the epidemiologic evidence linking chlorination by-products to bladder and colon cancer were to be increased through improved study methods, then the scales would be tipped toward efforts to decrease chlorination by-product levels, either through accepting some greater risk of waterborne infection or through more sophisticated and expensive engineering approaches. Similarly, toxicologic research demonstrating toxicity at lower levels of chlorination by-products than previously observed would tip the balance, as would engineering breakthroughs making alternatives to chlorination cheaper or more effective. In this realm of policy, changes in the epidemiologic evidence matter a great deal.

A counter example, no less controversial, in which refined epidemiologic evidence is unlikely to have significant policy influence is active cigarette smoking. While the full spectrum of health effects, dose–response relations, and responsible agents in tobacco smoke remain to be elucidated, the epidemiologic evidence of a monumental public health burden from tobacco use is clear. The policy controversies tend to focus more on uncertainty in the most effective measures to prevent adoption of smoking by teenagers, management of adverse implications for tobacco farmers, and issues of personal freedom. Refining the epidemiologic evidence linking tobacco use with disease is not likely to have a major impact on policy. The level of certainty for major tobacco-related diseases such as lung and bladder cancer and coronary heart disease is so high that minor shifts upward or downward from additional studies would still leave the certainty within a range that the epidemiology encourages policy that aggressively discourages tobacco use. Whether or not tobacco smoking causes leukemia or delayed conception is not going to have much effect on the overall policy. The epidemiologic evidence has, in a sense, done all it can with regard to the basic question of health impact of active smoking on chronic disease, particularly lung and other cancers and heart disease in adults. Nonetheless, the concerns with environmental tobacco smoke, potential impact of tobacco smoking on myriad other diseases such as breast cancer and Alzheimer's disease, the mechanisms of causation for diseases known to be caused by smoking, and measures for reduction in smoking call for additional epidemiologic research for these and other purposes.

Identifying policy decisions that would be affected by modest shifts in the epidemiologic evidence is one consideration in establishing priorities for the field. Those decisions that are teetering between nearly equally acceptable alternatives are the ones most likely to be tipped by enhancing the quality of the epidemiologic evidence, whatever the results of those additional studies might show. Strengthening or weakening the degree of support would have bearing on public health decisions. Research needs to continue even when the evidence is so limited that a strikingly positive epidemiologic study would fail to tip the balance, since such research is building toward future influence on policy. At the other end of the spectrum of knowledge, further understanding of well-established relationships may clarify biological mechanisms or help to point the way to discoveries involving other causative agents or other health conditions.

This framework suggests how epidemiologic evidence should be presented to be optimally useful in addressing specific public health issues or decisions. The goal is not to have epidemiologic evidence dominant over other scientific evidence or other considerations (Savitz et al., 1999), but rather to ensure that the influence of epidemiology is commensurate with its quality. Thus, the obligation on those who explain and interpret the evidence is not to provide absolute truth, but to accurately characterize the state of the evidence so that the epidemiologic research is weighed appropriately. Ideally, toxicologists, economists, and others will offer the same even-handed evaluation of the contributions from their disciplines. Much work is needed to better formulate explanations of epidemiologic evidence that serve this goal—for example, identifying the descriptive approach that would be most helpful to those who must use the information, whether policy experts or individuals making personal decisions about their lives. It is clearly not a service to oversimplify for the sake of clarity, even if it gives the consumer of the information illusory peace of mind. To treat probable evidence for an effect as certain or established or to treat weak evidence as no evidence may give temporary relief to those who must set and defend policy, but in the long run, the decisions that are made will not be as beneficial as if the uncertainty were properly quantified and accurately conveyed. Since epidemiologic research will continue, evidence presented prematurely as established may unravel, and evidence that is presently weak but misrepresented as absent may become stronger. The area of risk communication as applied to epidemiology is at an early stage of development, but represents an important interface between epidemiology and its applications.

One form of potentially useful information would be to provide an array of potential measures of effect and their corresponding probabilities of being correct. This probability distribution would presumably have some range of values designated as *most likely* and some distribution around those values. We could answer such questions as, "How likely is it that the true measure of effect is so close to the null as to be negligible?" with the consumer of the information having freedom to define negligible. Similarly, the user could ask, "How likely is it that the true measure of effect exceeds a given value?" Policy experts would welcome such insights, though less sophisticated audiences, including politicians, the media, and the general public may not. Part of the problem is that the descriptors that go along with quantitative probabilities are not used or interpreted consistently—one person's *negligible* is another person's *weak* evidence.

What such a characterization of the spectrum of possibilities and associated probabilities would do is to emphasize that there is some degree of uncertainty present (there is a range, not a point estimate), but also that the research has something to offer (not all outcomes are equally probable). Progress would be demarcated by higher peaks with less dispersion or lower probabilities for certain ranges of possible values. Even if the exact quantification of the uncertainty in the evidence were subject to error, the general shape and distribution of possible values would be informative.

This relevance to policy and life in general is both a blessing and a curse to the field of epidemiology. The opportunity to contribute to issues of societal concern and issues that affect people's daily lives is inspiring to practitioners of epidemiology and a principal incentive to fund research and disseminate the findings. On the other hand, the hunger for answers to the questions epidemiologists ask can also lead to public dissemination of incorrect findings, exaggerated claims of certainty, or unwillingness to accept evidence that is counter to otherwise desirable policy or lifestyle choices.

IDENTIFICATION OF KEY CONCERNS

Some efforts have been made to catalog all forms of potential bias in epidemiologic studies (Sackett, 1979), though such lists tend to become exercises in naming similar biases that arise in slightly different ways. Rather than serving as a checklist to ensure all concerns have been considered, they tend to serve more like a dictionary for looking up terms or as a demonstration of how fallible epidemiology is. Instead of such laundry lists of potential bias, a small number of concerns typically predominate in evaluating a specific study or set of studies. Rather than asking, without consideration of the specific phenomenon under study or the design of that study, "What are the ways that the results could be in error?," one needs to focus on the specifics of the phenomenon and design to determine the major threats to validity. Because a serious evaluation of a single source of potential bias is a painstaking process, involving a detailed, thoughtful examination of data from within and outside the study, consideration of more than a handful of such issues is impractical.

The uncertainty that limits conclusions based on the research is generally not evenly distributed among dozens of limitations, each accounting for a small amount of the potential error. More often, a handful of issues account for the bulk of the uncertainty, and perhaps dozens more each contribute in presumably minor, perhaps even offsetting, ways. Major concerns often include control selection in case–control studies or misclassification of disease or exposure. Among the myriad minor concerns are dishonesty by the investigators or data collectors, data entry errors, or programming errors—the potential is always present, but with reasonable attention, the probability of such problems having a sizable impact on the results is minimal. With an initial triage to identify the few critical concerns, resources can be brought to bear to examine the key problems in detail, and plans can be made for the next study of the phenomenon to improve upon one or more of the key limitations.

For the major sources of potential error, a critical review calls for speculation about the direction and magnitude of bias. A thorough assessment includes examination of the patterns of results within the study data, where possible, as well as consideration of results from other studies and methodological research on the topic. Where such an examination leads to the conclusion that the bias may well be present and of sufficient magnitude to have an important influence on the overall interpretation of the literature, further research may be needed to resolve the question of how important it is and ultimately take measures to mitigate its effect. While structural problems with studies can rarely be solved outright, they can almost always be elucidated to increase understanding or be better managed to reduce their impact.

Those who propose new research to advance our understanding have the burden of demonstrating that their efforts will do more than add another observation or data point. Epidemiologic studies are too expensive and time consuming to merely add another observation to a meta-analysis without having additional methodologic strengths that extend the literature that has come before. If a new study is merely as good as those that precede it, only random error is being addressed. Only if the current state of knowledge were faulty largely due to random error would another study of similar quality add markedly to the array of previous findings. Epidemiologic research is rarely limited solely or primarily by random error. The goal for a new study should be to identify a specific limitation of previous work, make the case that this limitation is likely to be consequential, and propose to improve the research methods in a manner that will refine our understanding by overcoming that limitation. When studies are based on such a strategy, progress is guaranteed as a result of the methods alone, regardless of the findings. If overcoming a strongly suspected source of bias has no impact on the findings relative to previous studies, then the credibility of the previous results is significantly bolstered. An important potential bias that reduced confidence in previous findings would have been put to rest. If overcoming a suspected bias does have a material effect on the results, then the credibility of preceding studies is substantially reduced. Not only does the new study advance the literature by being stronger than the one that preceded it, but when the specific reason that the previous study or studies were in error can be identified, the strength of the conclusion from the studies taken in the aggregate is markedly enhanced. Instead of two studies with differing results, or even a stronger study that contradicts a weaker one, we have an explanation of how the previous study went astray and an understanding of the impact of that error based on the later, superior one.

Sometimes the need is not for more substantive studies addressing the exposure–disease association directly, but rather for empirical methodological research. For example, the validity of a commonly used exposure measure may need to be examined in detail, or the relation between willingness to participate in studies and the prevalence of disease may warrant evaluation. Building such methodologic work onto substantive studies is one strategy, but often the methodologic issue can be addressed more optimally in isolation from the application to a specific exposure–disease association. Such research advances knowledge about the hypothesis of interest, where such issues are significant sources of uncertainty, and may actually advance many lines of investigation simultaneously if the problem has broader relevance. For example, a better appreciation of the quality of self-reported alcohol use would be potentially applicable to research on alcohol's effect on cardiovascular disease, oral cancer, fetal growth, and motor vehicle injury, as well as studies of patterns and determinants of alcohol use. Even studies of other sensitive, personal behaviors, such as drug use or sexual activity, may be enhanced by such research. Similarly, examination of biases associated with selecting controls in case–control studies through random-digit dialing would be pertinent to a wide range of exposures and diseases that have been based on that method of control selection.

INTEGRATED CONSIDERATION OF POTENTIAL BIAS

Even if we could successfully identify the small set of critical limitations, and accurately characterize the potential for bias associated with each of those concerns, we would still face the challenge of integrating this information into an overall evaluation of a study or set of studies addressing the same hypothesis. What we would really like to know is the probability distribution for the causal relation between exposure and disease, that is, a quantitative assessment of the probability that the causal impact of exposure on disease takes on alternate values. This assessment would integrate observed results with hypothesized biases. Information of this quality and certainty is not readily obtained, but there are simplified approaches to integration of evidence that move in that direction.

One simple but important question to address is the direction of bias most likely to result from the array of methodological considerations. If all the sources of bias are predicted to result in errors of a particular direction (overestimation or underestimation of the effect), the presumption would be that the effects are cumulative, and that more extreme biases may result than would be predicted from each factor operating in isolation. The overall probability that the measured value deviates from the true value in one direction is increased relative to the probability that it deviates in the opposite direction, and the probability that the magnitude of error is extreme would likewise be increased.

If the major sources of potential bias are in conflicting directions, some most likely to inflate the measure of effect, others likely to reduce it, then the integration may increase the probability assigned to values closer to the one that was observed. Because it is unknown which bias will predominate, there may be a range on either side of the observed value with relatively high probabilities assigned, but extreme deviations are less plausible if the biases counteract one another than if the biases act synergistically.

Only direction of bias has been considered so far, but of course the magnitude of bias is critical as well. In some instances, there may be absolute bounds on the amount of error that could be introduced; for example, if all nonrespondents had certain attributes or if an exposure measure had no validity whatsoever, these extreme cases would usually be assigned low probabilities. Quantification of the magnitude of individual biases more generally would be valuable in assessing their relative importance. Where multiple biases operate in the same direction, if one predominates quantitatively over the others, assessment of its impact alone may provide a reasonable characterization of the range of potential values. Where biases tend to compensate for one another, the overall impact of the combination of biases would likely reside with the largest one, tempered to only a limited extent by the countervailing biases.

The terminology used to provide the bottom line evaluation of potential bias is important to consider. The evaluation should incorporate benchmarks of particular concern for differing responses to the evidence. The observed measure of effect is one such benchmark, but others would include the null value and values that would be of substantial policy or clinical importance. If a doubling of risk associated with exposure would reach some threshold for regulatory action, for example, then information on the observed results and potential biases should be brought together to address the probability that the true value meets or exceeds that threshold. Short of generating the full probability distribution of true effects, some estimation of the probability that the observed measure is likely to be correct, the probability that the null value is accurate, or the probability that the measure of effect is in a range of policy or clinical relevance would be helpful in characterizing the state of the evidence.

INTEGRATION OF EPIDEMIOLOGIC EVIDENCE WITH OTHER INFORMATION

As discussed in Chapter 2, a comprehensive evaluation of health risks or benefits ought never be based solely on epidemiologic information. Other biomedical disciplines, including toxicology, genetics, and pathology have relevance to human health. An understanding of the pathophysiology of disease, even though not directly applicable to assessing causes in populations, is clearly pertinent to the evaluation of whether a hypothesized cause of disease is likely to be influential in populations. Even basic chemistry is applicable to assessing health consequences of exposure—for example, in assessing the risks or benefits of a compound with unknown consequences that bears a structural similarity to a chemical with known effects. In the study of environmental pollutants, information on the sources and pathways of exposure is important. All information that helps to assess the pathways through which an exposure might operate, drawing on knowledge from a range of basic and clinical sciences, helps to assess the potential for human health effects and will help in making a probabilistic judgment regarding health risks or benefits in populations.

Epidemiologists have to guard against being defensive and thus insufficiently attentive to evidence from other disciplines. Although basic biomedical disciplines often enjoy greater prestige and their practitioners sometimes fail to appreciate the value of epidemiology, epidemiologists should not retaliate by undervaluing those approaches. Critics from disciplines other than epidemiology (and some epidemiologists) may place excessive weight on the more tightly controlled but less directly relevant lines of research and insufficient weight on epidemiology in drawing overall conclusions. Similarly, epidemiologists and occasionally other scientists mistakenly believe an integrated evaluation of the array of relevant evidence should place all the weight on observed health patterns in populations (i.e., epidemiology), and none on other approaches to evaluating and understanding the causes of disease. The key point is that these other disciplines and lines of evidence are not done solely to assist in the interpretation of epidemiologic evidence, i.e., evaluating the plausibility of the epidemiology, but rather to help in making the broader evaluation of health risks and corresponding policy decisions.

An argument can be made that perfectly constructed epidemiologic information is the most relevant basis for assessing the presence or absence of human health effects in populations. Epidemiology alone examines the relevant species (humans) under the environmental conditions of concern (i.e., the actual exposures, susceptibility distribution, and concomitant exposures of interest). There is no extrapolation required with regard to species, agent, dose, etc. Epidemiologists alone have the capability of studying the people whose health is adversely affected. Even if the detailed understanding of mechanisms of disease causation requires other disciplines, the basic question of whether humans are being affected would be answered by epidemiology—if only it could be done perfectly.

Epidemiology alone however, is never sufficient for fully assessing human health risks. The principal limitation is the uncertainty regarding epidemiologic findings and the inescapable challenge and fallibility of inferring causal relations. The very strength of epidemiology, studying humans in their natural environment, imposes limitations on causal inference that are only partially surmountable. While perfect epidemiologic evidence would provide a direct indication of the true effects in human populations, epidemiologic evidence is never without uncertainty, whether it points toward or away from a causal association. In practice, the complementary strengths of epidemiology and more basic biomedical evidence always provide a clearer picture than could be generated by epidemiology in isolation. Even where epidemiology has been most autonomous, for example in identifying the substantial excess risks of lung cancer associated with prolonged, heavy cigarette smoking, confidence was bolstered by identifying the mutagenicity of tobacco combustion products and evolving knowledge of the pathophysiology of tobacco's effects on the respiratory system. In evaluating much more modest elevations in risk, the burden on these other disciplines is much greater to interpret whether the weak associations (or their absence) from epidemiology accurately reflect the role of the agent of concern. Evaluation of potential health risks from environmental tobacco smoke, with relative risks for lung cancer in the range of 1.2 to 1.5 draws heavily on other lines of research to make the assessment of whether a causal association is likely to be present.

Sufficiently strong evidence from toxicology that an agent is harmful, as exists for dioxin, for example, reduces the need for epidemiologic data to make decisions about regulation and control of exposure. At the extreme, the need for direct epidemiologic evidence as the basis for regulation may be negated. If the probability of harm to human health is sufficiently high independent of the epidemiologic evidence, then sound policy decisions can be made without awaiting such information. In contrast, for extremely low-frequency electromagnetic fields, for example, there is some epidemiologic evidence supportive of a weak association, but an absence of demonstrated mechanisms of disease causation or evidence of adverse effects in experimental systems (NRC, 1997). Because the epidemiology is both fallible and indicative of only small associations, when combined with the lack of support from other scientific approaches, the evidence for harm to human health is very weak.

The epidemiology and lines of evidence from other biomedical disciplines can be either parallel or truly integrative. Often, the epidemiologic observation is supported by mechanistic or biological evidence solely as another, independent indication that the agent may have health consequences. The agent is found to be associated with increased risk of disease based on epidemiologic data, and one or more reasonable biological pathways through which such an effect might be causal are suggested and have some empirical support. Human biology is sufficiently complex that imaginative, knowledgeable researchers can almost always derive reasonable pathways to explain an epidemiologic observation of an association, making candidate mechanisms of only modest value in bolstering the epidemiology. The credibility and empirical evidence supporting those pathways will vary, of course. Nevertheless, under this scenario, the information provided is parallel to the epidemiology, but not truly synergistic.

A more beneficial integration of the biological and epidemiologic evidence occurs when postulated mechanisms can be tested directly in the epidemiologic research and vice versa: there is a feedback loop of information across disciplines. Instead of merely lending credibility to the epidemiology, the biologic evidence suggests testable hypotheses for epidemiologists to pursue. For example, the proposed mechanism may suggest which forms of exposure should be most potent or which subset of disease a given agent should most directly influence. Ideas regarding intermediate outcomes or effect modifiers, including indicators of genetic susceptibility, may be generated. The value of such biologically grounded hypotheses is not that they are somehow inherently superior or more likely to be correct for having been built upon other disciplines. Rather, if the research bears out the suggestion, then the epidemiologic evidence itself will be much stronger (larger measures of effect, clear indications of effect-modification) and the coherence with the biological evidence will be stronger. Clues from mechanistic research should be scrutinized in planning epidemiologic studies to derive testable hypotheses, not merely to take comfort that such research exists (Savitz, 1994). In turn, the epidemiologic findings should provide feedback to laboratory investigators regarding hypotheses to pursue through experimental systems. If the epidemiologic observations are sound, then they can be a rich source of hypotheses to be examined through experimental approaches in the laboratory. When such epidemiologically driven studies are found to support the epidemiologic evidence then the overall coherence of the findings across disciplines and the cumulative evidence will be stronger.

CONTROVERSY OVER INTERPRETATION

Epidemiologists and often non-epidemiologists lament the controversy, sometimes bordering on hostility, which is common to many important topics for which the evidence is truly uncertain. Those who are not scientists can interpret this discord as a troubling barrier to knowing the right thing to do, focusing on the disagreement as the underlying problem rather than the lack of conclusive evidence as the basis for the disagreement. In some cases, the scientific evidence may be quite clear but there is disagreement over the appropriate policy or personal decision-making that cannot be answered even with perfect scientific information. Those who would like to fine tune their diets to minimize risk of chronic disease face variable interpretations of truly inconsistent research, but also indications that the very actions that may reduce risk of one disease may increase the risk of another. There is some tendency to blame the messenger in the face of such a dilemma.

Epidemiologists are sometimes troubled by the public disharmony as well. The implication that epidemiologists cannot agree on anything is viewed as discrediting the science, or implying that no matter how much research we do, we cannot uncover truth. Of course, the specific sides in such a debate will have their own criticisms of the logic or even integrity of the other side. Those who believe a causal association is present will lament that their critics are nitpicking, taking small or hypothetical problems and exaggerating their importance. It's been said that "epidemiologists eat their young" with regard to the unlimited ability to find fault with research. Those who believe that premature or false assertions of causality have been made, however, argue that harm is being done by misleading or worrying the public unnecessarily, and that these assertions will later be proven false, discrediting the field.

A more sanguine view is that thoughtful, non-rancorous debate is beneficial for the field and helpful, not harmful, in characterizing the current state of knowledge and its implications for policy. All sciences engage in such assertions and challenges, from physics to anthropology, and the underlying science is not and should not be called into question as a result. Nor should the controversy in epidemiology be viewed as evidence against the rigor and value of the discipline. Presentation of new research findings is a form of debate, using data rather than isolated logical arguments. New research is designed to enter into the ongoing debate, hypothesizing that the proposed study will shift the evidence in one direction or the other. Direct challenges in the form of debates at research meetings, in editorial statements, or face-to-face in informal settings can only stimulate thinking and move the field forward; if spurious issues are raised they can be put to rest as a result of being aired. Obviously, when the debate becomes personal or ideological, progress will be inhibited and objectivity compromised. If the benefit of controversy is clarity about the evidence and the identification of strategies for enhancing the quality of evidence, emotion and ego detract from the realization of such benefits.

In proposing principles for the evaluation of epidemiologic evidence, the intent is not to provide a framework that will enable all knowledgeable, objective epidemiologists to reach the same conclusions. That would imply that the truth is known and if we could just sit down together, have the same base of information available, and apply the same methodologic principles, we would reach the same conclusions. Because the information is always incomplete to varying degrees, we are extrapolating from what is currently known to what would be known if the evidence were complete. Even the methodologic principles do not ensure unanimity of interpretation, because the inference about potential biases is just that—an informed guess about what might be. The goal of applying the tools and principles summarized in this book is to change the debate from one based on global impressions and subjective biases to one that is specific, informed, and generates clarity regarding research needs, pinpointing issues for further methodologic development.

Starting from the premise that all bodies of research are inconclusive to some extent, the principal need is to determine precisely where the gaps are. Such statements such as "The evidence is weak" or "Studies are inconsistent" or "Something is going on there" invite disagreement of an equally subjective and global nature. A debate over conflicting, superficial impressions offers no benefit either in clarifying where the current evidence stands or in pinpointing what is needed to reach firmer conclusions. The basis for those conflicting inferences needs to be elucidated. If the evidence is perceived to be weak by some and strong by others based on, for example, differing views of the quality of exposure assessment, then we need to reframe the debate by compiling available evidence re-garding the quality of exposure assessment. We may find that validation studies are the most pressing need to advance this avenue of research. If controversy is based on adequacy of control for confounding, we have tools to address the plau-sibility of substantial uncontrolled confounding. Placing the controversy on more secure foundations will not produce agreement, and may even anchor both sides more firmly in their original positions. Again, the goal is not consensus, but an informative and constructive debate.

For the major issues that underlie differing conclusions (not all possible methodologic issues), the evidence needs to be dissected. The evidence from studies of the topic of concern, as well as ancillary methodological work and other sources of extraneous information should be brought to bear. Typically, there will be some support for each of the opposing sides, and a disagreement over the summary judgment may well remain after a complete examination of the issues. What should emerge, however, is a much more specific argument that helps to define empirical research that would alter the weight of evidence. Each side may bring the preconception that the additional research will confirm what they believe to be true, but making the argument specific and testable is a sig-nificant step forward.

THE CASE AGAINST ALGORITHMS FOR INTERPRETING EPIDEMIOLOGIC EVIDENCE

Identifying the specific points of disagreement about epidemiologic research in order to objectively and comprehensively scrutinize the study methods and re-sults and thus assess the potential for bias has been proposed as a useful strat-egy. Imposing this structure on the examination of evidence should lead to clar-ity and point toward the researchable bases for disagreement. It might be argued that formalizing this process further through the development of algorithms or checklists for the interpretation of epidemiologic evidence would be the next log-ical step. In its ultimate form, attributes of individual studies or collections of studies could be entered into a computer program and a measure of the certainty would be produced, along with a priority list of research needs to improve the certainty of that evidence, rank-ordered based on the evidence that would most influence the certainty score.

The only widely used checklist is that proposed by Hill some 35 years ago for assessing the likelihood of a causal relation based on observational data (Hill, 1965). A number of characteristics of epidemiologic study results are enumer-ated that are relevant to an assessment of causality, but even the author warned against any attempts to apply those guidelines as criteria that demonstrate causal-ity if attained or its absence if not completed. As discussed in some detail elsewhere (Rothman & Poole, 1996), the items that are enumerated provide clues to potential for bias and there would be greater benefit on focusing directly on the potential for bias than on these indirect markers.

Strong associations or those that show dose–response gradients, Hill's first two criteria, provide evidence against the association being entirely due to confounding, under the assumption that confounding influences are more likely to be weak than strong and not likely to follow the exposure of interest in a dose–response manner. Preferably, one can focus directly on the question of confounding, and gather all the evidence from within and outside the study to suggest the presence or absence of distortion of varying magnitude. In fact, a strong association may be influenced by confounding of modest magnitude and still remain a fairly strong association, whereas a weak association is more likely to be obliterated. Hill's rationale is very likely to be valid, but there are more strategies for assessing confounding than he offered, and all are potentially valuable.

Other considerations proposed by Hill—such as specificity, in which causality is more likely if there is a single agent influencing a single disease—are of little value, except as a reminder to be watchful for selection bias or recall bias that might produce spurious associations with an array of exposures or outcomes. One approach suggested in this book is the examination of whether associations are observed that are unlikely to be causal, and thus call the association of interest into question. The menu of strategies is much broader than Hill's brief list would suggest.

The linkage to biological plausibility and coherence looks to evidence outside of epidemiology for support, whereas the evidence from other disciplines should be integrated with the epidemiologic evidence for an overall appraisal, not merely used to challenge or buttress the epidemiology. Concern with temporal sequence of exposure and disease is a reminder to be wary of the potential for disease to influence the exposure marker, such as early stages of cancer possibly reducing serum cholesterol levels (Kritchevsky & Kritchevsky, 1992), leading to an erroneous inference that low serum cholesterol is causally related to the development of cancer.

Hill's criteria are of value in helping to remind the interpreters of epidemiologic evidence to consider alternatives to causality, even when a positive association has been observed. A preferable approach to evaluating a study or set of studies is to focus on sources of distortion in the measure of effect, isolating any causal relation from distortion due to bias or random error. That process overlaps directly with issues raised by Hill but attempts to be more direct in pinpointing sources of error that can then be tested. The Hill criteria were intended to assess causality when an observation of an association had been made, not to interpret epidemiologic evidence more generally. For null associations, for example, the Hill criteria are not applicable, whereas the results nevertheless call for scrutiny and interpretation.

More extensive, formal schemes for assessing epidemiologic methods and evidence have been proposed. In some instances, the goal is to enumerate attributes that make epidemiologic studies credible (Chemical Manufacturers Association, 1991; Federal Focus Inc, 1996), focusing on methods or on the description of methods. A recent proposal for the use of an "episcope" (Maclure & Schneeweiss, 2001) would be a welcome formalization of the evaluation of bias, very much concordant with the ideas expressed here. Encouragement to provide information that helps to make informed judgments of the epidemiologic evidence can only be helpful. As the focus turns to making sense of the evidence that has been generated, rigid application of the checklists becomes more problematic. A skeptical interpretation is that epidemiologists prefer to shroud their expertise in some degree of mystery to ensure long-term job security. So long as an epidemiologist, rather than a computer program, is needed to interpret epidemiologic research, we remain a valued and relatively scarce resource. There are more valid reasons however, that such approaches can serve at best as a reminder of the issues to be considered but not as an algorithm for judgment.

The universe of issues that could potentially influence study results is quite extensive, even though the considerations are often grouped into a few categories, such as confounding, selection bias, and information bias. Within each of these, the application to a specific topic, study, or set of studies involves dozens of branches, tending toward very long lists of specific manifestations. The relative importance of these concerns is based not on some generic property resulting from the nature of the bias, but rather depends on the specific characteristics of the phenomenon being addressed in a given study. The sociologic characteristics of the population, the nature of exposure and disease measurement, the details of study conduct, and the methods of statistical analysis all have direct bearing on the potential for bias. The use of ancillary information from other relevant studies adds yet another dimension to the evaluation, requiring inferences regarding the applicability of data from other studies, for example, based on similarities and differences from the population at hand. Integrative schemes require some approach to weighting that synthesizes the highly distinctive issues into scores, so that even if the menu of items could be stipulated, their relative importance could not. In contrast to any predesignated weighting scheme, each situation calls for examination of the key concerns and a tentative assignment of relative importance based on epidemiologic principles. In one set of studies, nonresponse may be the dominant concern and deserve nearly all the attention of evaluators; in other studies, exposure measurement error may dominate over the other issues. Any scheme that assigns generic relative weights to non-response and to exposure measurement error is surely doomed to failure.

The alternative to an algorithm for evaluating epidemiologic evidence is evaluation by experts. There is a loss in objectivity, in that one expert or set of experts may well view the evidence differently than another expert or set of experts. The goal throughout this book has been to identify the specific basis for such variation, specifying the considerations that lead to a final judgment. Ideally, experts attempt to examine the spectrum of methodologic concerns in relation to the results, identify sources of uncertainty, evaluate the plausibility and implications of that uncertainty, and reach appropriate conclusions regarding the strength of the evidence and key areas in need of refinement.

While discussions about epidemiologic evidence often focus on an assignment of the proper adjective, such as strong, moderate, or weak evidence, in reality, the assessment is made to determine whether a specific decision is justified. In purely scientific terms, the bottom line questions concern the validity of study results, distortions introduced in the measure of effect, and the probability that the true association takes on different values. In applications of epidemiologic evidence, the question is how the information bears on personal and policy decisions. One might ask whether the epidemiologic evidence is strong enough to impose a regulation or to modify one's behavior, taking other scientific and non-scientific considerations into account. This balancing of epidemiologic evidence against other factors makes the judgment even more complex, less suitable for checklists and algorithms, but it may be helpful in making the uses of the epidemiology more explicit. The practical decision is not between differing views of epidemiologic evidence, but rather between differing courses of action. The incentive to invoke weak epidemiologic evidence as strong, or vice versa, in order to justify a decision would be avoided, and epidemiologists could focus on characterizing the evidence without the distraction of how that assessment will be used. Clarity and accuracy in the presentation of the evidence from epidemiology must be the overriding goal, trusting that others will use the information wisely to chart the appropriate course of action.

REFERENCES

Chemical Manufacturers Association. Guidelines for good epidemiology practices for occupational and environmental research. Washington, DC: The Chemical Manufacturers Association, 1991.

Federal Focus Inc. Principles for evaluating epidemiologic data in regulatory risk assessment. Washington DC: Federal Focus, Inc, 1996.

Hill AB. The environment and disease: association or causation? Proc Royal Soc Med 1965;58:295–300.

Kritchevsky SB, Kritchevsky D. Serum cholesterol and cancer risk: an epidemiologic perspective. Annu Rev Nutr 1992;12:391–416.

Maclure M, Schneeweiss S. Causation of bias: the episcope. Epidemiology 2001; 12:114–122.

National Research Council. Possible health effects of exposure to residential electric and magnetic fields. Committee on the Possible Effects of Electromagnetic Fields on Biological Systems, Board on Radiation Effects Research, Commission on Life Sciences, National Research Council. Washington, DC: National Academy Press, 1997.

Rosamond WD, Chambless LE, Folsom AR, Cooper LS, Conwill DE, Clegg L, Wang C-H, Heiss G. Trends in the incidence of myocardial infarction and in mortality due to coronary heart disease, 1987 to 1994. N Engl J Med 1998;339:861–867.

Rothman KJ, Poole C. Causation and causal inference. In D Schottenfeld, JF Fraumeni Jr (eds), Cancer Epidemiology and Prevention, Second Edition. New York: Oxford University Press, 1996:3–10.

Sackett DL. Bias in analytic research. J Chron Dis 1979;32:51–63.

Savitz DA. In defense of black box epidemiology. Epidemiology 1994;5:550–552.

Savitz DA, Moe C. Drinking water. In Steenland K, Savitz DA (eds), Topics in Environmental Epidemiology. New York: Oxford University Press, 1997;89–118.

Savitz DA, Poole C, Miller WC. Reassessing the role of epidemiology in public health. Am J Public Health 1999;89:1158–1161.

Vainio H, McGee PN, McGregor DB, McMichael AJ (eds). Mechanisms of carcinogenesis in risk identification (IARC Scientific Publ. No. 116). Lyon, France: International Agency for Research on Cancer, 1992.

INDEX

Page numbers followed by *f* and *t* indicate figures and tables, respectively.

Abortion, spontaneous. *See also* Miscarriage
  alcohol and, 18–20
  anesthetic gases and, 129
  elective vs., 19
  epidemiologic evidence, inferences and,
    18–20
  error measurement and, 18
  gestational age and analysis of, 238
  heavy menstrual period and, 218
  pesticide exposure and, 60, 61*t*
Accuracy
  absolute v. relative, 194, 201
  of causal relations, 26–27
  diagnostic, 207–8, 226–28, 229*t*
  disease ascertainment and, 206, 226
  disease ascertainment, subgroups and,
    230–32, 233*t*–234*t*, 239
  disease outcome ascertained, inference
    restricted and, 232, 235, 236*t*–237*t*, 238
  evidence presented with, 302
  in exposure prevalence, 86
  informative and fallible degrees of, 37
  public health and, 18, 302
  severity of disease and, 232, 235, 238
Action
  causal inference and, 24–27
  epidemiologic evidence basis of, 25, 302
Adenomatous polyps, 230–31
Age
  back-calculating of, 91

comparison, 64, 65*t*, 67–68, 86, 101–2, 104,
  104*t*, 105, 109*t*, 123, 126*t*, 191*t*
confounding by, 15
gestational, 210, 238
selection bias with higher, 104
Aggregation (lumping)
  data pooling as, 264–65, 267
  disease misclassification and, 210, 211,
    225–26, 239
  excessive, 211
  of individual trials, 262
  random error and, 252, 262, 264
Air pollution, fine particulate, 71, 71*t*, 169,
  179–80, 180*f*
Alcohol, 293
  alterations in consumption of, 20
  breast cancer and, 111, 275–76
  epidemiologic evidence, inferences and,
    18–20, 217
  error measurement in use of, 18
  intake, 164
  mental retardation, pregnancy and, 211
  myocardial infarction and, 170, 188
  race and, 275
  smoking and, 276, 277
  spontaneous abortion and, 18–20
  timing of use of, 19
Algorithms, 55, 299–302
Anxiety, spontaneous labor/delivery and, 64,
  65*t*–66*t*

Ascertainment, disease, 208–9
    accuracy and subgroups of, 230–32,
        233*t*–234*t*, 239
    accuracy of, 206, 226
    inference restricted and, 232, 235,
        236*t*–237*t*, 238
    overascertainment vs. underascertainment
        and, 213–16, 220, 228, 232, 238, 239
    underascertainment, subgroups and, 232
Association(s). *See also* Causal relation
    absence of, 35, 45
    absence of causal, 10
    assessment of, 9
    bias influence on, 3, 193–95, 220
    causal implications of, 2, 300
    without (reflecting) causal relation, 46–47
    confounder-disease, 142–44, 153, 155–56
    confounder-exposure, 142–44, 155–56
    confounding, 22–23
    estimates of, 128
    inconsistency and, 274
    lack of, 10
    measure of, 9–10, 21, 37, 102, 104–5
    media/public interest influence on, 194–95
    non-response elimination and strong, 272
    positive vs. observed absence of, 2
    random error and, 110–11, 245
    selection bias to measures of, 102, 104–5
    statistical, 2, 10
    strong, 272, 300
    weaker, 143, 272, 300

Baris, D., 131, 175, 175*t*, 177*t*
Bayesian shrinkage, 255
Beta carotene, 169
Bias, 279, 281, 285, 291–92, 300. *See also*
        Selection bias; Subjectivity
    assessment of direction of, 291–92, 293–94,
        301
    association influenced by, 3, 193–95, 220
    certainty limited by, 23
    consistency, (multiple studies) and, 4, 263,
        277, 281–82
    disagreement and evaluator's, 31–32, 34
    disease misclassification and, 238–40
    eliminating, 119, 216
    episcope and, 301
    financial support, investigator and, 14
    hypothesis and, 23, 34, 36, 277, 282, 293
    identification and correction of, 36–37
    inconsistency, methodological limitations
        and, 276–77, 278, 279
    information, 19, 20, 95, 100, 206
    integrated consideration of potential, 133–34,
        238–40, 293–94
    limitations of knowledge about, 44
    magnitude of distortion of, 42–43
    in more advanced disease, 47

    non-response, 22–23, 42–44, 55, 93, 120–23,
        124*t*, 133–34, 245
    towards null value, 192, 213, 214, 216
    probability deviations evaluated for, 43,
        294
    quantitative assessment of, 33–39, 294
    random error, multiple studies and, 261–64
    recall with, 193–95, 300
    remediable, 281
    with risk ratio reduced, 140
    role of, 22–23
    sources of, 30, 31, 67
    specifying scenarios of, 41–44
    statistical procedures in removing of, 36
    subset of candidate, 40–41, 42, 76
    susceptibility to, 276–77, 279
    (nondifferential) underascertainment vs.
        overascertainment, cohort studies and,
        214–15
Bias, from loss of study participants
    case-control studies, exposure prevalence
        and, 120
    clinical setting and, 117, 118*t*
    cohort studies, un/exposed groups and,
        119–20
    conceptual framework for, 115–20, 118*t*
    eliminating bias/confounding, adjustments of
        measured attributes and, 119
    exposure–disease relation, selection basis
        and, 119–20
    imputing information, nonparticipants and,
        129–31
    increased response for, 120
    integrated assessment of potential of, 133–34
    magnitude of deviation and effect of,
        118–19, 120
    mechanisms of, 117–18, 118*t*
    missing data and, 118*t*, 129–31
    nonparticipants characterized/followed-up in,
        120–23, 124*t*
    random losses, less damage in, 116–17, 119
    recruitment gradation of difficulty in, 120,
        124–28, 126*t*
    smaller the loss for less erroneous results in,
        116
    stratify study base, markers of participation
        and, 128–29
    subject's refusal and, 117–19, 118*t*, 121,
        122, 133
    traceability difficulties with, 117–19, 118*t*,
        121, 122, 124–25, 127
Biologically effective exposure, 164–67, 172,
    174, 178, 179, 190, 195–97
Boice, J.D., Jr., 268, 270, 270*t*
Bonferroni correction, 252
Bradford-Hill, A.B., 278
Brain tumors, 195, 197–98
Breast cancer
    alcohol association with, 111, 275–76

association, DDT/DDE and, 46–47, 48, 49,
  165–67, 182–84, 183*t*
bias in more advanced disease of, 47
blood levels, DDT and, 165–66
chlorinated hydrocarbons and, 196–97
DDT, DDE and PCB exposure for, 44–49
lactation, DDT/DDE and, 47–49, 182–84, 183*t*
oral contraceptives association with, 190–91,
  191*t*
Breast cancer screening
  cancer reduction and, 17
  epidemiologic evidence, inferences and,
    16–18
  mortality rate and, 16–18
  participants vs. nonparticipants of, 16–17
  public health strategy for, 17–18
Brinton, L.A., 190, 191*t*
Bronchitis, smoking and, 70, 95

Cancer. *See also* Brain tumors; Breast cancer;
    Leukemia; Lung cancer
  bladder, 85–86, 138–40, 141, 143
  brain, 90, 93*t*, 198, 199*t*, 200*t*, 225–26, 226*t*
  cervical, 13–14, 230
  cholesterol and, 188, 189*t*, 197, 300
  depression and, 198, 199*t*–200*t*
  endometrial, 96, 97*t*, 98, 99*t*, 100, 228, 230,
    231*f*, 235
  lymphoma and, 212
  magnetic fields and, 90–91, 92, 93*t*, 104–5,
    112–13, 123, 124*t*, 131, 132*t*, 153,
    225–26, 225*t*, 265, 266*t*, 267, 267*f*
  oral, 276, 293
  pancreatic, 154
  prostate, 102, 103*t*, 104*t*, 186, 187*t*, 209,
    232, 235
  registries, 59, 90, 104, 154
  research, 286
Cancer Prevention II Study, 71, 71*t*, 179
Cardiovascular disease, 204, 209, 223, 286
  estrogen therapy and, 73, 75*t*
  fine particulate air pollution influence on,
    71, 71*t*, 169, 179–80
Case registries, 90
Case–control studies
  disease misclassification and, 213–14
  (nondifferential) overascertainment for,
    213–14
  study participant's loss, exposure prevalence,
    cooperativeness and, 125, 213
  (nondifferential) underascertainment for, 213
Case–control studies, selection bias in, 235,
    236*t*–237*t*
  association's measures adjustment for known
    sources of non-comparability in, 105–8,
    107*t*
  association's measures in relation to markers
    of potential, 102, 104–5

coherent controls vs. non-coherent controls
    for, 112–13
coherence of cases and controls for, 86–89,
    108, 112–13
cohort studies vs., 5, 52, 53, 81–82
control group in, 81–82, 83
control selection for, 81–89, 182
control's purpose in, 84
controls vs. study base in, 53
defined, 52, 81
of disease incidence, 52
of disease prevalence, 52
(accurate) exposure prevalence and unbiased,
    86
exposure prevalence in controls compared to
    external population in, 96, 98, 99*t*,
    100–101, 112, 115
exposure prevalence measurement in, 53, 85,
    88
exposure prevalence variation among
    controls in, 101–2, 103*t*, 104*t*, 120
exposure–disease associations confirmed in,
    108, 109*t*–110*t*, 110–11, 112
geographic areas with, 88–89, 91, 94, 106
(discretionary) health care for, 92–96, 97*t*
health outcome-dependent sampling for, 52
historical population roster for, 91–92
integrated assessment of potential for,
    111–13
non-concurrent vs. concurrent, 92
social factors, individual behaviors and, 85,
    86, 95, 101, 111, 182
socioeconomic status for, 93*t*, 101, 104–5,
    106, 123, 124*t*
study base controls with, 83–86
subject selection for, 81–83
temporal coherence of cases and controls
    with, 89–92, 93*t*
Categories, nominal and ordinal, 52
Causal inference, 11, 20–24
  action and, 24–27
  alternative explanations as subjective in,   23
  bias's role with, 22–23
  challenges to, 22
  data, evaluation and, 22
  definition of, 20
  descriptive goals and, 15–16
  drawing of, 21
  from epidemiologic evidence for similar
    policy implications, 25
  epidemiologic research for clearer/broader,
    21, 287
  multiple studies, inconsistent results and, 262
  non-causal explanations for observed
    associations excluded from, 20
  policy decisions, individual behavioral
    decisions and, 24–27
Causal relation, 279
  accurate estimation of, 12

Causal relation (*continued*)
  association without reflecting, 46–47
  error in, 10
  inferences about, 11
  limitations in measuring, 11
  measure of, between disease and exposure,
    9–12, 15, 19, 37, 41, 46, 48, 51–52, 55,
    81, 85, 102, 104–5, 108, 109*t*–110*t*,
    110–11, 112, 119–20, 142–43, 152, 163,
    164, 165, 167, 181–82, 184, 185, 186,
    188–89, 193–98, 199*t*–200*t*, 224, 228,
    232, 281, 292–93
  public health and accuracy of, 26
  statistical associations and, 10–11
  universal, 12
Causality
  alternatives to, 300
  assessment of, 21
  as benchmark for validity, 10
  consistency and, 4, 279
  counterfactual conceptualization of, 17
  epidemiologic evidence interpreted in
    assessing, 23–24
  epidemiologic research, associations and, 21
  hypothesis of, 23, 278, 279
  judging of, 1–2
Census sampling, 106–7*t*
Certainty
  biases limiting of, 23
  diagnosis, examined, 219–21, 222*t*, 223
  moving towards, 24
Chemical exposures, 14
Chlorination, 288–89
Cholesterol, 188, 189*t*, 197, 300
Clinical setting, 117, 118*t*
Clinicians, 13
Cocaine, 106, 277
Coffee
  bladder cancer and, 85–86, 138–40, 141
  miscarriage and, 168–69
  smoking, lung cancer and, 156–57, 158*t*
Cognitive function, 182
Coherence
  of cases and controls, 86–89, 108, 112–13
  non-coherent controls vs., 112–13
  restriction of cases/controls for, 87
  temporal, of case/controls, 89–92, 93*t*
Cohort studies
  disease misclassification and, 213–15
  (nondifferential) overascertainment for,
    214–15
  study participant loss, questionnaire and, 125
  (nondifferential) underascertainment for, 214
Cohort studies, selection bias in
  aberrant disease rates in, 64
  ascertainment protocols for, 59, 60, 62
  baseline differences in risk of diseases,
    assessing and adjusting for, 72–73, 74*t*,
    75*t*, 76, 82
  case–control studies vs., 5, 52, 53, 81–82

comparison group's purpose in, 53–55, 57,
    63, 78
confounding and, 55–58, 72–73, 74
cross-sectional studies as, 52
defined, 52, 81–82
of disease incidence, 52
of disease prevalence, 52
diseases known not to be affected by
    exposure, assess rates and, 70–72, 71*t*
diseases unrelated to exposure found to be
    related in, 70, 72
expected patterns of disease, assessing
    presence, and, 63–64, 65*t*–66*t*, 67
exposure groups' measurement in, 52–53
group's stratum free from, 67
integrated assessment of potential for, 78–79
lack of information as tool for, 58
markers of susceptibility, assessing pattern
    and, 67–70, 69*f*, 74
non-exposed group's poor choice in, 115
observational design for, 54
questionnaire for, 125
random error for, 54, 70
randomized controlled trials for, 54, 73–74,
    76, 82
sociodemographic factors and, 64, 65*t*–66*t*,
    123
stratifying groups according to distortion for,
    67
study designs for, 51–53
study group restriction, enhanced
    comparability and, 73–74, 76, 77*t*, 78
subject selection in, 81–82
unexpected patterns of disease, assessing
    presence and, 64, 67
unexposed disease rates compared to
    external populations in, 58–60, 61*t*, 62–63
un/exposed group, disease rate/incidence and,
    53–55, 58–59, 64, 82, 84, 119–20, 188
whole population, random choice and, 52
Colonoscopy, 230–31
Community
  controls, 98, 99*t*, 100
  sampling, 106, 125–26, 126*t*
Comparability, 20. *See also* Non-comparability
  enhanced, 73–74, 76, 77*t*, 78
Compatibility
  bounds of, 256
  for data pooling, 264–65
  meta-analysis and studies with
    methodological, 271
Conclusions, 11, 30–32, 285–86, 290
Confidence intervals, 45, 48
  confidence limit ratio and, 257, 267*f*
  for defining bounds of compatibility, 256
  as interval estimates, 256
  observational studies and, 248
  overlap in, coverage, 257
  probability (p-value) and, 248, 255–57, 258
  random error and, 46, 251, 255–57

random variation in data conveyed by, 256–57
relative risk and, 257
statistical significance testing vs., 256
(different) studies' precision compared with, 257
wide, 275
Confounder(s)
exposure vs. disease associations of, 142–44, 153, 155–56
key, 22, 23
lactation as, 48–49
partial adjustment to imperfectly measured, 108
potential, 45
specific, 138–39
Confounding, 41
by age, 15
association, 22–23, 142–44, 147, 300
bias from, 157
causality, empirical associations and, 11, 20
consistent, 278
counterfactual definition of, 137, 138
data pooling and, 267
definition of, 2, 3, 5, 56, 137–38
deviation of, 144
difficulty measuring, 146
direction of, 144
distortion from, 141, 144, 300
dose-response gradient and, 155–57, 158t
eliminating, 119, 142, 157, 159
evaluation of potential, 78, 145–57, 149t, 159–60, 299
exchangeability and, 138–39, 159
exposure of interest effect on, 3, 137–38
hypothesis, 145–46, 155, 160
inaccurate, measurement and its consequences, 146–52, 149t, 160
indirect associations for, 143–44
informed judgment of, 4
integrated assessment of potential, 157, 159–60
knowledge of, based on other studies, 152–54
maximize association of disease and, 147
misclassification and, 147, 150
negative, 140–41, 144
non-comparability and, 56, 57–58, 138, 145, 146–47
non-exchangeability and, 137–38, 140, 159
null value for, 140, 144, 155
origins of, 5
positive, 47, 140–41, 144
potential of, 3
quantification of potential, 141–45
quantitative speculation for, 150–51
random error and, 41–42, 155, 245
randomization in removing, 139, 141
research for narrowing uncertainty on impact of, 4

residual, 72, 151–52
risk factors unknown and assessment of, 154–55
risk of disease, statistically adjusted, and, 72
risk ratio (RR), 140, 141, 143, 144–45, 150, 151
selection bias, cohort studies and, 55–58, 72–73, 74
selection bias in case-control studies and, 85, 105, 108
socioeconomic factors for, 147, 149, 149t, 152
statistical adjustment of, 56–58, 139–40, 149–50, 151, 159–60
stratification of, 106, 139–40, 142
substantial, 144
susceptibility to, 263, 280
theoretical background for, 137–41
unadjusted vs. partially adjusted measures of, 150–52
uncertainty and, 23
unobservable conditions with, 138–39
variable, 138–39, 142, 143, 145, 154
weak, influences, 300
Congenital defects, 60, 168, 193
Consistency
bias and, 4, 263, 277, 281–82
causality and, 4, 279
compensating strengths across studies for, 278–79
credibility with, 278
definition of purpose of, 273
evolution of epidemiologic research and, 279–81
findings of, 277–78
inconsistent findings and, 273–77, 282
replication and, 278–79
weakness/wrongness as, 277.281–82
Consistency. See also Inconsistency
Contraception, barrier, 151
Contraceptives. See Oral contraceptives
Controls
alternative, 96
of associated factors, 139
chosen vs. ideal, 111
coherence of cases and, 86–89, 108, 112–13
community, 98, 99t, 100
comparable source population for, 94–95
hospital, 92–93, 112
idiosyncratic control sampling method and, 88–89
ill, 92–93
inability to identify sample, 88
means among cases vs., 45
non-case, 94–95
non-concurrent vs. concurrent, 92
requirements for enrollment as, 89–90
selection of, from study base, 83–86
temporal coherence of, 89–92
Coronary heart disease, 72–73, 209, 223, 286, 289

Counterfactual, 137
Criticism, 32–33

Dalton, S.O., 198
Data
  actual measurement of, 16, 18
  assessment/analysis, 29–30, 239
  burden of, 20
  collection, 20, 44, 254, 278
  coordinated comparative analysis of, 267–68,
    269f
  different applications of, 13–14
  dredging (fishing), 254–55
  exposure, quality, 181–84, 183t, 185t, 188,
    192
  generator vs. interpreter, 14
  hypothesis formulation and analysis of,
    253–54
  imputed, 129–30, 131
  incomplete, 193
  information bias and, 19, 20, 95, 100, 206
  laboratory, 170
  loss of access to, 116
  measure of associations with, 21
  missing, 118t, 129–30, 131, 166, 175, 175t
  multiple comparisons influence on, 252–53
  pooling, 264–65, 266t, 267, 267f, 270
  prior expectations and, 186–87
  random variation in, 256–57
  (biased) recall of, 193–95
  self-reported, 170, 172, 174, 176, 178–79,
    184, 185t, 188, 194, 202, 227–28, 229t
DDE. See DDT
    (Dichlorodiphenyltrichloroethane/DDE)
DDT (Dichlorodiphenyltrichloroethane/DDE)
  association, breast cancer and, 46–47, 48,
    49, 165–67, 182–84, 183t
  blood levels of, 165–66
  breast cancer and early-life and later-life,
    47–48, 196, 197
  breast cancer and exposure to PCB and,
    44–49
  breast cancer, lactation and, 47–49, 182–84,
    183t
  ideal measure of, 166
  three calculations for, 45–46
Dementia, 15
Demographic patterns, 14, 64, 65t–66t, 93t,
    101, 104–5, 106, 122–23
Depression, 188
  cancer and, 198, 199t–200t
  disability and, 76, 77, 77t
  spontaneous labor/delivery and, 64, 65t–66t
Diabetes, 62, 63, 110t
Diagnosis
  under, 208–9, 217
  accuracy verified, subset of study
    participants and, 226–28, 229t
  certainty examined, 219–21, 222t, 223

clinical classification vs. biological
    classification in, 209
  erroneousness, changing results and, 207–8,
    228, 230, 231t
  exposure-driven, 217–19
  false positives vs. false negatives in, 207–8,
    209, 213, 220, 227, 228
  "gold standard," 206, 210, 232
  non-need for comprehensive ascertainment
    of, 208–9
  self-reported, 227–28, 229t
  symptoms and, 209
  undiagnosed cases and, 213
Dichlorodiphenyltrichloroethane (DDE). See
    DDT
    (Dichlorodiphenyltrichloroethane/DDE)
Diet, 95–96, 101, 119, 139, 169, 171, 173,
    231–32, 233t–234t
Dietary retinol, 108, 109t–110t
Dilatation and curettage (D&C), 96, 97t, 98,
    99t, 100
Disability, 76, 77, 77t
Disease(s)
  aberrant, rates, 64
  absolute rate of, 214–15
  as abstract constructs, 11–12
  as all health variants of interest, 11
  assessing presence of expected patterns of,
    63–64, 65t–66t, 67
  baseline differences in risk, 72–73, 74t, 75t,
    76, 82
  baseline, rates, 63
  baseline, risk, 53–54, 76, 142
  confounder-, association, 142–44, 153,
    155–56
  definition of, 10, 11, 209
  development, 83
  distorting exposure, exposure's measurement
    and, 195–97
  exposure caused by, 197–98, 199t–200t
  exposure's causal relation to, 9–12, 15, 19,
    37, 41, 46, 48, 51–52, 55, 57, 81, 85, 102,
    104–5, 108, 109t–110t, 110–11, 112,
    119–20, 142–43, 152, 163, 164, 165,
    166–67, 181–82, 184, 185–86, 188–89,
    193–98, 199t–200t, 224, 228, 232, 281,
    292–93
  health event assessed in form of, incidence,
    51
  known not to be affected by exposure and
    assess rates, 70–72, 71t
  psychological impacts of, 95–96
  randomness as (nearly) unattainable goal for
    groups and, 95, 139
  rarity of, 88
  risk, 72–73, 74t, 75t, 76, 82, 138, 140, 190
  (few) standardized ascertainment protocols
    for, 59
  unexposed group and rate/incidence of,
    53–54, 58–59, 119–20

unrelated to exposure (then later) found to be related to exposure in, 70, 72
Disease grouping
  aggregations of subgroups for, 225–26, 225t
  alternative approaches to, 224–25, 226
  definition of, 223
  selection of, 223–24
Disease misclassification, 207–8, 228, 230, 231t. See also Diagnosis; Ascertainment, disease
  accurate ascertainment, subgroups and, 230–32, 233t–234t, 239
  biological condition and, 207–8, 209, 235
  case–control studies influenced by, 213–14
  clinical classification vs. biological classification in, 209
  cohort studies influenced by, 213, 214–15
  consequences of, 206, 219–38
  diagnostic accuracy verified, subset of study participants and, 226–28, 229t
  diagnostic certainty examined with, 219–21, 222t, 223
  diagnostic erroneousness, changing results and, 207–8, 228, 230, 231t
  dichotomy vs. continuum approach to, 206, 210, 213
  differential, 213, 215–19, 227, 228, 232
  disease grouping alternate methods and, 223–26, 225t
  disease outcome ascertained accurately, inference restricted and, 232, 235, 236t–237t, 238
  evaluation framework for, 205–6
  false negatives in, 227
  false positives in, 220, 223–24, 226–27, 232, 252
  false positives vs. false negatives (overascertainment vs. underascertainment) in, 207–8, 209, 213–16, 220, 228
  inappropriate categorizing for, 210–11
  integrated assessment of potential bias from, 238–40
  labeling and, 220, 221, 222t, 227
  lumping vs. splitting (aggregation vs. disaggregation) for, 210, 211–12, 225–26, 239
  nondifferential, 212–14, 216, 227, 232
  nondifferential underascertainment, subgroups and, 232, 239
  null value and, 213, 214, 215, 216
  overascertainment vs. underascertainment in, 213–16, 232, 239
  quantification of association, exposure and not, 212
  quantitative probabilities for, 219–20, 227–28
  restrictive case definition and, 220
  risk ratio and, 220, 221
  sources of, 206–12

specificity for, 220, 224
stage of severity, size and, 232, 235, 238
study design influence on, 213–16
subsets different, different etiologies and, 221, 223
Disease rates, unexposed
  external populations (in cohort studies) compared to, 58–60, 61t, 62–63
Distortion
  from confounding, 141, 144, 300
  direct vs. indirect, 143–44
  disease, exposure measurement and, 195–97
  of exposure prevalence, 113
  of exposures, 56, 193, 196
  magnitude of, 42–43, 246
  from non-random allocation of exposure, 54
  nonrandom sample and, 130
  non-response and, 42
  stratifying groups according to, 67
Dose-response gradient, 232, 267, 300
  confounding and, 155–57, 158t
  exposure measurement and, 181, 189–92, 191t
  selection bias in cohort studies and, 67
  study participants' loss and, 125, 127
Drugs, illicit, 106, 185–86, 277

Education, 123, 198, 201
Effect
  accurate measure of, 36–37
  estimation measures of, 34–37, 41, 42
  measure modification, 68, 275–76, 296, 297
Electrical power lines. See Magnetic fields
Employment, healthy worker effect in, 68–69, 79
Environmental contamination, 165–66
Epilepsy, 197–98
Episcope, 301
Error(s). See also Bias; Misclassification; Random error
  bias for small, 38
  candidate biases subset and, 40–41
  conceptual framework for evaluation of, 37–39
  conceptual problem vs. operational, 170
  in confounding, 147, 160
  in constituting study group, 55
  definition of, 5, 10
  detrimental aspect of, 15
  in diagnosis, 5, 207–8, 228, 230, 231t
  of exclusion, 111
  exposure, (differential misclassification) and pattern of, 192, 216, 219
  extrapolations, unstudied populations and, 12–13
  of inclusion, 111
  magnitude of potential, 29, 38, 39
  measurement, 5, 12, 18
  misclassification, 12

Error(s) (*continued*)
  multiple studies and shared, 263
  non-random, 38
  non-response, conceptual inaccuracy of
    measurement tools and, 40–41
  of over/underinterpretation, 24, 26–27
  quantifying sources of, 38–39
  in self-reported information, 170, 172, 176,
    194, 202
  simple (clerical), 206, 216, 278–79
  size of study and no impact on, 42
  source of measurement of, 41
  sources for potential, 2
  (primary) sources of, 39–41
  study group's construction as potential
    source of, 5
  systematic, 38, 41
  systematic evaluation of sources of, 30–32,
    249
  systemic vs. random, 244–46, 248, 251
  technically accurate data, inferences and, 14,
    15–16
  technology and, 172
Estimate(s)
  confidence interval, 256
  in direction of null value, 259
  random error and, 37, 255, 256, 259
  single pooled, 271
  of uncertainty, 35
Estrogen therapy
  endometrial cancer and, 96, 97*t*, 98, 99*t*,
    100, 228, 230, 231*t*
  postmenopausal, 73, 74*t*, 75*t*, 107
Evidence, epidemiologic. *See also* Data
  accuracy of, 302
  (case against) algorithms for interpreting,
    299–302
  applications of, 13, 287–91
  as basis of action, 25, 302
  biological and, 296–97
  causality assessed in interpreting, 23–24
  clinicians use of, 13
  conclusions from, 30–32, 285–86, 299
  debate of merits of, 27
  effectiveness of, 7, 12, 23
  error, systematic evaluation of sources and,
    30–32
  error's evaluation, conceptual framework
    and, 37–39
  error's (primary) sources and, 39–41
  estimation of measures of effect for, 34–37
  extrapolation from, 298
  flaws of, 9
  future studies influenced by effectiveness of,
    23
  hypothesis formulation and (prior), 253–54
  inference from, and efficacy of breast cancer
    screening, 16–18
  inference levels from, and attendant
    concerns, 7, 8*t*

integrated with other disciplines, 9, 294–97
intellectual understanding of, 31
interpretation issues over, 1–3, 11, 26–27,
  297–99
limited, 33
multiple studies and aggregate evaluation of,
  281–83
multiple studies, patterns and integration of,
  261–62
multiple studies, synthetic/exploratory meta-
  analysis and, 268, 270–73
objective assessment of, 32–34
other scientific disciplines and, 9, 25–26,
  290, 294–97
persuasive or inconclusive, 7
policy decisions and inconclusive, but
  helpful, 287–90
policy decisions, subjectivity and, 32–33,
  285–86, 291, 297, 302
probability of correctness of, 290
public health improvement, nonscientific
  concerns and, 7–8
published, as valid, 27
scrutiny can be lacking for, 2
sufficient, 25
as suggestive, strong or weak, 286, 298–99,
  302
validity/evaluation of, 29–30, 34–35, 37
weak vs. no or counter, 25, 26, 27
weighed appropriately, 290
Exchangeability, 138–39, 159, 263
Experts, 31
  conclusions different for, 31–32
  subjectivity, objectivity and, 301–2
  summary judgment of, 30
Exposure(s)
  as abstract constructs, 11–12
  assessment, 279
  attributes of, 11
  chemical, 14
  classic concern of, 95
  confounded by indications of, 74, 142–43, 146
  confounder-, association, 142–44, 153,
    155–56
  continuous scale for, 53
  definition of, 9–10, 51, 163–64, 192
  developmental stage for, 168
  different timing of, 168, 172
  disease rate and, 59
  disease's causal relation to, 9–12, 15, 19, 37,
    41, 46, 48, 51–52, 55, 57, 81, 85, 102,
    104–5, 108, 109*t*–110*t*, 110–11, 112,
    119–20, 142–43, 152, 163, 164, 165,
    166–67, 181–82, 184, 185–86, 188–89,
    193–98, 199*t*–200*t*, 224, 228, 232, 281,
    292–93
  disease's known not to be affected by, and
    assess rates, 70–72, 71*t*
  disease's unrelated to exposure (later) found
    to be related to, 70, 72

distortion from non-random allocation of, 54
free from bias, 74
group, comparison, 52–55
occupational, 217–18
overascertainment and, 213–14
pesticide, 60, 61f, 82–83
prevalence before and after, 60
randomization, exchangeability and, 139, 263
randomized, assignment, 74, 139, 141
subgroups of, 74, 76, 100, 101
underascertainment and, 213
Exposure, measurement of, 18, 52–53, 111–12, 301
absolute vs. relative accuracy for, 194, 201
benchmark of validity for, 164
biochemical markers for, 176, 179
biological, 164–67, 172, 173, 174, 178, 179, 190, 195–97, 201
(known) consequences evaluated with, 187–89, 187t
data quality's variance for, 181–84, 183t, 185t, 188
differential exposure misclassification's mechanisms for, 193–95
(disease) differential misclassification, exposure status and, 213, 215–19, 228, 239
differential vs. nondifferential misclassification with, 192
diluted, 166
disease causing exposure and, 197–98, 199t–200t
disease distorting exposure and, 195–97
disease's strong relation to ideal, 166–67
dose-response gradient and, 181, 189–92, 191t
exposure aggregation's optimal level for, 168–69
exposure misclassification as differential or nondifferential, 192–202
exposure misclassification's consequences with, 163, 168, 172–92, 201–2
form of exposure and, 190
gold standard, 131, 172, 174, 175, 176, 178–79, 181, 196
ideal vs. operational, 164, 166–67, 170–72, 174, 191–92
lifetime markers of, 171
loss of information and, 166, 175
methods of, 164
multiple indicators of, 176, 178–80, 180f, 191, 192, 195
nondifferential exposure misclassification and, 192, 198–201
operational, 170–72
potential relevance of, 166
(known) predictors evaluated with, 185–87, 187t
qualitative vs. quantitative, 174–75, 189

range of, 163–64
risk of disease and, 190–91
routine compared to superior, 173–76, 175t, 177t, 179, 182
self-reported information on, 170, 172, 174, 176, 178–79, 184, 185t, 188, 194, 202
sensitivity of, 178–79
short-term vs. long-term, 176, 178
social factors and, 165, 182, 186, 187t, 198, 201
socioeconomic status and, 181–82, 184, 185t
subgroups with nondifferential exposure misclassification and, 198, 201
subsets of populations examined with differing exposure data quality and, 182–84, 183t, 185t, 187t
technology, errors and, 166, 172
temporally relevant, 167–68, 171, 172, 176, 201, 300
Exposure prevalence, 53, 60, 82, 83, 84, 85, 88, 90
disease misclassification and, 213–14
distortion for, 113
external population compared to (in case–control studies) of, 96, 98, 99t, 100–101, 115
non-coherent controls and, 113
over/understating of, 100–101
sampling, large disparities and, 100–101, 112
stratified sampling, selection bias and, 105–6, 112
study participant's loss and, 113
unbiased selection bias and accurate, 86
variation among controls for, 101–2, 103t, 104t, 120
External populations
comparability across, 62
exposed disease rates and, 59
exposure prevalence (in case–control studies) compared to, 96, 98, 99t, 100–101, 112
unexposed disease rates (in cohort studies) compared to, 58–60, 61t, 62–63
Extrapolations
errors, unstudied populations and, 12–13
of findings for generalizations, 12–13, 298
from subgroups, 122

Fruits, 231–32, 233t–234t, 235

Gender differences, 11, 15, 64, 65t, 187t
Genetic markers of susceptibility, 276, 297
Geographic areas
case–control studies, selection bias and, 88–89, 91, 94, 106
confounding and, 155, 158t
county averages and, 165

Geographic areas (*continued*)
exposure measurement and, 165, 186, 187*t*
loss of study participants and, 128, 131,
132*t*, 175–76, 175*t*, 177*t*
residential, 91–92, 112–13, 151–52, 265,
266*t*, 267, 270*t*
Gold standard
diagnosis/classification, 206, 210, 232
exposure, measurement and, 131, 172, 174,
175, 176, 178–79, 181, 196
study participant loss and, 131
Greenland, S., 3
Groups. *See also* Study group
algorithm for generating comparison, 55
cohort studies, selection bias, and
comparison, 53–55, 57, 63, 78
comparability of, 20
control, 82
excessive subdivision of (subgroups of), 211
non-comparability of, 56–58, 105–8, 146–47
non-exposed, 115
randomization process for, 54, 73–74, 76
stratifying, according to distortion, 67
subgroup's aggregation of, 225–26, 225*t*
subgroups, extrapolating from, for, 122
subgroups, highly selected, for, 68
subgroups of exposure for, 74, 76, 100, 101,
182–84, 183*t*, 185*t*, 198, 201
subgroups with accurate ascertainment,
disease misclassification and, 230–32,
233*t*–234*t*, 239
subgroups with nondifferential
underascertainment, disease
misclassification and, 232, 239

Head trauma, 195
Health care, 88. *See also* Hospitals
access, 163
alternative control groups for, 96
comparable source population with, 94–95
diet and, 95–96
enrollment, unambiguously defined source
population, and, 94
geography not determine, 94
hospital controls for, 92–93, 112
insufficient, 118
medical surveillance and, 96
non-case controls in, 96
particular, 94
seeking, 217
treatment, diagnosis and, 92
Health event
in form of disease incidence, 51–52
Health outcome, 56, 70, 78, 139, 147, 163,
179, 206
Health outcome-dependent sampling, 52
Health, public. *See* Public health
Health-related behaviors, 24–27, 85, 86, 95,
101, 111, 117, 118*t*, 119

Heat waves, 223
Hill, A.B., 2, 299–300
Hip fracture, 108, 109*t*–110*t*
Hodgkin's disease, 184, 185*t*, 212
Hormone replacement theory (HRT), 110*t*. *See
also* Estrogen therapy
Hospital(s)
controls, 92–93, 112
reasons for particular, 9
registry, 106
suitable, controls, 92–93
Hulka, B.S., 96, 230
Hypertension, 181–82, 209–10
Hypothesis
bias and, 23, 34, 36, 277, 282, 293
causal, 23, 278, 279
confounding, 145–46, 155, 160
consistency for, 273
data fishing in support of, 254–55
ex post facto, 254
formulation, 253–54
inconsistency with, 273–74
primary and secondary, 254
a priori, 253–54
refinement of, 272
testable, 23, 34, 36, 296–97

Illness. *See* Disease
Inconsistency, 279
across laboratories, 273–74
agent differing from populations in, 275–76
associations and, 274
bias, methodological limitations and,
276–77, 278, 279, 282
definition of, 273
effect modification and, 275–76
findings of, 274–77, 282
genetic markers of susceptibility and, 276
heterogeneity and, 276
random error produced by, 274–75, 278
statistical significance and, 275
variability and, 274–75
Individual variables, measure of associations
vs., 37
Inference(s), 143. *See also* Causal inference
about causal relations, 11
descriptive goals and causal, 15–16
drawing of, 21
from epidemiologic evidence, 7, 8*t*, 16–20
epidemiologic evidence, alcohol,
spontaneous abortion and, 18–20
epidemiologic evidence, efficacy of breast
cancer screening and, 16–18
from epidemiologic research, 11, 12–14
ordinal, 219–20
technically accurate data, error and, 14
Infertility, 208–9, 221, 222*t*
Information, bias, 19, 20, 95, 100, 206
Information. *See also* Data

Insurance, 94
Interest, measurement of
  common language vs. statistical jargon for,
    35–36
  primary, 34
  quantitative, 36
International Agency for Research on Cancer,
  286
Interpretation, 23–24
  (case against) algorithms for, 299–302
  challenges in, 4, 301
  conclusions and, 11
  issues in, of evidence, 3, 297–99
  over, 26–27, 248–49, 258
Intuition
  examined by, 228
  incorrect, 101

Jacobsen, B.K., 157, 158t

Kaufman, J.S., 147, 149t

Labeling, 220, 221, 222t, 227
Labor/delivery, spontaneous, 224–25
  anxiety, depression and, 64, 65t–66t
  sociodemographic/biomedical characteristics
    of pregnant women and, 64, 65t–66t
Lactation, 47–49, 182–84, 183t
Language, statistical jargon vs. common, 35–36
Leukemia
  acute lymphocytic, 56–57, 224
  acute myeloid, 224
  childhood, 90–91, 92, 93t, 104–5, 123,
    124t, 153, 175, 175t, 177t, 265, 266t,
    267, 267f
Lifestyles, 95, 117, 157, 158t
Loss. See Bias, from loss of study participants
Lubin, J., 268, 270
Lumping. See Aggregation (lumping)
Lung cancer, 95, 152, 218
  coffee, smoking and, 156–57, 158t
  fine particles and, 70, 71, 71t, 179–80, 180f
  radon and, 268, 269f, 270t
  smoking and, 111, 142, 147, 153, 156–57,
    158t, 167, 186, 187t, 188–89, 289, 295–96

Magnetic fields, 90–91, 92, 93t, 104–5,
  112–13, 123, 124t, 131, 132t, 153, 175,
  175t, 177t, 225–26, 225t, 265, 266t, 267,
  267f, 296
Mail surveys, 125–27, 126t, 129, 193
Matthews, K.A., 73
Media, overinterpretation and sensationalism
  of, 26–27
Medical examinations, 217
Medical interventions, 74

Medication
  assessment of, 186, 187t, 193, 195, 235,
    236t–237t
  side-effects, 146, 197–98
Melanoma, 70–71, 84–85
Melhaus, H., 108
Menopausal status, 275–76
Mental retardation, 210–11, 221
Meta-analysis, 268, 282
  compatibility of methods studies for, 271
  data pooling compared to, 270
  definition of, 5
  exploratory, 271–73
  meta-regression and, 272–73
  narrative review of studies and, 273
  observation of individual study with, 270
  potential determinants of, 271
  single pooled estimate for, 271
  statistical significance and, 271
  synthetic, 270–71
  variability sufficient for, 273
Miettinen, O.S., 87
Migraine headaches, 106
Miscarriage, caffeine and, 168–69
Misclassification, 15, 19, 38, 41, 96. See also
  Disease, misclassification
  algebra of, 163
  confounding and, 147, 150
  consequences of, 206
  definition of, 2, 205
  differential exposure, 193–95, 216–19, 227,
    228, 232
  differential vs. nondifferential exposure,
    192–202
  direct distortion by, 143–44
  error in implementing chosen approach for
    conceptual, 170
  exposure, 163, 168, 172–92
  loss information and, 166, 174–75
  nondifferential, 46, 198, 201, 212–15, 216,
    227, 232
  quantification of, 40
  routine exposure approximating superior
    exposure measurement for less, exposure,
    174
Morgenstern, H., 51
Mortality rate
  breast cancer screening and, 16–18
  heat waves and, 223
  lung cancer, heart disease and, 71, 71t, 169,
    179–80, 180f
Musculoskeletal disorders, 69, 69t
Myocardial infarction, 101–2, 104, 105, 168,
  170
  alcohol and, 170, 188

National Center for Health Statistics, 100, 130
National Health and Nutrition Examination
  Survey, 100, 102

Neural tube defects, 57
Non-comparability
    association's measures adjustment for known
        sources of, 105–8, 107*t*
    as comparable as possible, 147
    confounding and, 56, 57–58, 138, 145,
        146–47
    of groups, 56–58, 105–8, 146–47
Non-exchangeability, 137–38, 140, 159
Non-response, 40–41, 301
    bias, 22–23, 42–44, 55, 93, 133, 245
    bias, from loss of study participants, 120–23,
        124*t*, 133–34
    distortion and, 42
    not known for certainty, 44
    random error and, 245
    reasons for, 43
    selective, 267
    strong association and elimination of,
        272
Null hypothesis, 10, 35, 43, 213, 300
    positive vs., 255
    random error and, 38, 141, 252, 255
    statistical significance testing and, 249–50,
        252, 256, 258
Null value, 215, 252, 255
    bias towards, 192, 213, 214, 216
    confounding and, 140, 144, 155
    disease misclassification and, 213, 214, 215,
        216
    estimates in direction of, 259
    relative risks above/below, 275
Nurses Health Study, 227
Nutritional epidemiology, 169, 171

Objectivity, subjectivity vs., 32–33, 301–2
Observational studies
    confidence interval boundaries and, 248
    designed trial vs., 247
    exposure through implicit allocation method
        for, 246
    flawed nature of, 2
    probability values and, 248, 250
    random allocation, potential imbalances and,
        247, 250
    random error and, 246–48
    random sampling lacking in, 246, 250
    smaller vs. larger, 247
    true replications unlikely in, 263
Occupational disease, 68–69, 139
Occupational exposures, 217–18
Odds ratio, 214, 215, 225*t*, 237*t*
    adjusted, 45, 233*t*–234*t*
Oral contraceptives, 279
    breast cancer and, 190–91, 191*t*
    medical examines with, 217
Organochlorides, 44–45, 196
Osteoporosis, 63, 64, 93–94, 95, 107, 110*t*,
    168

Pap smears, 230
Parkinson's disease, 82–83
Participants, nonparticipants vs., 16–17, 22
PCB. *See* Polychlorinated biphenyls (PCB)
Pelvic inflammatory disease, 151
Pesticide exposure
    Parkinson's disease and, 82–83
    reproductive outcomes compared to, 60,
        61*t*
Physical activity, 109*t*, 158*t*
    cholesterol and, 188, 189*t*
    depression and, 188
    disability of, 76, 77, 77*t*
    myocardial infarction and, 101–2, 104, 105,
        168
    osteoporosis and, 168
Physiologic parameters, 221
Policy decisions, 285
    causal inference, individual behavior and,
        24–27
    disagreement over, 297–98
    epidemiologic evidence as inconclusive, but
        helpful for, 287–90
    modest shift in epidemiologic evidence
        influencing of, 289
    objectivity, subjectivity and, 32–33, 285–86,
        291, 297, 302
Polychlorinated biphenyls (PCB), 44–45
Pooling, data, 266*t*, 267, 267*t*
    compatibility across studies for, 264–65
    definition of, 5
    meta-analysis compared to, 270
    random error reduced in, 265, 267
Population. *See also* External populations;
        Study population
    accurate representation of study, 18
    agent differs from, 275–76
    exposure data quality and subsets of,
        182–84, 183*t*, 185*t*, 187*t*
    free-living human, 116
    laboratory, 116
Pregnancy, 277. *See also* Abortion,
        spontaneous; Labor/delivery, spontaneous
    clinical setting, losses from studies, preterm
        birth and, 117
    (inaccuracy of) identification of early, 18
    induced hypertension, 87
    loss, 238
    mental retardation and, 211
    preterm birth and, 117, 224–25
    sexual activity and preterm birth in late, 76
    sociodemographic/biomedical characteristics
        of, 64, 65*t*–66*t*
Prevalence, disease, 52
Prevalence of exposure. *See* Exposure
        prevalence
Prevalence measure, 37, 100
Prevalence ratio, 69
Probability, 249
    bias and, 43, 294

disease misclassification, 219–20, 227–28
sampling, 86
Probability values (p-values)
    confidence interval and, 248, 255–57, 258
    critical, 263
    random allocation and, 263
    statistical significance testing and, 250–51
Proof, definitive vs. more probable than not, 24
Public health. *See also* Policy decisions
    accurate measurements and, 18
    breast cancer strategy with, 17–18
    causal relations' accuracy and, 26–27
    change in clinical practice and consequences
        to, 13
    disease, variants of interest and, 11
    epidemiologic research for improvement of,
        7–8, 33, 288, 290
    epidemiology, other scientific disciplines
        and, 9, 25–26, 290, 294–97
    extrapolations of findings for generalizations
        for, 12
    goal of, 8
    nonscientific concerns, scientific disciplines
        and, 8
    planning and allocation of, 15
Pulmonary diseases, 217–18, 223, 227–28,
    229*t*
P-value. *See* Probability values (p-values)

Questions, family of, 38–39

Race, 1–4*t*, 98, 99*t*, 100, 101–2, 103*t*, 104*t*,
    149, 149*t*, 187*t*, 275
Radon, 268, 269*f*, 270*t*
Random. *See also* Sampling
    disease/groups and (nearly) unattainable
        goals at, 95, 139
    losses as rarely, 132
    losses for less damage, 116–17, 119
Random error, 5, 15, 20
    aggregation (pooling) and, 252, 262, 264,
        265
    association and, 110–11, 245
    cohort studies and, 54, 70
    confidence intervals and, 46, 248, 251
    confounding and, 41–42, 155, 245
    control experimental conditions for isolating,
        40, 41
    definition of, 243–44
    estimates and, 37, 255, 256, 259
    hypothesis formulation, data and, 253–55
    ill-defined random processes with, 41
    inconsistency produced by, 274–75, 278
    misallocation of attention in, 40
    multiple comparisons, related issues and,
        251–55
    multiple studies, bias and, 261–64
    non-response bias and, 245

not act in all-or-none fashion, 248
null hypothesis/value and, 38, 141, 255
observational studies' special considerations
    for, 246–48
overall assessment of, 258–59
overinterpretation, bias and, 248–49, 258
pattern of deviation but not effect predicted
    for, 244
probability and, 141, 248, 250–51, 263
prominence of, 245
quantifying of, 39, 251, 255
random allocation for, 243–44, 247
sampling for, 43, 243–44, 246–47, 278
(increase) size of study and decrease of
    impact of, 38, 42, 141, 245, 253, 255,
    265
small deviations more probable than large
    deviations for, 244, 246
(false) splitting and, 226
statistical significance testing and, 248–52
symmetrical around true value and, 42, 48,
    259, 263
systemic error vs., 244–46, 248, 251
uncertainty of, 244, 259
Randomization, 54, 73–74, 76, 82
    confounding and, 139, 141
    exchangeability, exposure and, 139, 263
    trials, 263
Reaven, P.D., 188, 189*t*
Refusal, subject, 117–19, 118*t*, 121, 122, 133
Regression techniques, 130, 142, 149
Replication(s), 4
    consistency and, 278–79
    multiple studies, random error and, 261–62
    observational studies as unlikely true,
        263–64
Reproductive outcomes, pesticide exposure
    compared to, 60, 61*t*
Research, epidemiologic, 1, 44–49. *See also*
    Studies
    applications of, 287–91
    for broader causal inference, 21
    change in clinical practice and effect on, 13
    consistency and evolution of, 279–81
    for contribution to resolve uncertainty, 1
    debate and new, 298
    demonstration of need of future, 292
    empirical methodological, 292–93, 297
    epidemiology, other scientific disciplines
        and, 9, 25–26, 290, 294–97
    exposure and disease causal relation in,
        9–10, 46
    flaws of, 9
    goals of, 7–10, 11, 12, 15–16
    inferences from, 11, 12–14
    interpretation controversy over, 297–99
    key concerns about, 291–93
    producing leads from, 9
    public health improvement with, 7–8, 33,
        288, 290

Respiratory disease, fine particulate air
    pollution influence on, 71, 71*t*
Risk
    baseline, 60, 76, 142, 263, 275
    baseline disease, 53–54, 76, 142
    communication, 290
    disease, 72–73, 82, 138, 140, 190–91
    exposure type and, 190
    factors, 108, 109*t*–110*t*, 110, 154–55
    relative, 47, 48, 154, 157, 191, 217, 220–21,
        223, 228, 230, 257, 269*f*, 270, 275
    unknown, 154–55
Risk ratio (RR)
    confounding, 72, 140, 141, 143, 144–45,
        150, 151, 152, 180*f*
    disease misclassification and, 220, 221
    inconsistent findings and, 275
Rothman, K.J., 3, 10, 167

Sampling. *See also* Surveys
    biased, 85, 86, 105–6
    census, 106–7, 107*t*
    community, 106, 125–26, 126*t*
    control, 86, 107
    exposure prevalence, selection bias and
        stratified, 105–6, 112, 125
    health outcome-dependent, 52
    idiosyncratic control, 88–89
    interview, 193, 227, 278
    mail surveys as, 125–27, 126*t*, 129, 193
    observational studies and, 246–47, 250
    over, 52, 86
    from particular area, 89
    probability, 86
    random, 84, 88, 95, 111, 211, 250
    random digit dialing (telephone), 106–8, 107*t*
    random error and, 43, 243–44, 246–47, 278
    stratified, 85, 86, 105–6, 112, 125
    theory, 43, 247, 255
    unbalanced, 85
Selection
    factors and measurement errors, 40
    issues within group, 20
    subject, 15
Selection bias, 15, 38, 41. *See* Bias, from loss
        of study participants
    confounding vs., 5
    definition of, 2, 4, 56, 88
    direct distortion by, 143–44
    freedom from, 19
    incorrect causal component with, 20
    non-comparability and, 56, 58
    non-participation and, 5
    from non-response, 22–23
    prone vs. free of, 249
    source of, 108
    study group influence on, 5, 115–16
Selection bias, in case–control studies, 235,
        236*t*–237*t*

association's measures in relation to markers
        of potential, 102, 104–5
    coherent controls vs. non-coherent controls
        for, 112–13
    coherence of cases and controls for, 86–89,
        108, 112–13
    cohort studies vs., 5, 52, 53, 81–82
    confounding and, 85, 105, 108
    control group addressing exposure and bias
        in, 84–85
    control selection for, 81–89
    control's purpose in, 84
    (accurate) exposure prevalence and unbiased,
        86
    exposure prevalence in controls compared to
        external population in, 96, 98, 99*t*,
        100–101, 112, 115
    exposure prevalence variation among
        controls in, 101–2, 103*t*, 104*t*, 120
    exposure-disease associations confirmed in,
        108, 109*t*–110*t*, 110–11, 112
    (discretionary) health care for, 92–96, 97*t*
    idiosyncratic control sampling method and,
        88–89
    imperfect markers for partial adjustment of,
        108
    inability to identify sample controls from
        study base in, 88
    integrated assessment of potential for, 111–13
    intentional, 85
    non-concurrent vs. concurrent, 92
    social factors, individual behaviors and, 85,
        86, 101, 111
    study base controls with, 83–86
    subject selection for, 81–83
    temporal coherence of cases and controls
        with, 89–92, 93*t*
    underascertainment and, 213
    undiagnosed cases and, 213
Selection bias, in cohort studies
    ascertainment protocols for, 59, 60, 62
    baseline differences in risk of diseases,
        assessing and adjusting for, 72–73, 74*t*,
        75*t*, 76, 82
    case–control studies vs., 5, 52, 53, 81–82
    comparison group's purpose in, 53–55, 57,
        63, 78
    confounding and, 55–58, 72–73, 74
    diseases known not to be affected by
        exposure, assess rates and, 70–72, 71*t*
    diseases unrelated to exposure found to be
        related in, 70, 72
    dose-response gradient in relation to, 67
    effect measure modification across strata
        relation to pattern of, 68
    empirical evaluation for, 68
    expected patterns of disease, assessing
        presence, and, 63–64, 65*t*–66*t*, 67
    exposure groups' measurement in, 52–53
    group's stratum free from, 67

integrated assessment of potential for, 78–79
lack of information as tool for, 58
markers of susceptibility, assessing pattern
    and, 67–70, 69t, 74
origins of, 72–73
residual, 72
severity of, 69–70
sources of potential bias for, 58
specific candidate source of, 76, 78
as specific exposure-disease association of
    interest, 57
stratified sampling, exposure prevalence and,
    105–6, 112
study designs for, 51–53
study group, error in constituting, and, 55
study group restriction, enhanced
    comparability and, 73–74, 76, 77t, 78
subject selection in, 81–82
unexpected patterns of disease, assessing
    presence and, 64, 67
unexposed disease rates compared to
    external populations in, 58–60, 61t, 62–63
un/exposed group, disease rate/incidence
    and, 53–55, 58–59, 64, 82, 84, 119–20
Self-esteem, 32
Sensitivity analysis, 125, 127, 129, 130
Serum lycopene, 102, 103t, 104t
Serum selenium, 186, 187t
Sexual activity, 139
    in late pregnancy, 76
Sexually transmitted disease, 151, 277
Smoking, 25, 109t, 119, 126
    alcohol and, 276, 277
    bladder cancer and, 86, 138–40, 141, 143
    brain cancer and, 198, 199t–200t
    bronchitis, lung cancer and, 70, 71t, 95
    exposure history of, 217, 218
    exposure measurement and, 171, 173, 176,
        179
    infertility and, 221, 222t
    interpretations of problems with, 33
    lung cancer and, 111, 142, 147, 153,
        156–57, 158t, 167, 186, 187t, 188–89,
        295–96
    pancreatic cancer and, 154
    policy decisions for, 24–25
    related diseases, research and, 289
Social factors. See also Demographic patterns
    case–control studies, selection bias and, 85,
        86, 95, 101, 111, 182
    cohort studies, selection bias and, 64,
        65t–66t
    confounding and, 157, 158t
    exposure measurements and, 165, 182, 186,
        187t, 198, 201
    loss of study participants and, 117, 118t,
        123, 124t, 125, 126t, 129, 133
Socioeconomic status
    case–control studies, selection bias and, 93t,
        101, 104–5, 106, 123, 124t

confounding and, 147, 149, 149t, 152
exposure measurement and, 181–82, 184,
    185t
loss of study participants and, 123, 124t, 133
Specificity, 220, 224, 300
Speculation, intelligent, 21
Statistical associations, 2, 10
Statistical dependence, 1–2
Statistical jargon, 35–36
Statistical methods, 2
    bias removal from, 36
    causal relations and, 10–11
    confounding and, 56–58, 139–40, 149–50,
        151, 159–60
    multiple studies, synthesis and, 262–63, 264
    probability and, 141
Statistical significance testing
    (examining of) association's increased for
        increase of results of, 252
    confidence interval vs., 256
    dichotomous decision and, 250, 251, 258
    inconsistency and, 275
    individual trials too small for, 262
    meta-analysis and, 271
    null hypothesis and, 249–50, 252, 256, 258
    overinterpretation encouraged by, 248–49,
        258
    parallel approach to systemic error with, 249
    positive vs. negative, 249
    probability of obtained results with, 249
    probability values contrived with, 250–51
    random error and, 248–51
    systemic error, random error and, 248–49,
        251
Stensvold, I., 157, 158t
Step function, 256
Strawbridge, W.J., 76, 77t
Studies. See also Case–control studies; Cohort
        studies
    complete documentation of methods of, 116
    confidence intervals for comparing precision
        of different, 257
    consistency vs. bias in, 4
    consistency vs. causality for, 4
    as continuum, 37
    cross-sectional, 52
    deficiencies and previous, 31
    effectiveness of evidence influencing future,
        23, 31, 44
    hypothesis formulation, data analysis and,
        253–54
    key concerns about, 291–93
    lumping of, 210–11, 225, 239, 252
    non-randomized, 74
    random error's decrease with increase size
        of, 8, 42, 141, 245, 253, 255, 265
    randomization process for, 54, 73–74, 76,
        82, 139, 141, 263
    resources vs. yield of, 121
    revealing/assessment of methods of, 22

Studies (*continued*)
    size of, 38, 42, 141, 211, 214, 245, 253, 255
    small vs. large, 173, 215, 246, 247, 255
Studies, multiple
    aggregate evaluation of evidence in, 281–83
    causal inference, inconsistent results and,
        262
    compatibility of, 264–65
    consistency, inconsistency and, 262, 263,
        273–81
    coordinated comparative analysis of, 267–68,
        269f, 270t
    counting of positive/negative associations of,
        275
    data pooling and, 264–65, 266t, 267, 267f
    evolution of research and, 279–81
    heterogeneity and, 276
    integration of evidence, patterns across,
        261–62
    (synthetic and exploratory) meta-analysis
        with, 268, 270–73
    narrative review of, 273
    random error, bias and, 261–64, 265
    replication of, 261–62
    single study vs., 279
    statistical power, random error and, 262–64
Study base
    calendar time, case registries for, 90
    controls from, 83–86
    definition of, 83, 84, 94
    exposure prevalence for, 98
    inability to identify and sample control from,
        89
    past or continual (stable) residence as basis
        of, 91–92, 112–13
    primary, 87
    (defined) probability sampling from, 86
    random sampling of, 84
    sample controls of, 87
    sampling from particular, 89
    secondary, 87
    for selection of coherent cases and controls,
        87
Study group(s). *See also* Groups
    cohort vs. case–control, 5, 52, 53
    construction of, 5
    definition of, 115
    error in constituting, 55
    non-concurrent vs. concurrent, 92
    restriction, to enhance comparability, 73–74,
        76, 77t, 78, 105
    selection bias and, 55, 73–74, 77t, 78, 105,
        115–16
    well-defined, 111
Study participants, diagnostic accuracy verified
        and subset of, 226–28, 229t
Study participants, loss of
    case–control studies, exposure prevalence
        and, 120

case–control study, exposure prevalence,
        cooperativeness and, 125
clinical setting and, 117, 118t
cohort studies, questionnaire and, 125
cohort studies, un/exposed groups and,
        119–20
conceptual framework for, 115–20, 118t
deviation and effect of, 118–19, 120
dose-response function and, 125, 127
early respondents vs. all respondents and,
        125–27, 126t
eliminating bias/confounding, adjustments of
        measured attributes and, 119
elimination of non-response and, 133
exposed vs. non-exposed nonrespondents in,
        125
exposure-disease relation, selection basis
        and, 119–20
free-living human influence on, 116, 118t,
        131–33
geographic areas and, 128, 131, 132t, 133t,
        175–76, 175t, 177t
gold standard measure of exposure and,
        131
imputing information, nonparticipants and,
        129–31, 132t
increased response for, 120
integrated assessment of potential of bias
        for, 131–34
mail surveys and, 125–27, 126t, 129
mechanisms of, 117–18, 118t
missed appointments and, 127
missing data with, 118t, 129–31
nonparticipant's characterized/follow-up in,
        120–23, 124t
non-participation, measure of effect, and,
        128–29, 133
nonrespondent vs. respondent for, 124–25
nonrespondents vs. reluctant respondents for,
        127–28
non-response bias from, 120–23, 124t
percentage of, 131
random losses, less damage in, 116–17,
        119
as rarely random, 133
recruitment's gradation of difficulty in, 120,
        124–28, 126t
refusal by subject for, 117–19, 118t, 121,
        122, 133
rescued participants, non-response bias
        estimated and, 133–34
self-selection unlikely as random with, 130
smaller loss for less erroneous results in,
        116
social factors and, 117, 118t, 123, 124t, 125,
        126t, 129, 133
socioeconomic status and, 123, 124t, 133
stratify study base, markers of participation
        and, 128–29

traceability difficulties with, 117–19, 118*t*,
  121, 122, 124–25, 127
Study population, accurate representation of, 19
Study products, 35–36
Subjectivity
  alternative explanations, causal inference
    and, 23
  objectivity vs., 32–33, 301–2
  public policy and, 32–33, 285–86, 291, 297,
    302
Sunscreen, 70–71
Surveillance, Epidemiology, and End Results
  (SEER) Program, 59
Surveys, 100, 101, 102, 125
Susceptibility
  to bias, 276–77, 279
  to confounding, 263, 280
  genetic markers of, 276, 297
  selection bias in cohort studies relation to
    markers of, 67–70, 69*f*, 74
Susser, M., 11

Tobacco. *See* Smoking
Toxicology, 26, 290, 296
Tumors, 195, 197–98, 235, 236*t*–237*t*

Uncertainty, 1
  confounding and, 23
  magnitude and estimates of, 35
  of random error, 244, 259

Validity
  assessment of, 47
  of associations, 9–10
  of epidemiologic evidence, 29–30, 34–35, 37
  measurement of effect and, 34–35, 37
  published works and, 27
Value(s)
  center vs. periphery of interval, 206, 256
  null, 140, 144, 155, 192, 213, 214, 215, 216
  true, 206, 256, 263, 302
  true vs. measured, 43, 244, 245, 293, 294
Vegetables, 231–32, 233*t*–234*t*, 235
Villeneuve, P.J., 225, 225*t*

Water, drinking, 288–89
Wertheimer, N., 153
Wolff, M.S., 44, 45, 47, 48, 49

Ye, W., 154

Ruffin v. Commonwealth, 225–28, 230, 237, 241–42
Ryan, Charles, 189–90

Sandin v. Connor, 202, 206–8
Sartre, Jean-Paul, 121–24
Scalia, Antonin, 180, 233, 240
Schor, Naomi, 120
Schultz, Vicki, 180
Segregation, 21–22; and *Brown v. Board of Education*, 7, 21, 166, 168, 182, 250, 264–77, 281; in prisons, 199–200; and Self-referentiality, 120
Separatism, 251
Sex discrimination, 17–18, 131–82
Sexuality, 47–52; abyss of, 72–73, 81; and the trials of Flaubert and Baudelaire, 115–16
Shauer, Frederick, 4
Shuler, Robert, 306
Signifiers, liberated, 119
Simi Valley trial, 39, 61
Simpson, O. J., 15, 25–26, 30–93
Sixth Amendment, 214
Sixty Minutes, 185
Slavery, 19–21; abolition of, 146–47; and prison systems, 19–20, 183–84, 202–4, 229, 231, 241–43; and sex discrimination, 131, 135–37, 144, 146–47; and stigmatization, 251–59, 272, 278
Socialism, 124
Spectatorship, 60–62
Speech, 30, 85–88, 283–317
Stevens, Thaddeus, 147, 204–5, 228, 241
Stewart, Terry, 190–91, 200, 244, 249
Stigma, 21–22, 205, 249–81
Stowe, Harriet Beecher, 255
Sumner, Charles, 227
Superintendent v. State of Arizona Improvement Company, 231
Sutherland, George, 156
Symington, Fife, 184
Symptoms, of meaning, 28

Taboos, 16, 89
Taft, William Howard, 157
Taney, Roger Brooke, 21, 250, 255–64, 270, 274
Taxation, 158
Taylor, Telford, 98
tenBroek, Jacobus, 266–67
Thelen, David, 11
Thirteenth Amendment, 226–29, 255–59, 261–66, 271–72, 278–80
Thomas, Clarence, 240–43, 271
Tolstoy, Leo, 15, 25–26, 30
Tomlins, Christopher, 145
Tourgée, Albion W., 264–65, 266, 281
Transcendence, 118, 121, 124, 126–27
Transgression, 115, 124, 126
Trauma: abyss of, 75–79; and the cross-legal nature of trials, 39–41; Felman on, 14–16, 25–93; perception of, 38, 39–41
Triangular relationships, 50–51
Trinity Methodist Church v. Federal Radio Commission, 306–8
Trujillo, Ernest J., 224
Trumbull, Lyman, 256–57
Truth, 10, 11, 26; Felman on, 26, 54, 70, 78, 83, 88; historical search for, 97; integrity of, 78; and the literary text, 99
Truth-claims, 97–99
Turner v. Safley, 220, 223–24
Tussman, Joseph, 266, 267
20/20 (news program), 185

Uncle Tom's Cabin (Stowe), 255
Unconscious, structural, of law, 28–33
United States v. Rhodes, 256
University of California v. Bakke, 131, 136–37, 251, 271, 273, 275, 277

Van Buren, Martin, 255
Verdits, 55–56
Victims, 2, 38
Victory, poetic, 122

Voting rights, 17–18, 131–82

Warren, Earl, 230, 269–70, 272
Westbrook v. The State, 231, 233
West Coast Hotel, 7
West Indian slave laws, 183, 202
White, Byron, 204
White, Lucie, 14, 18–19
Whitley, Harol, 200
Whitley v. Albers, 232–33
Wieneke, Kathleen L., 222
Wilkerson, Isabel, 77

Willens, Jonathan, 200
Williams, Medria, 88
Wisdom, John Minor, 250–51
Wolff v. McDonnell, 199–200
"Woman question," 17–19, 131–82
Women's Suffrage: The Reform against Nature (Bushnell), 149
World War I, 310
World War II, 96, 135, 279, 292, 316

Zelenak, Anthony, 195–96